Animal in Biomedical Research: Theory and Practice

Animal in Biomedical Research: Theory and Practice

Gaurav Tyagi

RANDOM

RANDOM PUBLICATIONS

NEW DELHI (INDIA)

Animal in Biomedical Research: Theory and Practice

ISBN 978-93-5111-788-9

Published in 2016 in India by

RANDOM PUBLICATIONS

4376-A/4B, Gali Murari Lal, Ansari Road
New Delhi-110 002
Phone : +9111-43580356, 011-23289044, 011-43142548
e-mail: sales@randompublications.com,
info@randompublications.com, randomexports@gmail.com

Reprinted 2026

Type Setting by : Friends Media, Delhi-110089

Preface

Research on animals also has led to countless treatments, techniques, and medical technologies. Animal research was indispensable to the development of immunization against many diseases, including polio, mumps, measles, diphtheria, rubella and hepatitis. One million insulin-dependent diabetics survive today because of the discovery of insulin and the study of diabetes using dogs, rabbits, rats and mice. Organ transplantation, considered a dubious proposition just a few decades ago, has become commonplace because of research on mice, rats, rabbits and dogs.

The use of animals in biomedical research has a lengthy history. Early Greek writings (circa 500 B.C.), for example, describe the dissection of living animals by physician-scientists interested in physiological processes. These early vivisections appear to have been done mostly for exploratory purposes, however, to describe the inner workings of animals. Later, Roman physicians--including perhaps the single most influential figure in the emergence of the medical sciences, the physician Galen--began to perform what we would now regard as the first genuine experiments involving animals. Using vivisections to test specific hypotheses and explore competing explanations of biological phenomena, these early physician-researcher were among the first advocates of the idea that the use of animals in research was morally justifiable in light of the potential health benefits associated with those experiments.

Biomedical research is essential to the health and well-being of our society. Advances in biomedical research have dramatically improved the quality and prolonged the duration of life throughout the world. However, the ability of the scientific community to continue its efforts to improve personal and public health is being threatened by a movement to eliminate the use of animals in biomedical research. This movement is spearheaded by groups of radical animal rights activists whose views are considered to be far outside mainstream public attitudes and whose tactics range from sophisticated lobbying, fund-raising, propaganda and misinformation campaigns to violent attacks on biomedical research facilities and individual scientists. These violent attacks are carried out by a relatively small number of activists compared with those who use peaceful means of protest, but they have profound and wide-ranging effects.

Specially bred rats and mice are the mammals used most often in medical research. Because rats and mice have so many biological similarities to humans, they make up 90–95% of the mammals in biomedical research. Some strains of rats and mice are susceptible to diseases such as cancer or high blood pressure. In addition, rodents develop diseases over a span of days or weeks instead of months or years. In the 1980s, major research discoveries made it possible to create strains of mice whose genetic make-up has been altered so that they carry specific disease-causing genes.

Present book has been complete to cater to the requirements of the teachers, researchers and students.

– Author

Contents

1

Introduction

Animals are used to understand basic biology, as "models" for studying human biology and disease, and as test subjects for the development and testing of drugs, vaccines, and other biologicals (i.e. antibodies, hormones, ingredients in vaccines, etc.) to improve and advance human health. As models, scientists aim to produce artificially, a condition in an animal in a laboratory that may resemble the human equivalent of a medical disease or injury. Animals are used in all capacities of research: for example, a rabbit's sensory system may be studied in basic research; she may be used as a model for eye and skin disorders, or used in eye and skin irritancy tests for environmental toxicity testing.

The exact number of animals used in biomedical research is unknown, particularly since government statistics do not include mice, rats, birds, and fish; some estimates place the total number of these species in research to be in the tens to hundreds of millions. The use of genetic engineering—manipulation of an animal's DNA or genes—is prevalent throughout many fields of research, particularly biomedical. "...[T]he mouse has become the flagship of animal testing, especially useful with genetic modifications, gene knockouts [genes are removed], and knockins [genes are added]. In 2003, NIH [National Institutes of Health] launched the Knockout Mouse Project and has awarded more than $50 million with the goal of creating a library of mouse embryonic stem cells lines, each with a gene knocked out."

While most animals are purposely bred for research, others, like cats and dogs, may be acquired through different sources, such as auctions, advertisements, or from pounds and shelters (known as "pound seizure"). Of the many species used in biomedical research, specific animals are preferred in certain areas. Dogs, typically young purpose-bred beagles, are commonly used in cardiovascular studies, heart and lung research, genetic studies, age-related research, pulmonary studies, cancer research, and orthopedics, such as the development of prosthetic devices for hip and knee replacements, vertebral fusion models, cervical disc degeneration, etc. Cats "have long been a mainstay of NIH-funded studies of neurological, cardiovascular, and respiratory diseases, and the immune system." Researchers also use cats in cancer research, genetic disorders, and eye, ear, and infectious disease research. Nonhuman primates are used in research on vaccines, infectious, cardiovascular, and neurological diseases, aging, reproductive biology, gene therapy, drug addiction, xenotransplantation (cross-species transplants), and vaccine and toxicity testing. The two most common primate species used by far are Rhesus and Cynomolgus macaques—also known as crab-eating macaques. Of the nonhuman great apes, chimpanzees are currently the only species used in biomedical research.

Researchers frequently use rabbits in toxicity and safety testing of medical devices, vaccines, and drugs. In 2009, over 222,000 rabbits were used in research, more than any other species covered under the Animal Welfare Act (AWA), followed next by guinea pigs and hamsters, who are both used a great deal in toxicity testing and as models for infectious, cardiovascular, and neurological diseases, and drug abuse research. Both mice and rats are heavily used in vaccine and drug research and testing, and birds are used in research on organ development and deformity, visual impairment, muscular dystrophy, and nutrition, among other things.

BASIC RESEARCH

Basic research is exploratory research, an open-ended search for more information for knowledge's sake. "Basic biological research has traditionally studied life at the most basic level; what the cell is, what it is made of...what everything is built of and so forth." A wide variety of animals are used in basic research, with mice being the most common. Rats, birds, amphibians, and fish are also used, and invertebrates such as fruit flies and worms are heavily used in genetic research.

"Historically, animal use in research was synonymous with basic research. It was easy to dissect or vivisect animals without any particular end in mind." In many ways, this is still true today. Stated in a 2010 review on the use of animals in basic research, "According to figures from the NIH, basic biomedical research receives more funding than all other forms of research, [and] uses animals more often than not..."

While basic research does not set out to find cures for human diseases, "much current [basic] research [is] being done under the guise of applied research because it increases the likelihood that the project will be funded by a granting institution."6 In a 2009 review of animal models in research, the authors list several NIH-funded research grants that are basic research, but described under the pretense of applied research by claiming clinical relevance for humans. By claiming potential clinical applications, a slippery slope is created that allows any and all animal research to be justified in spite of contrary evidence to its applications for humans. As stated in a 2011 science news article, "With an annual budget for NIH of more than $30 billion, the problem is not the amount invested in medical research, but how it is used. Right now we're operating under the assumption that somehow there's a yet-to-be-discovered silver bullet, and that if we just spend more money on fundamental science, researchers will discover that silver bullet and all will be well. It's not going to work that way."

ANIMAL MODELS

For practically every known human disease, researchers attempt to induce similar aspects of the disease in animals to create an animal "model" of that disease. Supposedly predictive, animals "are used with the aim of discovering and quantifying the impact of a treatment, whether this is to cure a disease or to assess the toxicity of a chemical compound." This is how animals are "used in the context of drug testing and studying human disease."9 Areas of disease research involving animals include neurological, infectious, digestive, genetic, connective tissue, and chronic diseases. In these areas, animals are used as models of traumatic brain injuries, spinal cord injuries, congenital blindness, Parkinson's, Alzheimer's, AIDS, diabetes, cancer, obesity, and so on.

In order to create these models, animals are subjected to invasive procedures, which can include surgeries, traumatic injuries, burns, force-feeding, blood draws, biopsies, food, water, and social deprivation, dart gun sedation, prolonged restraint, behavioral and environmental manipulations, viral and bacterial infections, and exposure to toxic drugs and chemicals.

Examples include, "creating heart attacks, heart failure, abnormal heart rhythms, strokes, and other cardiovascular traumas in monkeys, dogs, pigs, and other animals; inducing symptoms of migraines in cats and primates through brain stimulation and manipulation with chemicals; implanting electrodes into the intestines of dogs to induce motion sickness and vomiting; implanting electrodes into the brains and eyes of monkeys and cats to conduct neurological and vision experiments; and dropping weights onto rodents to produce spinal cord injuries and paralysis."

DRUG AND VACCINE DEVELOPMENT

Millions of animals and taxpayer dollars are used in the production and testing of biologicals, such as vaccines and antibodies. For example, a complete batch test for a therapeutic protein can involve 12,000 mice and cost $2.4 million; 2007 estimates for the cost of drug development and to bring it to market range from $800 million to $1.7 billion. Potential drugs are often required to be tested in at least two animal species in preclinical trials before moving on to human clinical trials. Yet "only around 5% of drugs that show potential in animal studies ever get licensed for human use.

" Potency tests of such products as vaccines are still based routinely on the principle of protection, i.e., survival or death after exposure, which was first introduced in the 1890s. Many of these tests are exceptionally cruel, involving high levels of pain and distress for a range of species from rodents to nonhuman primates (including chimpanzees). According to 1998 USDA statistics, more than 60 percent of the animals reported to experience unrelieved pain were used for vaccine testing.

BIOMEDICAL APPLICATIONS

There are fewer welfare problems with biomedical applications as there are few secondary modifications (although phenotypic problems can still occur). Also, as these animals have high value, their care is undoubtedly better than that of farm animals.

BIOPHARMACEUTICALS

The proteins or substances secreted in the physiological products should not have any effects on the organism of the secreting transgenic animal. If the substance is carried in the circulation and is biologically active in the animal's organism, it can cause certain physiological dysfunctions which can cause pain and discomfort. Secretion of the substance should be confined to the expressing tissue, but this is difficult to control. It has been reported that the early expression of a transgene can cause the premature development of the mammary gland and render any subsequent lactation painful.

Xenotransplantation

No phenotypical abnormality has been noted in pigs produced for xenotransplantation, so there are no problems of animal welfare, even though the efficiency of the microinjection technique used to obtain such transgenic pigs is low. As regards animal health, modification of their cell structure could render pigs susceptible to infection from human viral disease. The special conditions of husbandry also raise concerns about the pigs' welfare. The isolation needed for pathogen-free pigs and while awaiting organ donation causes abnormal behaviour among pigs which are extremely sociable animals.

Other

Problems of welfare (and ethics) arise in connection with genetically engineered farm animals that are created to study human diseases or the toxicity of medical drugs or other substances. Standard testing procedures need to be drawn up to avoid all stress and suffering.

The impact of genetic engineering on the health and welfare of animals is a major public concern. Perception of animal welfare varies widely because determined by cultural attitude to animals, and involves ethical judgements. Biotechnologies can cause suffering, physical and psychological stress, behavioural and physiological abnormalities and/or problems of health among animals, whatever their intended use or function. On the other hand, they also have the potential to reduce or eliminate such problems, which also arise under intensive animal production practices.

GENETICALLY MODIFIED INSECTS

TRANSGENIC INSECTS

Insect biotechnology is used to create genetically modified insects that are useful for pest control, especially in agriculture, and for the control of vector-borne animal or human disease. One of the major objectives of transgenesis is in fact to control the transmission of vector-borne diseases such as malaria. The vectors can be controlled by the usual methods, involving insecticides, actions against vector home environments or means of protection, such as mosquito nets, but these methods are only relatively effective because of growing resistance to insecticides and the physical limitations of the methods themselves.

The only course of action is then to eliminate the vector itself. Biotechnology can be used to reduce or even eliminate vector insect populations, or to reduce the capacity of an insect to carry and disseminate a parasite or pathogen. Various methods have been proposed: the use of sterile males, the introduction of a lethal gene or the introduction into the insect vector population of a gene that gives resistance to infestation by human or animal pathogens.

Use of Sterile Males

Sterile males are used to reduce vector population density and sterilization can be done by chemical or physical irradiation. However, such methods reduce mosquito viability as the irradiation causes lesions in all insect tissues. Biotechnology can improve the sterility of males without damaging their viability and can therefore improve the effectiveness of control programmes and reduce the number of released insects. The use of sterile males requires sexing so that females are not released.

Distinguishing male from female is easy in species that permit visual sexing on the basis of size of pupae, but can be a real challenge in others. Proposed methods include the use of a dominant gene associated with a female-specific promoter which would render the females dependent on a high concentration of tetracycline for survival and would therefore render them unviable in a natural environment.

The males would simply carry this gene which they would introduce into the wild population. Such a gene could however be a major problem if it were to establish itself among wild communities of non-targeted insects. The use of sterile males is effective if the females mate with them. However, the females of some species of mosquito are monogamous so this system would lose effectiveness under the massive inflow of already fertilized females. Depending on the target species, it would therefore seem best to combine methods, notably with another genetic technique.

Particular Characteristics

The production of Anopheles mosquitoes resistant to *Plasmodium* infection (malaria) is an interesting concept, but the gene in question has to be closely linked to the dissemination mechanism. However, the "resistance" trait would appear to depend on several genes. It has also been shown that 100% effective resistance is needed in areas with high prevalence and dissemination of the pathogen.

The problem is that the creation of selection pressure based on *Plasmodium* could eventually lead to the emergence of resistant *Plasmodium*, which has led to the idea of introducing several independent genes resistant to the pathogen. This is a major problem as biotechnologies are used for traits that are regulated by a single gene and cannot be used where a trait stems from a complex set of genes.

Linking and transferring the set of genes is also complex. Another example is the sterilization of male ephemera larvae infesting cotton bolls using irradiation, which has not been 100% effective despite the high cost. Scientists have thought of inserting a gene capable of blocking the development of fertilized eggs, to help reduce the wild populations.

DIRECT PROBLEMS

Stability and Effectiveness of the Inserted Gene

Insertion needs to be stable and effective. Once the desired trait has been identified, the responsible gene needs to be defined and the inserted transgene needs to express itself at the right time and in the appropriate tissues. The resulting insect is then studied and can be reproduced in large volumes if observations are satisfactory. Dissemination models need to be prepared and trials conducted in confined areas.

Cost of Biotechnologies

The control of insect vectors of animal and human disease is a controversial subject. Traditional methods need to be seen to be ineffective if biotechnologies are to be introduced, and this for two basic reasons: the high cost of obtaining transgenic insects and the time and resources needed to conduct GMO risk analysis. A cost-benefit study is required.

The Problem in Human Health Terms

In the case of the control of certain vector-borne diseases, the elimination of the parasite within the vector population could result in an increase in population, which could foster the propagation of other vector-borne human or animal diseases. For example, mosquitoes rid of *Plasmodium* could become more susceptible to other human or animal pathogens. Tests are therefore required, especially for parasitic worms (Anopheles mosquitoes are vectors for filaria) and numerous viruses, including HIV. For the time being, mosquitoes do not seem to be carriers of the HIV virus, but it would be disastrous if they were to become so. Virologists see this as totally inconceivable but public opinion appears to see it as a major concern. Data need to be found to prove that this is not possible.

Problem of "Driver" Mechanisms

Three mechanisms are proposed:

1. *The use of transposable elements (which replicate and disseminate)*: Present know-how renders this mechanism too uncertain, and the risk of horizontal transfer of an uncontrolled transgene means that it is forbidden.
2. *Wolbachia infection in mosquitoes*: This mechanism is still under development and thus untested.
3. The use of complex mechanisms using two complementary lethal genes that counteract one another. Hybrids only possessing one of these genes would be unviable which would benefit the animals carrying the two genes. Bonding the gene for resistance would enable it to implanted among the target population.

Without a driver mechanism for dissemination, the method would be seriously restricted by the migratory movement of vectors, notably female mosquitoes. Combining these methods with the use of sterile males would be more effective as they would eventually lead to a reduction in the wild population.

Problem of Bonding

This is a major problem, for it is impossible to envisage creating insect resistance to infestation by a pathogen if there is no guarantee of complete bonding between the driver mechanism and the transgene. There would be crossings and hybrids, without bonding, and those with the driver mechanism would not be effective for control.

RISKS TO THE ENVIRONMENT

Problems of Insect Confinement and Release

Insects have high mobility and considerable potential for colonization of new environments. They must therefore be confined to permit study without risk to the environment.

This is important to avoid the propagation of a transgene in a wild population, especially in the case of biopharmaceutical insects. Transgenic insects should be confined in a laboratory, as there is no way they can be detected after release into the environment, especially if they proceed develop in an unexpected manner.

Two guides with differing emphases have been drawn up for insect confinement:

1. A classification of risks to the environment and of GMOs, with specific procedures for each. A distinction is made between different kinds of GM insect and corresponding levels of confinement.
2. Recommended practices of the US Animal and Plant Health Inspection Service (APHIS) which constitute a single standard procedure without distinction between transgenic insects, and highlighted by the OECD in 1998.

At present, each laboratory develops its own procedures for the confinement of GM animals, without uniformity. The thorny problem of insects created for biopharmaceuticals is not taken into account. Some observers argue that confinement requires time and investment at the expense of pure research, but the release of genetically modified insects could feasibly have damaging and more or less irreversible consequences for the environment.

HORIZONTAL TRANSFER OF A TRANSGENE

The risk of horizontal transfer of a transgene is regularly emphasized and, if this were to happen, could have significant consequences for the environment. The insertion of genetic material into wild populations, such as genes resistant to antibiotics (markers) or to insecticides, is highly undesirable. Such an occurrence is impossible to evaluate as we lack information on horizontal transfer mechanisms and related frequencies.

There has been very little study, but horizontal transfer would appear to be possible between conspecifics. The underlying mechanism is unknown, but this phenomenon has been known to occur with small fruit flies.

High plasmid exchange is also possible between insects and intestinal bacteria, which are then found in faeces and thus the environment. The impact of such gene transfers is unknown, but close links exist between insects and other organisms (pollinizers, preys or predators, vectors, etc.) which means negative impact on an insect population could have a major impact on all ecosystems.

CONTROL AND REGULATORY BODY

National regulations often tend to forget transgenic insects. No regulations or international recommendations exist for the confinement of transgenic insects. However, their release is subject to authorization in most countries. There are sometimes several regulatory bodies at national level and control procedures can be complex.

In the US, several different federal and national institutions need to be consulted before GM or non-GM insects can be released. Some commentators would also like to see the health agencies involved. So far, the only releases of transgenic insects that have taken place in the US have been for short duration trials. Their subsequent destruction, or at least total recovery, are prerequisites for authorization to conduct such trials.

NEED FOR RISK ANALYSIS

Risk analysis should be conducted prior to any release of transgenic insects and should include studies on:

- The stability of the transgene
- The possibility or not of horizontal transfer of the transgene
- The present and potential geographic distribution of the gm insect
- The different traits transferred to the gm insect and their impact on the ecosystem
- Possible unforeseen side effects on the environment.

The traits and fitness of a transgenic insect appear to be easily verifiable. On the other hand, the horizontal transfer of the transgene and short-, medium- or long-term side effects on the environment are more difficult to determine. A large number of scientific uncertainties need to be cleared before transgenic insects can be released into the natural environment.

DETERMINING THE LEVEL OF RISK

There are three possible scenarios:

1. A field or controlled-environment trial permitting the recovery or destruction of all the insects;
2. The release of sterile insects for biological control; this poses less risk than insects meant to establish themselves among the wild population as they cannot breed.
3. Insects for permanent establishment in the environment and crossbreeding between GM insects and wild insects to disseminate the transgene.

We can identify the risk but assessing the likelihood of risk is virtually impossible. Domesticated insects are virtually incapable of surviving alone in the environment (*e.g.* silk worms).

The risk of dissemination of these insects is thus very low. Sterile insects represent the same low risk of dissemination because horizontal transfer is very rare. The case of bees would appear to be more uncertain as bees are half domesticated, so have higher potential for survival and dissemination in the environment.

Risk analysis models for transgenic insects do exist, but have limitations as designed on the basis of possibly biased theoretical data. There are too many known and unknown interactions between the different factors (population dynamics, genetics, environment and space, etc.)

Transgenic insects require proper risk analysis if reliable risk-benefit analysis is to be conducted. The possibility of finding alternatives to the costly and time-consuming production of GMOs needs to be looked into, as do the objectives of producing transgenic insects and the achievements to date. Negative impacts need to be studied and reduced, which will mean standardizing the risk analysis to be carried out before any release of GM insects. Retrospective studies following the introduction of these animals will also be needed.

ANIMAL HEALTH AND WELFARE

Reproductive Biotechnologies and Techniques

All reproductive manipulations, including semen collection, repeated artificial insemination, embryo collection and transfer, or the inducement of superovulation can cause stress to animals during constraint and handling. These methods are not specific to GM animals and few have been studied from the perspective of animal welfare. The intensity of violation during artificial insemination and embryo collection varies according to the species. These two techniques are relatively uninvasive for cattle and are done with local anaesthetic.

On the other hand, for smaller species such as sheep, goats and pigs, they entail invasive surgical intervention (laparotomy or laparoscopy) and thus cause operative and post-operative pain. Cows carrying an embryo are subject to amniocentesis to check the genotype. Cows carrying nontransgenic embryos or male embryos are aborted and have another embryo inserted.

This limits the number of recipient females used to give birth to transgenic animals, but it also raises welfare concerns as these animals are regularly exposed to stress and pain.

At the same time, they can be prone to slow or difficult calving (dystocia) requiring increasingly frequent caesarean sections. Abnormalities in the offspring can also raise concern for an animal's welfare. Alternatives to such methods causing stress and pain are sometimes suggested, such as the removal of ova in the slaughterhouse, non-invasive embryo collection or techniques of cloning and in vitro culture to reduce the number of recipient animals.

In Vitro Culture

In vitro culture tends to extend the gestation period and to produce higher birthweights, resulting in difficult deliveries and frequent surgical intervention. These animals have more congenital malformations (skeletal malformation, incomplete development of the vascular system or urogenital tract, immune system dysfunction, brain lesions) and high perinatal mortality.

The mechanisms responsible for these abnormalities are not known, but chromosomal anomalies, abnormal regulation of gene expression during embryo development and problems of communication between foetus and mother have been implicated. Culture conditions also appear to be directly associated with the level of developmental abnormalities and perinatal mortality.

Efficiency of Biotechnologies

Efficiency varies according to technique. Microinjection is particularly inefficient, with reported successful transgenic offspring of only 1%. Embryo mortality stands at 80% to 90% and there is high perinatal mortality. In addition, few animals possess the inserted gene at birth and many show anatomical, physiological or behavioural abnormalities. The efficiency of methods used also depends on the species modified. Efficiency has a direct bearing on the number of attempts needed for success and the number of animals used.

While several embryos can be implanted into mice and pigs to offset embryo mortality and thus considerably reduce the number of recipient females, this does not seem possible with cattle because of the phenomenon of freemartinism. Transgenic animals do not necessarily pass the transgene to their offspring. It has also been reported that offspring can have a limited lifespan, a variety of malformations and general or specific malfunctions. This is attributed to so-called "mosaic" transgenic animals that do not carry the transgene uniformly in all their cells.

Gene Expression

The random insertion of transgene sequences in the genome of a target cell can have major consequences, especially in the expression of certain genes. Numerous abnormalities have been noted among transgenic animals, depending on the function of the transformed gene.

Recessive silent abnormalities can be expressed during breeding between transgenic animals, and their homozygous offspring could present a number of abnormalities. Controlling genetic expression is variable and difficult requiring the use of appropriate promoters and regulatory sequences. Many abnormalities are still observed among resulting animals, both mammals and fish (physiological and morphological problems, sensitivity to disease and stress, behavioural problems, etc.). These will undoubtedly lessen as techniques improve.

Benefits to Animal Welfare and Integrity

Biotechnologies are also promoted as improving animal welfare and health, with reduced mortality and morbidity because of greater resistance to disease and parasites; the elimination of phenotype characteristics such as horns; the adaptation of animals to intensive production; a reduced sensitivity to suffering and stress.

They also help control the sex ratio among animal populations, especially chickens, thus avoiding the slaughter of male chicks. Others also argue that animals with greater genetic value receive better care which can only enhance their welfare. However, a problem of animal health does arise. The shrinking gene pool and the uniformity of genomes could weaken animal populations and make them more susceptible to disease.

Nuclear Transfer

The method of somatic cell nuclear transfer is relatively new and inefficient. The failure rate is high, as is prenatal and postnatal mortality, and there are many abnormalities causing problems of health and welfare from the immediate postnatal period: respiratory distress, lack of suckling reflex, physiological and morphological abnormalities, behavioural problems.

The cause of these problems has not been identified with any certainty (stages of the technique itself, difficulty in genetically reprogramming the inserted nucleus, etc.). Study findings do however vary considerably and many transgenic animals have been successfully produced. Further studies are required.

BIOMEDICAL VERSUS AGRICULTURAL RESEARCH REQUIREMENTS

For research results to be applicable to commercial agriculture, the animals have to be handled and housed in conditions similar to those on commercial farms. In these situations, many of the animals may not be accustomed to close contact with people, and commercial handling equipment such as cattle squeeze chutes and other specialized equipment will be required. In another type of research, an agricultural animal may be used for biomedical research and housed in small indoor pens that are not similar to commercial conditions. Biomedical researchers have conditioned and trained animals to cooperate with injections, restraint, and other procedures.

Primates, pigs, and sheep can be easily trained to voluntarily enter a restraint device or hold out a limb for various procedures. Hutson reported that providing food rewards to sheep made them more willing to move through a handling facility in the future.

Training animals to cooperate greatly improves welfare, and removes some effects of restraint stress on physiological data. Low levels of cortisol and glucose were obtained from unsedated antelopes that had been conditioned to enter a restraint box and voluntarily stand still for blood tests. Training animals to voluntarily cooperate with injections, blood sampling, and other procedures is definitely recommended for biomedical settings where a few animals are used for medical experiments. However, it is often not practical for agricultural research in which large numbers of animals are handled.

FLIGHT ZONE AND BEHAVIOUR PRINCIPLES

People who are handling cattle, bison, sheep, horses, and other grazing animals should have knowledge of flight zone principles. The flight zone concept does not apply to animals that are trained to lead with a halter or otherwise conditioned to close human handling. The flight zone varies depending on whether cattle or other livestock have been extensively or intensively raised.

Extensively raised cattle may have flight zones up to 50 m, but intensively raised cattle may have flight zones only 2 to 8 m. The size of an alley can change flight zones. Sheep in a 2-m wide alley had a smaller flight zone than sheep in a 4-m wide alley. An approximation of the flight zone can be made by approaching the animal and noting at what distance the animal moves away. When the handler is outside of the flight zone, cattle will turn and face the handler. Flight zones can be exploited by handlers to move cattle and other livestock efficiently and quietly.

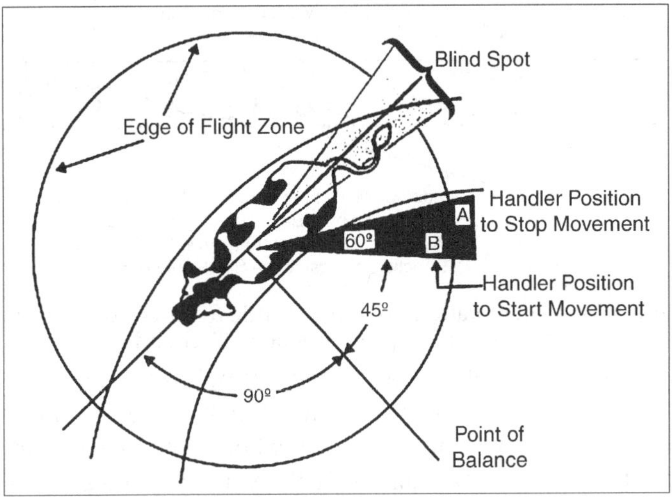

Fig. Flight Zone Diagram Showing the Most Effective Handle Positions for Moving an Animal Forward. Reproduced with Permission of T. Grandin.

For example, handlers should be positioned at the edge of the flight zone and behind the point of balance to move cattle forward. A common mistake made by many handlers is to stand in front of the shoulder and attempt to make an animal go forward by poking its rear.

This gives the animal conflicting signals. To move the animal forward, the handler should be behind the point of balance; Figure presents the concept of flight zone and point of balance.

Figure shows how to move an animal forward in a chute by walking quickly past the point of balance at the shoulder in the opposite direction of desired movement. To cause cattle to stop or back up, handlers should be positioned ahead of the point of balance.

Too deep a penetration of the flight zone may cause extensively raised cattle to bolt or run away or rear up in a chute. Animals will often stop rearing if the handler backs up and gets out of the flight zone.

Personnel working with cattle should be trained to use flight zones correctly. Extensively raised grazing animals that arrive at a research facility may have a large flight zone. The size of the flight zone will gradually diminish if they are handled calmly and have frequent contact with people. Farm animals are social and a lone animal separated from its herdmate often becomes severely agitated. Many injuries to both people and animals occur when a single lone animal runs into a fence or charges.

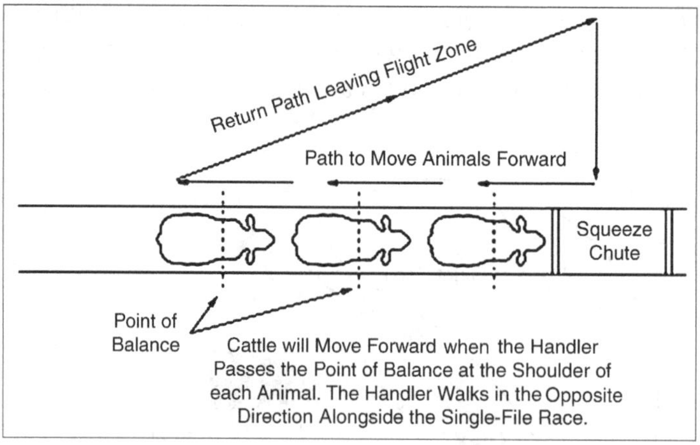

Fig. Handler Movement Pattern to Induce Cattle to Move Forward in a Race. Reproduced with Permission of T. Grandin.

An agitated lone animal can be calmed by putting some other animals in with it. Cattle and sheep will follow a leader. When one of the animals starts to move, the others will follow. Natural following behaviour can be used to facilitate calm movement of animals. If animals are calmly moving in the desired direction, the handler should back up and stop putting pressure on the flight zone. Continuous pressure on the flight zone may cause animals to start running, which is undesirable.

AIDS FOR MOVING ANIMALS

Animals in properly designed facilities may be moved using their natural behaviour and without the use of any aids. The goals of movement should be to minimize stress to each individual animal, reduce fear, and maintain calmness in all animals. All handlers should be trained in the natural behaviour of the species including their flight zone and in proper handler movement and interaction, and be able to recognize any signs of distress, anxiety, or behaviours that may result in injury or stress to the animals.

When necessary, nonelectrical driving aids such as paddles, flags, and panels may be an adjunct with the use of natural behaviour and handling skills. Handlers should be trained in the proper and effective use of each driving aid, which is appropriate to the species. An electric prod should only be picked up and used in a specific situation where it is needed and then put away.

Handlers have a better attitude towards the animals when electric shocks are not used. Data collected at meat plants indicate that most cattle and pigs could be moved throughout an entire handling system without electric prods.

On a ranch or feedlot, the use of electric prods should be limited to 10% or less of the cattle. When an electric prod needs to be used, it should be applied to the hindquarters of the animal. Usually 1 to 3 brief shocks are needed.

If the animal does not respond, the use of the electric prod should be discontinued immediately. It should never be applied to sensitive areas of the animal such as the eyes, ears, genitals, udder, or anus. Battery-operated prods are recommended because they administer a localized shock between 2 prongs. Electric prods should not be used on newborn animals, debilitated weak animals, nonambulatory downed animals, or emaciated animals.

Electric prods are highly stressful to pigs. Repeated shocks greatly increased the percentage of nonambulatory pigs. Multiple shocks and aggressive handling significantly increased blood lactate and other indicators of metabolic stress compared with gentle handling. Pigs that become nonambulatory because of fatigue or porcine stress syndrome should not have electric prods used on them.

Some examples of the use of an electric prod as a last resort or if human or animal safety is in jeopardy are listed below:

- To move an animal after repeated attempts with nonelectrified driving aids such as a plastic bag on the end of a stick, flags, slappers, rattle paddles, or streamers tied to the end of a stick have failed; the use of an electric prod is preferable to beating, ragging, pushing, or hard tail twisting of animals. If excessive slapping or electric prodding is required routinely, then the personnel involved may be too anxious or inadequately trained in proper animal handling or the facility may need modifications. Smaller animals may be gently lifted or rolled onto a transport mechanism.
- To get a downed animal in a truck that is located at a truck stop on the side of a highway. In this situation, opening up the truck gates or unloading the animals is not possible. 3 For cattle that are choking in a head stanchion or headgate or become jammed in a chute or other equipment.

ANIMAL PERCEPTION

Hearing

All species of grazing animals have sensitive hearing. Cattle and horses have hearing that is more sensitive compared with humans to high-pitched sounds. The human ear is most sensitive at 1000 to 3000 Hz and cattle are most sensitive to 8000 Hz. Handlers should not yell or shout at cattle because shouting may be just as aversive as an electric prod. In another experiment, the sounds of people yelling caused a greater increase in heart rate than the sounds of gates clanging. Intermittent or high-pitched sounds caused greater behavioural reactions and increased heart rate in pigs compared with steady or low-pitched sounds. Intermittent sounds and rapid movements are also more likely to cause cattle to react. Handlers should be observant of the position of an animal's ears. Horses and cattle will point their ears directly towards things that attract their attention.

Vision

Cattle, sheep, and horses have wide-angle vision and they can see all around themselves without turning their heads. Grazing animals have depth perception when they are standing still with their heads down. Depth perception is probably poor when the animals are moving with their heads up. This explains why they stop and put their heads down when they see a shadow on the floor. Grazing animals are dichromats. The retinas of cattle, sheep, and goats are most sensitive to yellowish-green; and bluish-purple light.

The dichromatic vision of the horse is most sensitive at 428 and 539 nm. Dichromatic vision and the absence of a retina receptor for red may explain why livestock are so sensitive to sharp contrasts of light and dark such as shadows or shiny reflections on handling equipment. Poultry appear to have excellent vision.

Chickens and turkeys possess 4 cone-cell types in the retina giving them tetrachromatic colour vision, compared with the human trichromatic vision based on 3 cone-cell types. Moreover, the spectral sensitivity of chickens is greater than that of humans from 320 to 480 nm and 580 to 700 nm.

Their maximum sensitivity is in a similar range to humans. The broader spectral sensitivity of poultry may make them perceive many light sources as being brighter than a human would see. Poultry may be more docile during handling in blue light spectra.

Lighting conditions have a large effect on chicken behaviour when the birds are shackled for slaughter. During handling of poultry, the occurrence of flapping should be minimized. Changes in lighting may be used as one tool to keep birds calmer during handling.

EFFECTS OF VISUAL DISTRACTIONS AND HANDLING

Livestock of all species will often refuse to move through a chute or other handling facility if they see distractions such as shadows, reflections, or people ahead of them. Removing distractions that cause animals to balk and stop will facilitate animal movement. A calm animal will stand and point its eyes and ears towards distractions that attract its attention.

If the leader is allowed to stop and look at a distraction, it will often move forward and the other animals will follow. If the animals are rushed, they may turn back and refuse to move forward when they see a distraction. Distractions are most likely to cause balking or other handling problems if the animals are not familiar with the facility. Experienced dairy cows will often ignore a distraction such as a floor drain, but new, inexperienced heifers will balk at it.

Table. Visual Distractions that may Cause Animals to Balk and Refuse to Move

- Sudden changes in floor structure or surface such as drain grates, objects on the floor or change in flooring material.
- Shadows, puddles, and shafts of light; seeing light through a slatted floor.
- Animals may refuse to enter a dark place. Use indirect lighting to facilitate movement towards the light. Animals tend to move from a darker place to a more brightly illuminated place, but they will not move into blinding light.
- Reflections on a wet floor or shiny metal. Move lights to eliminate the reflection or use non-reflective surfaces.
- Moving people in front of approaching animals. People should stand where approaching animals do not see them.
- Jiggling chains, coats on a fence, flapping plastic, or swinging ropes. Remove these distractions.
- Animals see people, moving objects such as vehicles or objects with high colour contrasts outside of the chute. Improve movement by installing solid sides.

Table contains a list of distractions that may cause animals to balk and refuse to move. This list can be used as a guide for modifying handling facilities where excessive use of electric prods is occurring. In facilities where animals move easily and quietly and electric prods are seldom used, removal of distractions may not be needed.

FACILITY DESIGN PRINCIPLES FOR ALL SPECIES

Flooring

For all species, nonslip flooring is essential. Animals often become agitated when they start slipping. Handling and restraint will be safer and animals will remain calm if animals have nonslip flooring. Handling facilities should have nonslip floors and good drainage.

Equipment Maintenance

Surfaces that contact the animals must be smooth and free of sharp edges that could injure animals. Sharp edges will cause bruises and injury. Managers should routinely inspect equipment and have a programme of regular maintenance based on use. Special attention should be paid to latches on restraint devices.

Sanitation

Managers should regularly inspect facilities to ensure cleanliness. When new facilities are being designed, ease of cleaning is an important part of the design. Concrete curbs can be used to direct manure to a drain. Hoses, shovels, and other tools that are needed for cleaning should be readily available. Sanitation equipment should be removed after routine cleaning. Animal handling facilities should be regularly cleaned after use and maintained in good working condition.Injuries and accidents can happen to animals and handlers from equipment lockup or other problems that can occur with buildup of filth, breakage, or wear and tear. Managers should routinely inspect the facilities to ensure cleanliness and to maintain a regular maintenance schedule based on use.

GENERAL PRINCIPLES OF RESTRAINT AND HANDLING

Training of animal care personnel in handling procedures should include consideration of the well-being of the animals. During the handling and restraint of animals, care should be exercised to prevent injury to animals or personnel. Animals should be handled quietly but firmly. Properly designed and maintained facilities operated by trained personnel greatly facilitate efficient movement of animals. Prolonged restraint of any animal must be avoided unless such restraint is essential to research or teaching objectives.

The following are important guidelines for the use of animal restraint equipment:

- Animals to be placed in restraint equipment ordinarily should be conditioned to such equipment before initiation of the project, unless the preconditioning itself would increase the stress to the animals.
- The period of restraint should be the minimum required to accomplish the research or teaching objectives.
- Electrical immobilization must not be used as a method of restraint. It is highly aversive to cattle and sheep. Electrical immobilization must not be confused with electrical stunning that causes instantaneous insensibility or electric prod use that does not immobilize animals.
- Restraint devices should not be considered normal methods of housing, although they may be required for specific research and teaching objectives.
- Attention should be paid to the possible development of lesions or illness associated with restraint, including contusions, knee or hock abrasions, decubital ulcers, dependent edema, and weight loss. Health care should be provided if these or other serious problems occur, and, if necessary, the animal should be removed either temporarily or permanently from the restraint device. Animals should be handled and restrained in facilities and by equipment appropriate for the species and procedure.

Some aggressive behaviours of larger farm animals pose a risk to the health and well-being of both herdmates and human handlers. These behaviours may be modified or their impact reduced by several acceptable restraint devices and practices. Only the minimum restraint necessary to control the animal and to ensure the safety of attendants should be used. Care should be exercised when mixing animals to minimize fighting, especially when animals are grouped together for the first time. Animals should be handled and restrained in facilities and by equipment appropriate for the species and procedure. For cattle, for example, a chute facility should be available. Unless they are very young or tame, calves restrained for routine procedures should be handled by means of a calf chute equipped with a calf cradle.

PRINCIPLES TO PREVENT BEHAVIOURAL AGITATION DURING RESTRAINT FOR ALL SPECIES

The following guidance is provided to prevent behavioural agitation:

- Nonslip flooring should be provided. Repeated small rapid slips may cause agitation.
- Avoid sudden jerky motion of either people or equipment. Smooth movements will keep animals calmer.
- When an animal is raised off the ground, during restraint, it will usually remain calmer if its body is fully supported.
- Even pressure over a wide area of the body has a calming effect. The Panepinto sling for small pigs and cattle squeeze chutes use this principle.
- A calm, confident tone of voice will help keep livestock calmer.
- *Optimum Pressure*: Not too loose and not too tight. An animal needs to be held tight enough to feel the feeling of restraint, but not so tight that it feels pain. Excessive pressure will cause struggling.
- *Blocking Vision:* Using a blindfold made from a completely opaque material will often keep cattle and horses with a large flight zone calmer. Solid sides on cattle chutes or a fully enclosed dark box have a calming effect.

2

Animal Breeding: Research Theory and Practice

The science of Animal breeding is defined as the application of the principles of Genetics and biometry to improve the efficiency of production in farm animals. These principles were applied to change animal populations thousands of years before the sciences of genetics and biometry were formally established. The practice of animal breeding dates back to the Neolithic period, when people attempted to domesticate wild species such as reindeer, goats, hogs and dogs.

Domestication was performed through controlled mating and reproduction of captive animals which were selected and mated based on their behaviour and temperament. Judging from cave paintings that have survived, selection was also applied to some qualitative traits such as coat colour and the absence or presence of horns. Without written records, there is no certain knowledge of the evolution of animal breeding practices, but written documents dating back more than 4000 years indicate that humans appreciated the significance of family resemblance in mating systems, recognized the dangers of intense inbreeding, and used castration to prevent the reproduction of undesirable males. Progress in the performance of domesticated animals through these selection practices was very slow; improvements were mainly due to animals adapting better to their environments.

Robert Bakewell, an English animal breeder of the 18th century, is considered the founder of systematized animal breeding. He was the first to emphasize the importance of accurate breeding records, introduced the concept of progeny testing to evaluate the genetic potentials of young sires, and applied inbreeding to stabilize desired qualitative traits. He also promoted concepts such as "like begets like," "prepotency is associated with inbreeding" and "breed the best to the best." Bakewell and his contemporaries in Europe pioneered the development of diverse breeds of Beef cattle, Dairy cattle, Sheep. Colour, conformation, geographical origin and some production characteristics were the main factors that differentiated these breeds. Wide geographical redistribution of animal populations was also an important factor in the formation of new breeds, as invading armies, migrating people and traders transported livestock to new lands. Animal breeding as a modern science belongs to the 20th century. Although numerous geneticists and biometricians have made significant contributions to the development of this science, J.L. Lush of Iowa State University is considered the father of the modern science of animal breeding. Lush and his students developed major scientific procedures applicable to the genetic improvement of farm animals.

BENEFITS OF EACH TYPE OF BREEDING

By definition, purebred dogs have a smaller gene pool to draw on than mixed breed dogs. That smaller gene pool gives the breed its individual characteristics, such as physical appearance and temperament. It is what makes a poodle a Poodle and a Golden Retriever a Golden Retriever. But there is considerable controversy with regard to whether the gene pools of the modern pure-bred have become too small.

Inbreeding

In-breeding is more likely to help "set" or "fix" a particular trait within a breed or a line by narrowing the gene pool to favour those traits. So if a breeder is looking to set a particular desirable feature of their line then in-breeding and choosing the offspring most strongly possessing that trait can be beneficial. In the first pedigree Sydney is the maternal son of Annie, thus doubling on Annie's genes. Or another way to look at it is Annie is both Sydney's mother and Grand-mother. In the second example we have a full brother/sister in-breeding so we are doubling up on the genes from both Kiley and Annie.

In-breeding can also help identify those bad genes that exist within a line. Dogs possessing the bad genes can be eliminated from a breeding programme and carriers also identified. Intermittent in-breeding within a line or breed is not damaging to the long term health of the animals. However, in-breeding over successive generations can lead to reduced fitness and fertility problems among the offspring, resulting in phenomena known as In-breeding Depression. It can take many generations to show up depending on the traits involved. To use this method responsibly a breeder would not want to in-breed on animals with known genetic disorders, temperaments not in keeping with its given breed, or known serious structural faults, or to in-breed frequently even on healthy-superior specimens.

Line-Breeding

Line-breeding is another way to help "set" or "fix" desirable traits. With line-breeding we breed animals that are related, but we are also routinely introducing genes from other lines into the genetic mix. It takes longer to fix the desirable traits this way, but doing so lowers the risk of those problems associated with repeated in-breeding. Loose line-breeding over successive generations will result in more variations of physical appearance than would in-breeding or tight line-breeding, but will keep the physical look and structure within the same general size and shape, it also carries fewer long term risks. *According to geneticists:* Line-breeding can be carried on for many many generations without deleterious effects on the line or breed as long as the individuals involved have few hidden genetic disorders.

Out-Crossing

Out-crossing in terms of pure-bred dogs is the breeding of unrelated dogs. On a pedigree no names will be repeated within the first 5 generations. This type of breeding has both advantages and disadvantages. Which as it turns out are flip sides of the same argument. The greatest genetic diversity are maintained by out -ccrossing, but this also leads to the least consistency in terms of physical appearance and other traits.

Out-crossing does not guarantee that the animals won't develop genetic disorders, but it does tend to reduce the numbers of affected offspring. Best chance of getting an animal that is less prone to developing a genetic disorder comes more from finding a conscientious breeder that screens their animals for hereditary disorders and breeds for the betterment of the breed. All three methods of breeding have their place in a long term, well thought out breeding programme.

Talk to the breeder, ask questions as to what their goal is in doing a particular breeding. Ask about the risks and what problems are known to that line. And all lines have some because the perfect dog and the perfect lines are still goals of the future for all breeders.

ANIMAL BREEDING AND GENETICS – IP PROTECTION

The broad area of biotechnology encompasses many of the patent applications in our field and the US Supreme Court has established guidelines that apply to this technology (Nebel *et al.,* 2002). The Court made it clear in *Brenner v. Manson* that patent utility implied usefulness and not just "any invention not positively harmful to society." The Court expressed reservations regarding a monopoly on compounds with unknown functions, and that utility must extend beyond proving that the product is a result of scientific research (Nebel *et al.,* 2002).

Technologies in the field of animal breeding that may require (or qualify for) IP protection include, but are not limited to: statistical methods for genetic improvement, DNA markers for genetic improvement, transgenic and cloned animals and methods to produce them, new methods to measure traits, methods to identify animals, computer software and other written materials.

Patent coverage in not just confined to genetic markers. Lines of pigs or chickens have been patented and can be viewed as a specialized extension of early breed development or trademarking for protection of this IP. Other patents exist for methods involving cellular and animal manipulation and involve processes like stem cell development, transgenic production (*i.e.*, US 6,271,436) and cloning (*i.e.*, US 6,215,041 or US 6,258,998). Several advances related to mechanical or electronic devices have been made and include new A.I. or embryo transfer tools, advanced ultra-sound equipment, formulas and methods to measure backfat and other traits in livestock (*i.e.*, see early patent US 4,359,055 and more recent US 5,717,142). The increasing need for traceability of animals and animal products has spawned a number of inventions including electronic ID tags and retinal scanning methods and devices.

Considerable discussion has ensued recently from a patent entitled "Method of Bovine Herd Management" granted in the U.S. in 1994 and later in Canada (Schaeffer, 2002). The invention is for the "test-day model" and includes the gathering, mathematical treatment, and the use of the modified data by dairy producers.

The novelty and unobviousness of the patent has been seriously questioned. It was pointed out that the practices of gathering, manipulating and using data by dairy producers have existed for nearly 100 years. The patent therefore claims rights to a practice that has been public knowledge for a long time. The novel idea within the patent was the specific mathematical model and procedures that Everett and co-workers developed for the analysis of test day yields.

Everett was also not the first researcher to apply a model to test day records and as has been demonstrated, the model as described in the patent, is not necessarily the best model that could be applied (Schaeffer, 2002). This patent generated considerable discussion.

It has been argued "what would the field of animal breeding be if the selection index or Henderson's BLUP had been patented?" Yet while quantitative geneticists see the thought of such protection as sacrilege, molecular scientists accept (but may not like) that in a similar way the foundation patent for PCR exists and royalties must be paid for its use.

OTHER LEGAL CONSIDERATIONS

In the US and some other countries, there is no clear exception to infringement for research use of patented inventions, even in non-profit or educational institutions. Researchers are required to obtain a license or permission from the patent owner to use a protected invention for research purposes. In other countries, there is either an exemption for educational or non-commercial research or research on improving the invention. Research using the invention, however, is not allowed.

Researchers should also be concerned with possible claims for "contributory infringement," *i.e.*, assisting someone else to infringe on a patent. For example, due to a claim of possible contributory infringement, the US Genome Coordinators were asked to halt the practice of supplying primers for microsatellite analysis to other researchers. To resolve the issue the Coordinators began buying the primers from a company with a research license.

ETHICAL, SOCIAL AND ECONOMIC ISSUES

Many ethical and social issues have been raised related to patenting of animals and genes (Bent, 1989; Brody, 1989; Dresser, 1988; Evans, 2002). These include: 1) patenting of animals or genes will be destructive to nature and allows man to play "God"; 2) patenting will devalue animal life and hence human life; 3) patenting will increase animal suffering; 4) patenting will lead to a decline in genetic diversity of animals and threaten species; 5) patenting speeds the trend towards commercialization of academic research and 6) patenting will undermine conventional farming and lead to increased industrial farming systems. Early humans domesticated animals and master breeders and geneticists have transformed them into productive species. Was this playing "God" or interfering with nature? The use of transgenics for making specialized animal lines for disease research is certainly adapting nature but does it devalue life and is it unethical or immoral? These are value judgements that most in society have decided are acceptable (Brody, 1989). Certainly some lines have been (and need to be) drawn to delineate what is acceptable and unacceptable. For example, most people and governments have concluded that while cloning of animals is acceptable (at least for research purposes), cloning of humans, for whatever reason, is immoral, unethical and to be avoided.

Animal welfare and animal rights issues continue to be at the forefront of livestock production and biomedical research (Evans, 2002). Individuals who believe that animals have "rights" will likely be opposed to patenting any invention derived from animal research. The most commonly cited examples are those relating to transgenic animals (*i.e.*, early transgenic pigs) in which some animals had health problems. Production and patenting of specialized lines of rodents for biomedical research that have a tendency to develop specific diseases is also considered unethical by animal rights activists (Brody, 1989). If, however, individuals believe that animal rights are subordinate to those of humans, but that they deserve proper care and welfare then the issue of patenting is much less of a concern.

It has been suggested that through the use of gene markers and highly selective breeding, or through the use of transgenics and cloning, that genetic diversity will be greatly reduced. Certainly these methods have the potential to remove within-line variation but they are likely to increase between-line variability. However, it may be argued that the patent system in fact encourages diversity as it promotes and helps establish, via patent-related deposits of biological materials, a broader genetic diversity (Bent, 1989). Related to this issue is the issue of patenting of products from animals or plants from developing countries. Should companies be allowed to sample and alter wild stocks and to subsequently earn great sums of money by then selling them to both developed countries and back to the countries from where they were obtained? Some individuals say this so-called biopiracy is encouraged by patenting and some countries are moving to address these concerns (Evans, 2002). An extension of this is the issue of species integrity. The development of transgenic pigs for xenotransplantation and other species with human genes for human protein production threatens the genetic lines that determine species. While consideration of xenotransplantation has slowed due to fears of retroviruses and diseases like mad cow disease and AIDS, as Evans (2002) points out this dispute over species integrity "is not empirical" but it is tied up in the individual and societal views on nature and "the notion of awe and wonder." It is likely, no matter how repugnant this process is to some, there will be development of transgenic lines of animals for biomedical research (not food production) and applications that do encompass genes from other species.

In a perfect world, public support of research would be 100 per cent of required funding and all IP would be publicly available in the country of origin. Many US public institutions are now funded at about 40 per cent of total budgets and pressures to obtain outside funding are growing. Companies supplying funding expect to "own", through licensing agreements or otherwise, the IP that results. Protection of IP can provide research partners a greater basis for trust and exchange of ideas and help insure that public institutions focus research on areas of high relevance and payoff. Commercial relationships also aid in technology transfer, employment opportunities for students and may allow for research opportunities not available in the public sector. Fretz and MacKenzie (2002) have suggested that: 1) such activities serve the public good; 2) short term, low quality research should not be favoured in order to obtain funding; 3) managing of IP must be a balance of serving the institution, funding agency and public; 4) independence of the researcher and institution must be maintained; 5) the mission of the public institution is not altered and 6) conflicts of interest should be avoided. Institutions must be proactive in balancing funding, IP protection and commercialization.

Does patenting increase the likelihood of "industrial farming?" Economic and governmental issues certainly play a role in the size of the average farm and the level of commercialization of farming. It can be argued that if large companies have exclusive licensing arrangements for genetic tools then small breeders will be disadvantaged. Market pressures related to size of operation and efficiency of production are much larger influences on the industrialization of farming and livestock production than patenting.

Other issues regarding patenting that have an economic basis can be discussed. Langinier and Moschini (2002) provide an excellent review of the economics of patenting and the benefits and costs that are derived. While inventors would prefer broader claims, limited claims encourage competition and further innovation. Complex products often require building on other patents. Unfortunately, development does become blocked by other patents (especially at the leading edge) and this has negative effects on both the developer as well as the public. Licensing of patents exclusively to one company may benefit that company and segments of the public but might also limit further innovation and not be in all the public's best interest. Langinier and Moschini (2002) concluded "that continued efforts are required to improve the workings of the patent system" to improve the economic performance of the system.

PATENTING OF GENETIC INNOVATIONS IN ANIMAL BREEDING

While herdsmen have practiced the art of animal breeding since the beginning of domestication of livestock, the science of animal breeding is just now entering its second century. From its roots in Mendelian inheritance to the developments in quantitative genetics our field has now grown to include modern molecular sciences. The practical applications of the field have been to genetically improve the animals that produce meat, milk and other products of economic value.

Animal breeding as commerce has always "protected" its endeavors commercially by developing breed societies and using pedigrees to protect the intellectual property developed by the master breeders. The advent of molecular biology, sequencing of genomes and the development of cloning, have brought with them large additional investments. These developments have come with the expectation of increased rewards by investing companies and the reality that technical improvements must be protected in order to obtain sufficient return. The purpose of this paper is to discuss forms of intellectual property, in particular patents and patent law, and to suggest ways it might impact the field of animal breeding and genetics.

FORMS OF INTELLECTUAL PROPERTY

Intellectual property (IP) is the property resulting from the creative or "inventive" work of an individual or individuals. The protection of IP is described in a large body of law that includes copyrights, trademarks, trade secrets, and patents. Copyrights protect IP such as articles, books, web pages, computer software and music. Copyright protection applies when the work is in a publishable form. The ã symbol is not required, but recommended and enforcement of rights is made easier by federally registering the mark. In trademark law, the Ô claims common law trademark rights, while the ® indicates federal registration.

Trademarks are used primarily to identify the source of the owners' goods, products or services. Examples include "Le Label Rouge", "American Berkshire Gold" and the gene marker *HAL*-1843 ä that is associated with the gene test for porcine stress syndrome. A trade secret represents IP that is not divulged by the owner and confers some competitive advantage.

Trade secrets can last as long as the information is kept secret. An example of a trade secret might be specific information to make specialized synthetic lines or calculate breeding values. Trade secret law (in the US called the Uniform Trade Secret Acts) helps protect a technology from theft but the degree of protection is dependent on the type of technology and the means used to keep the information secret.

Patents represent the largest form of IP and their development is rooted in a large body of law both in the US and abroad. Such laws and their interpretation are subject to change, especially when new technology is introduced. The descriptions that follow are meant to be general in nature. Patents were developed to "promote the progress of science and useful arts, by securing for limited times, for authors and inventors, the exclusive rights to their respective writings and discoveries" (Article 1, Section 8, US Constitution) in return for making details of inventions available to the public. Patenting was developed in order to support the development of science and innovation. A patent, once granted, represents a legal monopoly granted by the respective country's government to an inventor (specific to that country), permitting the patent owner to prohibit anyone else from making, using, or selling this invention for a specific period of time (now generally 20 years). Infringement of a patent is a civil wrong and the owner may sue for economic damages or injunction to stop infringement. Patents are intended to protect but not withhold technical information. Patents are very different from published papers. Inventors, unlike coauthors, must take part in the inventive process, not just participate in the research. Patents are not peer-reviewed but instead are assessed by patent examiners to determine the application's patentability.

A patent application must disclose sufficient detail to enable "one of reasonable skill in the art" to duplicate the invention. The application must be unobvious, *i.e.*, not a simple, obvious extension of existing technology. Novelty is the next criteria and refers to something created that is new. Lastly, the invention must be useful. The scope of patent rights is determined by the claims. Some patents, like gene marker patents, may enjoy very wide coverage across species while others may be limited to single polymorphisms in one breed. Patents may be related to a process, a product produced by a process or dependent on another patent. Patents are open to interpretation by both examiners and lawyers. In the US, patents can be applied for up to one year after publication or public disclosure but this is not allowed in other countries. Patents in and of themselves do not ensure income. They must be promoted and protected and can be viewed as tradable assets and licensed or assigned to third parties. Confusion often exists relative to "international" patents (see http://www.cambiaip.org), which actually do not exist. Under the Paris Convention Treaty, a group of countries agreed to work with each other to provide a unified examination process and to make filing in its member countries easier by forming the World Intellectual Property Office (WIPO). In unison they adopted the one-year period in which to file an application in one of the other countries without losing the benefit of the original filing date. Using this procedure avoids the citation against the applicant of any "art" that became known after the original filing date in the country of origin, but before the filing date in another country. Under this Patent Cooperation Treaty (PCT), an applicant is allowed one year to file at the WIPO office and, by designating member countries, holds the legal rights and original filing date in those designated countries without having to file in each country or pay the national expense up front. Although there are fees associated with the PCT application, they are less than one would pay for the foreign national filings at a later date. To obtain a patent in these countries, the application does eventually need to be filed in the national patent offices, fees paid, translations done and the laws and regulations of each country office followed. The applicant may have additional time from the national filing date to request examination, depending on particular country requirements. Delaying examination may provide the time desired to continue development and/or commercialization, however, during this period, fees called "annuities" must generally be paid. Due to the expense involved, applications are generally filed only in countries where protection is really needed.

A BRIEF HISTORY OF PATENTS

The early protection of intellectual property rights can be traced back to Venice in the Middle Ages when master craftsmen in guilds prohibited competition from former apprentices for a period of 20 years (Waltersheid, 1994). Such laws had considerably different economic effects for the master craftsman, the apprentice and the general public. For livestock, early breed societies were developed and monitored pedigrees to protect the IP of the master breeders.

The first modern patent act is often thought of as The US Patent Act of 1790. There was similar legislation in France in 1791. Patents related to living matter are relatively new. One of the earliest patents for living matter was granted to L. Pasteur for a yeast strain but this was done under the belief that it was an inanimate object and not living (Lesser, 2002). The first specialized patent law applied to living organisms was that of the Plant Protection Act of 1930 in the US and provided what is commonly referred to as Plant Breeders Rights (PBR) to propagate new varieties by asexual methods. In 1961, a similar law was passed in France called the UPOV (International Union for the Protection of New Varieties of Plants - Union Internationale pour la Protection des Obtentions Végétales; http://www.upov.int).

Protection in the US was expanded in 1970 with the Plant Variety Protection Act to include sexually reproduced plants. The UPOV was revised in Europe in 1991. Under these laws two principles, "breeder's rights" which allows breeders to use protected varieties without permission of the owner and "farmer's privilege" which allows farmers to collect seeds from their crops and use them, were developed (Lesser, 2002). For years many seed companies have attempted to halt this latter practice by asking farmers to sign contracts prohibiting it. Recent technology, like the "terminator" technology (Kaiser,

2000), biologically prohibits the practice. Santaniello *et al.* (2000) provides an excellent review on all aspects of patent protection for plants.

The dawning and blossoming of the molecular age presented real problems for the protection of IP related to living organisms other than plants. In 1975, a French company failed to patent a "dwarf, egg-laying chicken hen produced by a process" involving a sex-linked recessive gene (Bent, 1989). In 1980, the United States Supreme Court in a 5-4 decision (*Diamond v. Chakrabarty)* declared that "anything under the sun that is made by man" is patentable. This case concerned the patenting of genetically engineered bacteria that destroyed oil sludge. In 1987, the US Patent trade office issued a pronouncement of the patentability, in principle, of non-human multicellular organisms that were not naturally occurring (Bent, 1989). This was quickly followed in 1988 by the landmark patent on the so-called "Harvard mouse" which was engineered to be susceptible to cancer. In Europe, similar laws were passed allowing patenting of animals and animal-related inventions. From 1995 to 2001, a total of 45 animal patents were granted in the US (Lesser, 2002). While these changes in patent law had large economic implications, the social and moral ramifications were also enormous.

3

Liquid Transport in Animal Body

We may begin with the exchange of gases, which in our own case we call breathing. In simple animals like jellyfish and many worms there are no special organs for this purpose.

Dissolved oxygen soaks through their skins from the water in which they live, and dissolved carbon dioxide soaks out. In somewhat more complicated creatures like the earth-worm there is a special fluid, the blood, one of whose functions is to carry oxygen from the skin to the internal organs, and carbon dioxide back.

In the most advanced water-dwellers we find special tufts of thin skin, the gills, into which blood is pumped by a heart or hearts, so as to expose it to water with which it may exchange gases. Gills may be naked, as in the young tadpole, but usually, as they are very delicate, they are protected by lids or pouches, as in fish or lobsters, where they lie behind the head on each side.

In air-breathing animals there are two quite different kinds of breathing organ. In insects and spiders, air is carried to every part of the body by tiny branching tubes called tracheae, which open by numerous pores, mainly on the sides of the abdomen.

In air-breathing vertebrates and molluscs the blood is exposed in the lungs to air which is continually renewed by the act of breathing. Some animals combine several methods.

Thus a frog can use its skin alone for breathing so long as it does not need much oxygen, but it normally employs its lungs as well.

The human lungs are elastic organs of a spongy texture, consisting of millions of very small cavities which open into stiff tubes called bronchi. These in turn open into the windpipe in the front of the neck. Since air cannot enter the space between the lung and the chest-wall, the lungs expand when the chest is expanded.

This can happen in two different ways. In the first place the diaphragm, a sheet of muscle separating the chest and belly, and bulging upwards into the former, may contract and force the contents of the belly downwards and outwards.

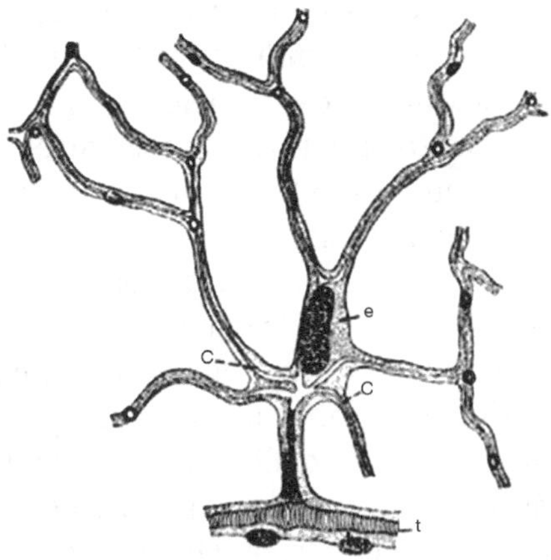

Fig. Final Ramifications of Tracheae in a Caterpillar.

This pulls the bases of the lungs down, and draws air into them. Or the muscles which lie between the ribs may contract so as to bring the ribs, which normally slope downwards, into a more horizontal position. The breast-bone is thus pushed away from the vertebral column, while at the same time the diameter of the chest from side to side is increased, and the lungs expand to fill the extra volume.

Muscles acting in the opposite direction force the air out again if necessary; generally the elasticity of the lungs is sufficient. Thus the air to which the blood in the lungs is exposed is constantly being changed.

The inspired air contains 21 per cent. of O_2 and only 0.03 per cent. of CO_2, whilst the expired air (after being dried) contains about 17 per cent. of O_2 and 3 per cent. of CO_2. To understand how this change occurs we must study the circulation of the blood. The blood flows to and from the heart, as we have seen, through a closed system of tubes known as arteries, veins, and capillaries. It leaves the heart by the arteries, which are comparatively thick-walled, and seldom near the surface, and returns by the veins, which have thinner walls, and often lie just below the skin.

It passes from the arteries to the veins by the capillaries, which are too small to be seen with the naked eye, but are found in almost every tissue. The most easily felt arteries in man are those of the wrist and temple, the most easily seen veins those on the back of the hand and foot. Finally, the heart, which pumps the blood round, is a hollow muscle with four chambers, lying between the lungs, and about as large as the two fists together. The blood from all parts of the body except the lungs enters the heart from behind, near the right-hand top corner, and flows into a chamber called the right auricle.

This contracts rhythmically (the average rate in a grown man at rest is about seventy times a minute) and forces its contents into a thicker-walled chamber lying below it, the right ventricle. As soon as this is full it contracts in its turn. The blood is prevented from returning into the auricle by a valve, called the tricuspid. It therefore finds its way out through the pulmonary artery, which leads it to the lungs. The semilunar valves at the base of the artery prevent it from flowing back into the ventricle when this relaxes at the end of its stroke. In the lungs it has to pass through capillaries in the walls of the air-sacs, so that it is only separated from the air by a very fine membrane, and can easily lose its carbon dioxide and take up oxygen.

It returns from the lungs by the pulmonary vein, this time to the left auricle, which contracts at the same time as the right auricle, and fills the left ventricle. The left ventricle, which is assisted by valves not unlike those on the right side of the heart, forces the blood into the largest artery, an elastic tube called the aorta, from which it is distributed all over the body by the other arteries.

One way of forcing it round through the narrow capillaries would be to have a cistern at the top of the head from which it flowed down again, but this arrangement would clearly not work when its owner lay down. In reality, a fairly steady pressure is kept up by the fact that the walls of the aorta and the arteries are always stretched, and continue to squeeze the blood along between the strokes of the ventricles.

The pressure in man is about that of a column of blood 1.7 metres high, i.e. equal to the head of blood which would be obtained from a cistern 1.7 metres above the heart. The heart of a grown man at rest delivers about 8 litres per minute, or just over 100 cubic centimetres per beat.

During exercise the heart may deliver three or four times as much per minute, mostly as the result of an increased number of beats per minute. The beat of the heart which is felt below the fifth rib on the left side is due to the left ventricle striking the wall of the chest each time it contracts and stiffens. The blood is squirted along the arteries at a rate which may be as high as 50 centimetres a second, and each fresh wave causes a pulse in the artery.

If an artery is cut, the blood comes in a series of spurts from the side nearest the heart, and can be stopped by pressure on the heart side of the cut. It is easy (and safe) to stop the pulse in the wrist by pressing on the same artery higher up, either inside the elbow or inside the upper arm just below the armpit, where it can be felt. The blood flows through the capillaries very slowly, at about half a millimetre per second. Their average length is about a millimetre, while their diameter may be less than 0.01 millimetre. Their very thin walls allow water, gases, and dissolved substances to be exchanged between the blood and the tissues with great ease. From the capillaries the blood oozes gently into the veins.

They have no pulse, and a comparatively small pressure and rate of flow. A cut vein bleeds steadily and the flow can be stopped by compressing the side away from the heart. The flow of blood in the veins is assisted by the presence of valves in them, which only allow it to move towards the heart. If the finger-tip be run along one of the veins of the forearm away from the heart, the vein will dilate on the heart side of each valve.

When therefore the contraction of various muscles squeezes the veins, the blood can only flow towards the heart. If a man stands quite still the blood tends to accumulate in the veins of his legs, and he is liable to faint from failure of the supply to his brain. When he starts walking the blood is at once squeezed out of these veins. The only veins in man which do not lead straight back to the heart are those from the digestive canal and some other abdominal organs, which pass into the liver.

Here the food absorbed by the blood from the gut is dealt with. As the liver needs oxygen, it has also a supply of fresh arterial blood. In most other animals the circulation is somewhat different. Thus in a fish the blood only goes once through the heart in a complete journey, instead of twice, and it all passes through the gills before going on to the tissues. In the frog, in keeping with its two ways of breathing, we have a condition almost half-way between that found in fish and men. The blood entering the right side of the heart by the main vein flows into *R.A.*, the right auricle; thence, through a valve, into *R.V.*, the right ventricle, which pumps it, through a valve, down *P.A.*, the pulmonary artery, to the lungs, *Lg.*

The blood here flows in capillaries, and is then gathered up into the pulmonary vein, *P.V.*, and taken to the left side of the heart, entering the left auricle, *L.A.*, then (through a valve) the left ventricle, *L.V.*, and by this being pumped out (again through a valve) into the aorta, *Ao.* Some of the blood (A^1) goes to the head and anterior extremities, whence it is returned by the anterior venae cavae (V^1), into which discharges the main trunk of the lymphatic system, the thoracic duct (*Th.D.*). The rest (A^2) goes to the trunk and hind limbs.

That which supplies the digestive tube (*Al.*) passes to the liver (*Lr.*) by the hepatic portal vein (*V.P.*); the liver also receives arterial blood direct by *H.A.*, the hepatic artery. The hepatic vein, *H.V.*, joins the veins from the other posterior regions, V^2, and flows to the heart in the inferior vena cava, *V.C.I.* *Lct.* denotes the lacteal lymphatic vessels from the intestinal wall, *Ly.* ordinary lymphatics. We must now consider how the blood acts as a carrier of oxygen and carbon dioxide.

Water at body-temperature will only take up one two-hundredth of its volume of oxygen from air; if the blood were no better than this we should need a heart working forty times as fast as the one we have. Actually the oxygen is carried round in loose chemical combination with a body called haemoglobin. This is a protein, but contains iron as well as the usual carbon, hydrogen, oxygen, nitrogen, and sulphur. It is of a purple colour, but becomes red on combining with oxygen, which it readily takes up from the air.

Thus the blood in the veins is purplish, but if exposed to air either in the lungs or by opening a vein, it at once becomes red. The haemoglobin which it contains enables blood to hold 18 volumes of oxygen per cent., which is 6/7; of the amount contained in the same volume of air, and about 40 times what the blood could carry without haemoglobin. Since blood carries dissolved solids as well as gases, a single set of capillaries supplies the tissues with all that they need for activity, growth, and repair, besides removing most of the waste products.

The carbon dioxide produced in the tissues is mainly carried, not in solution as such (CO_2), but in combination as sodium bicarbonate ($NaHCO_3$). If we look at a drop of blood under a microscope we see that it consists of a clear fluid full of little reddish-yellow biscuit-shaped bodies about 0.007 millimetre in diameter. They can just be seen with a powerful hand-lens. A cubic millimetre of blood contains about five million, and as a man has about 4 litres of blood the total number in his body is about 20 million million, or far more than the number of men who have lived since history began, or probably at all. Their total surface is about 1,500 times the surface of the body.

All the haemoglobin of the blood is contained in them, and they therefore carry round the oxygen from the tissues. Their huge surface area renders this exchange easy. They are cells which have lost their nucleus and are therefore not fully alive, but act as passive carriers of oxygen. They are always being produced in large numbers in the bone-marrow, and destroyed in the spleen and liver when worn out.

For every 500 or so of these red corpuscles there is one white corpuscle. They are true cells with nuclei, and some of them are capable of active movements. There are at least six different kinds with different functions, mostly of a protective character.

Thus one kind eat up parasites found in the blood, another kind burrow through the walls of capillaries in inflamed areas, and remove dead or injured tissue and disease-germs, often forming collections of 'matter' or pus. Others produce substances which kill disease-germs, and so on. The blood also contains non-cellular bodies called platelets, which are smaller than the corpuscles and are concerned in clotting and in immunity; there may also be tiny drops of oil after a fatty meal. Besides the blood-vessels, all vertebrates possess another system of vessels which open into the veins, but contain clear fluid called lymph.

The lymphatic vessels slowly drain away fluid from the spaces between the cells. On the course of the vessels the fluid passes through small lymph-nodes or glands, which may be felt under the skin in the neck, armpit, or groin, before entering the blood. The lymph contains white corpuscles which are largely produced in these glands, and abnormal bodies from the tissues are dealt with in them. Thus if the arm is inflamed, the lymph-nodes of the armpit are generally enlarged, as they are busy destroying poisons or bacteria from the inflamed tissue.

The lymphatics also play a part in digestion, which we shall study later. We must now see how the cells obtain the food-stuffs which they require. In simple animals such as polyps every cell is so close to the digestive cavity that it can obtain food thence directly. In most higher animals, however, the cells which line the alimentary canal and its glands are highly specialized for the purpose of breaking up the food-stuffs into soluble forms and passing them rapidly into the blood or other body-fluids.

This process is called digestion. A few internal parasites like the tapeworm have no gut, but absorb their food through their skin, relying on their host to break it up for them. The course of digestion in man is as follows. The food is chewed in the mouth, where it is also moistened by saliva, a fluid secreted mainly by three neighbouring pairs of glands. Two pairs of these lie between the tongue and the lower jaw, the third pair (whose inflammation causes mumps) lie below the external ear, mainly inside the lower jaw-bone.

Besides moistening the food, saliva contains an enzyme, ptyalin, which breaks up starch into an easily soluble sugar called maltose. Enzymes play a much larger part in digestion than do mechanical processes. Each digestive enzyme is a definite substance with the property of bringing about, or enormously speeding up, a particular chemical reaction.

Pepsin from the stomach will split up half a million times its weight of protein, but will not alter starch or fat. So delicately is an enzyme adjusted to the substrate on which it acts, that as most food molecules are asymmetrical (as we know from their rotation of the plane of polarized light and their asymmetrical crystals) so are the enzymes that act on them.

Enzymes have been compared to keys which open certain locks only. But they are like 'Yale' rather than ordinary keys. For we can make in the laboratory a sugar or peptide (part of a protein molecule) which only differs from the natural variety in that its molecules are related to the natural molecules as a left hand to a right or an object to its image in a mirror. Enzymes will not act on these artificial substances, though they digest their mirror-images which occur in nature. So Alice, who went through the looking-glass in the story, could not have digested the looking-glass proteins and carbohydrates.

She would have had to get her energy from fat and alcohol, whose molecules are symmetrical, and would finally have died of protein starvation. Enzymes are not alive, and can still work when removed from the body; but they are generally destroyed by boiling. The action of ptyalin can easily be shown. A solution of boiled starch gives a blue colour with iodine.

If saliva is allowed to act on it for a few minutes at body-temperature or a few hours in the cold, the starch is broken down to sugar and loses this property. If the saliva is first boiled no change occurs. When the food is swallowed, it is passed into the gullet or oesophagus. To get there it must pass over the mouth of the wind-pipe, and when any falls down this we choke.

To prevent this, the breathing is stopped while we swallow, and the cartilages at the top of the wind-pipe which are concerned in voice-production are brought together so as to close the top of the larynx. It is further protected by a cartilaginous lid at the back of the tongue called the epiglottis, which is pressed backwards over it by the food during swallowing. The movements of the laryngeal cartilages can easily be felt. As the food leaves the mouth it passes out of the control of consciousness and will. The movements of our digestive canal, except at the two ends, are carried out by smooth or involuntary muscle and are controlled by a special part of the nervous system over which the mind does not preside.

The food or drink on leaving the mouth is seized by the smooth muscle of the oesophagus, which contracts behind it and relaxes in front, thus passing it rapidly down into the stomach. Owing to this gripping action one can eat or drink while standing on one's head.

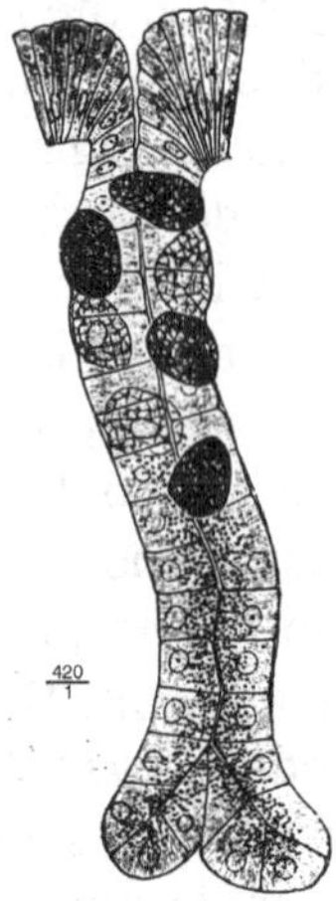

Fig. A Simple Gland From The Stomach of a Bat.

The narrow duct opens above into the cavity of the stomach, among columnar cells. The main part of the gland is a simple tube, formed of a single layer of cells; these secrete pepsin. A few darker-stained cells are seen near the outer side of the tube; these probably secrete hydrochloric acid.

The human stomach is a bag of smooth muscle lined with a membrane consisting mainly of microscopic glands. When expanded it will generally hold about 2 litres. The gastric juice is a clear fluid containing about ½ per cent. free HCl, and several enzymes, of which the most important is pepsin. In presence of acid (though not in a neutral or alkaline fluid), pepsin causes proteins to break up into bodies called peptones and proteoses, which have very much smaller molecules than the proteins from which they are derived, and are more soluble.

Some carbohydrates are attacked by the hydrochloric acid. Thus each molecule of cane-sugar is split into one of glucose and one of fructose, and inulin, a starch-like body found in many plants, is broken up into fructose. Fats are less affected in the stomach. A meal remains in the stomach for a time—generally between one and four hours—which depends on the nature and quantity of the food taken. All this time the muscular walls of the organ are contracting in such a way as to mix the food thoroughly with the gastric juice. Hardly any absorption occurs in the stomach.

When its contents are fully mixed the muscular ring surrounding the lower orifice of the stomach, the pylorus, opens, and a jet of its contents is squirted into the duodenum, the top portion of the small intestine. After a heavy meal the stomach may take several hours in emptying itself.

The human small intestine is a tube about 6 metres long and 3 cm. in diameter when relaxed. It is lined by fine projections of the mucous membrane, the villi, which give it a velvety texture, and increase tenfold the surface available for absorption. Between the bases of the villi are the mouths of numerous microscopic glands, and just beyond the pylorus open the ducts of two large glands, the liver and pancreas.

The liver, among its other functions, secretes bile. This contains substances which have the property, possessed in a less degree by soap, of lowering the surface-tension of water in which they are dissolved. Drops of oil or melted fat tend to join up so as to have as small a surface as possible. This tendency of the surface to shrink is prevented by the bile in the intestine, so when fat-drops are broken up there they do not coalesce again, but form a milky emulsion. Hence the fat-splitting enzyme made in the pancreas can act on a vastly greater surface of fat than would otherwise be available. A man with jaundice from a blocked bile-duct can digest milk, whose fat is already broken up, but not suet or butter, which form big drops.

The bile also contains pigments formed from the haemoglobin of worn-out red corpuscles. These are excreted in the faeces and give them their yellow colour. In jaundice the bile-duct is blocked, and accordingly the skin becomes yellow and the faeces white. Bile is stored in the gall-bladder till required.

The pancreas secretes a juice containing a number of enzymes. One of these, like ptyalin, breaks down starch into maltose. Others break down maltose to glucose, and lactose (milk-sugar) into glucose and galactose, a very similar substance. Another breaks down fat into glycerol and fatty acids, which partly combine with alkali to form soap.

In every case the molecules formed will pass more easily through a membrane than those of the food. If the juice contained a protein-splitting enzyme it would probably digest the pancreas itself and its duct. However, it contains a substance which, on mixing with the secretions of the intestinal glands, yields trypsin, an enzyme which attacks proteins and the products of peptic digestion, breaking them down into amino-acids. These enzymes will not act in an acid fluid, so the bile and pancreatic and intestinal juices contain enough sodium bicarbonate to neutralize the acid of the gastric juice. The secretion of the intestinal glands, besides the substance which helps to form trypsin, contains an enzyme which will break down peptones, though not whole protein molecules, into amino-acids.

There are also enzymes which break down milk-sugar and cane-sugar to sugars containing only six carbon atoms. So far as we know, no animal more complicated than a snail produces an enzyme which will break up cellulose.

But grass consists very largely of cellulose, and to digest it hoofed animals and other plant-eaters employ bacteria which grow in their digestive canal. In cud-chewers like the cow and sheep these bacteria live in special compartments of the stomach; in the horse in the large intestine, which may have a capacity of 200 litres.

The bacteria can get very little oxygen, so they cannot oxidize the cellulose, but they turn a good deal of it into methane, which is wasted, and leave much undigested. The rest, however, is broken up into small molecules which the animal can absorb. In man, cellulose is not digested, but it is useful in giving bulk to the faeces and preventing constipation, which easily occurs when the food leaves no indigestible residue. The food is thus broken up into easily soluble constituents, and is ready to be absorbed. This is done by the epithelium of the small intestine. The passage through is not a mere filtration. For example, the blood contains one part of sugar per thousand, and if sugar merely filtered across from gut to blood, it could never quite disappear from the gut as it in fact does.

Actually, during the absorption of food, the absorptive cells perform work, for which they need an extra supply of oxygen. The fats are, in part at least, put together again from glycerine and soap, and passed as a fine milky emulsion into the lacteals, as the lymphatics of the small gut are called. These join together to form the thoracic duct, which runs up through the chest and empties into the jugular vein at the base of the neck.

The blood may be noticeably milky after a heavy meal of fat. The rest of the products of digestion are passed into the capillaries, and dissolved in the blood. All the veins from the gut run to the liver, and here the food is further dealt with. Thus sugar, if not needed immediately for oxidation, is stored as a starchy body called glycogen, discovered by Claude Bernard, and gradually liberated as required later on.

Some of the sugar and most of the fat are stored elsewhere. Part of the sugar is stored as glycogen in muscles, but much of it is made into fat and stored under the skin and round some of the internal organs, along with fat from the food. In the frog fat is stored in special fat-bodies. The stored glycogen is later split up into glucose for use in the body by an enzyme, which continues to work after death, and the sugar thus liberated gives liver its well-known sweet taste. Absolutely fresh liver is not sweet. Again, ammonia, which is formed in the digestion of many proteins, is, in the liver, mostly combined with carbon dioxide to form urea ($2\ NH_3 + CO_2 = CON_2H_4 + H_2O$).

Urea is a very innocuous body, but ammonia rather poisonous if it gets to the brain, so that if the blood from the gut is short-circuited into the vena cava instead of going into the liver, a heavy meal of meat may cause convulsions. The liver also deals on the same sort of lines with any excess of amino-acids in the blood and with various poisons; its most important function is thus the regulation of the blood's composition, and not the secretion of bile. During starvation the body lives on its stores of fat, and the liver takes on the new duty of converting the stable fats such as those of suet into oils like that of linseed, which are very easily oxidized. The unabsorbed residue of the food from the small intestine passes into the large intestine, where it remains in man for a day or so, and is acted on by bacteria.

These are of little or no value to man, though very valuable to some animals. In man little but water is absorbed there. By this removal of water the bulk of the waste food is reduced by about nine-tenths. The large intestine also excretes poorly soluble salts, such as calcium phosphate, from the blood. These would clog up the urinary passages if they were excreted by the kidneys. The active tissues take oxygen, sugar, fat, and aminoacids from the blood, and use them for oxidation, growth, and repair. Into the blood they empty waste-products, of which the most important are water, carbon dioxide, and urea, but other soluble waste-products of protein metabolism include sulphuric and phosphoric acids, creatinine, and uric acid.

The last two contain C, H, O, and N. They are all excreted by the kidney except the carbon dioxide and some of the water, which go out by the lungs, and, in the case of water, the skin. The kidneys consist of a mass of tubules (about a million on each side in man) each beginning in a capsule containing a tuft of capillaries, and ending, after a winding course, in the central cavity of the kidney.

The capillary tuft seems to act as a filter, and the fluid that soaks through it is blood minus corpuscles and minus a few of the large molecules, such as the proteins concerned in clotting. As this filtrate runs down the tubules, the cells lining them reabsorb valuable constituents of the blood, such as sugar, and probably add unwanted ones such as urea, ammonia, uric acid, creatinine, and sulphates. The urine trickles down the ureters into the bladder, whence it is emptied from time to time. An adult man produces on an average about 1.5 litres of urine per day, containing 30 grams of urea, 15 of sodium chloride, and 10 of other soluble waste-products. The blood is thus the medium of exchange between the different parts of the body. The heart keeps it moving, the lungs and gut supply it with fresh oxygen and foodstuffs, other organs get rid of waste products, and all the tissues of the body take from it according to their needs. The life of every part of the organism therefore depends on an adequate supply of blood of proper composition.

THE NERVOUS SYSTEM

The activities so far described may almost all be found in machines, but a complicated machine needs human control if the parts are to work harmoniously. The body to a large extent runs itself. The diaphragm and heart contract with the appropriate force and rhythm, the pancreas begins to secrete as food reaches the duodenum, and so on. Many of its activities are unconscious: consciousness and will only play a part where our past experience is likely to be of value in influencing our behaviour.

The unconscious responses of the nervous system are called reflex actions, or reflexes; though of course it is also responsible for voluntary actions. The nervous system controls striped muscle, heart muscle, smooth muscle, and glands, but with very few exceptions it is only the striped muscles that the will can influence, and even they are often moved by reflexes.

In every reflex or voluntary action three organs are always concerned, first a receptor organ which is appropriately stimulated, then a longer or shorter path in the nervous system, and finally an effector organ. The latter is always a muscle or gland in man, though other animals have electric and luminous organs under nervous control. In the case of voluntary action the delay in the central nervous system may be very long, but there is always some external motive for a voluntary action. The nature of reflex and voluntary action will be made clearer by a few examples.

	Action.	*Receptor.*	*Effector.*
1.	Speeding up of the heart on increasing its supply of blood.	Nerve-endings in right auricle.	Heart muscle.
2.	Contraction of pupil in strong light.	Retina of eye.	Smooth muscle of iris.
3.	Reddening of skin after a scratch.	Pain spots of skin.	Smooth muscle of small vessels which open.
4.	Secretion of saliva on smelling food.	Olfactory organ in nose.	Salivary glands.
5.	Knee jerk.	Nerve-endings in tendon.	Extensor muscles of thigh.
6.	Blinking on eye being struck at.	Retina of eye.	Eyelid muscles.
7.	Breathing.	Respiratory centres in brain.	Muscles of chest and diaphragm.
8.	Sneezing.	Nerve-endings in nose.	Muscles of chest and diaphragm.
9.	Answering a bell.	Organ of Corti in ear.	Leg muscles.

All but the last are reflexes. The first three are entirely independent of will or consciousness. They are performed by smooth muscle. The fourth involves consciousness but not will. It can, however, be influenced by voluntary attention. The next four are performed by striped muscle, and are partly under voluntary control. The last is a very simple voluntary action. The line between reflex and voluntary action is not sharp. Only an experienced schoolmaster can tell voluntary from reflex coughing.

It will be seen that the receptor organs are generally, but not always, sense-organs, that is to say, their stimulation produces consciousness as well as reflex action. We can learn a great deal about the properties of nerve by taking a muscle with its motor nerve out of a recently killed animal. If we stimulate the nerve by electrical or chemical means, or mechanically (e. g. by pinching), the muscle will contract. This irritability continues for many hours, though the muscle is very easily fatigued unless it has a proper oxygen supply. The muscle may be made to work a lever which writes on a moving sheet of paper, and the effects of different stimuli can thus be compared.

We can also measure the heat or electrical changes produced. By such means we learn the following facts about nervous conduction. Each fibre conducts independently of the others. It conducts not a steady stream, but a series of nervous impulses. An impulse is not an electric current, but an activity of the nerve-fibre producing an electrical effect and a little heat as it goes along. It travels at about 30 metres per second or 70 miles per hour in man.

Thus a man, hit by a car going at 80 miles per hour, will probably feel nothing because his brain is destroyed before any nervous impulses from his skin reach it. After the passage of an impulse the fibre needs a rest of one-thousandth of a second or more before it can transmit another.

All impulses in the same fibre are normally of the same intensity. Thus, from this point of view, we may compare a nerve to a bundle of telegraph wires, down which electrical waves of the same intensity pass at varying intervals, but not to a bundle of telephone wires, in which the intensity of the waves is variable. Finally, the energy of a nervous impulse is so small that about four million impulses (which would take several hours to pass) would be needed to heat a nerve 1° C. A voluntary muscle responds to one nervous impulse by a twitch, to a rapid series by a steady contraction. A contracting human muscle is getting about forty-five impulses per second. The energy liberated in a gram of contracting muscle is several hundred thousand times greater than that in a gram of the nerve which supplies it. This ratio is about the same as that of the energy developed by a thirty H.P. motor-car running for twelve hours, to that used by the man who turns the starting-handle for a minute.

Muscles can be made to contract by weak artificial electric currents as easily as by those produced by the nerve. We are not yet sure of the details of how a muscle contracts, though it seems that the lactic acid formed causes microscopic fibrils to contract, as many proteins do when placed in weak acid.

A muscle is not a heat engine, for it has a very high efficiency such as is only found in heat engines one part of which is very much hotter than the other. Its chemical energy is converted directly into work without first passing into heat. The actual process of contraction may have an efficiency of 90 to 100 per cent., but an amount of energy greater than the work done in contraction is wasted as heat during the re-synthesis of the lactic and phosphoric acids, so that the whole process has an efficiency of only about 40 per cent.

Moreover, a good deal of energy is needed for the extra breathing and heart action during exercise, besides the basal metabolism which goes on all the time. So, considered as a machine, a man never has an efficiency of more than 25 per cent. At best, he turns three times as much energy into heat as into work. Moreover, a muscle heats up while keeping up a steady contraction, as in standing, supporting a weight, or pushing at a closed door. Striped muscles become quite flabby when their nerves are cut, but heart muscle and smooth muscle remain active.

Striped muscles have probably only one set of motor nerves which make them contract. Involuntary muscles have two sets: stimulation of one set causes increased activity, of the other set rest or lessened activity. The effects of stimulating a nerve-fibre depend mainly on its connexions in the body, to some extent on the quantity and rhythm of the stimulus, but not at all on where in its course it is stimulated. These facts were first discovered by Müller in 1826. Thus a blow on the 'funny-bone' or just above it is felt in the ring and little fingers because the nerve from them runs near the surface at this point, and irritation of the nerves in the stump of an amputated leg will give a man pain which he feels in toes that he may have lost forty years ago.

Again, when the nerve to the face muscles has been destroyed, the power to move them may sometimes be regained by grafting the nerve supplying certain neck and shoulder muscles into the old track of the facial. But when connexion has been made the patient, in order to move the face, must will to move the shoulder. The most accessible receptor organs are those of the skin.

They can easily be studied in an area where they are scattered, as on the side of the knee. If the skin is shaved we find that only parts round the hair roots are sensitive to gentle touch with a bristle.

Each root is surrounded by a network of nerve-fibres which are easily stimulated. The small hairs act as levers, and render the 'touch spots' more sensitive. In hairless parts, such as the palm, sole, and lips, there are special receptors for touch. Similarly if we go over the skin with a warm blunt metal point, we find that warmth is only felt at a second set of points (not those sensitive to touch), cold at another set, and pain at a fourth.

Many areas on the thigh are quite insensitive to pain, as they have no pain-spots. It is characteristic of receptor organs to be specially sensitive to one kind of stimulus, which may be physical, as with the skin organs, or chemical as with those of taste and smell.

They will, however, generally respond to inappropriate stimuli, if these are strong enough. Thus mustard will stimulate first the heat and then the pain-spots. A blow or pressure on the eye will make one see stars, and so on. On the other hand each receptor organ, with the paths leading from it to the brain, can generally only give rise to one kind of sensation. This, however, depends on the part of the brain to which it leads, not on the organ which is stimulated. There is no fundamental difference in the nature of the impulses in different nerves, as there is in their effects. If we stimulate the optic nerve, even after the loss of the eye, we get visual sensations, and so on. If we put the right hand into hot water, and the left into cold for a minute, and then both into lukewarm water, this feels cold to the right hand and hot to the left.

This is characteristic of the senses. They tell us more about differences of intensity in their stimuli than about their absolute intensity. When we look at a candle in sunlight we find it hard to believe that we can see by it, or even be dazzled by it, at night. We go into a dark room, and see nothing at first, but soon adapt ourselves, and see the things in it instead of a uniform blackness.

After half an hour in a sound-proof room one finds the noise of one's own heart and breathing unpleasantly loud, though normally one cannot hear them. The fineness of discrimination for touch depends mainly on the closeness of touch-spots. Thus, on the palm, where they are very numerous, we can distinguish two points from one if they are 1 centimetre apart. On the back, where there are few touch-spots, this distance must be increased seven times or more. Under the skin are receptors of many kinds. Some respond to deep pressure, and others to pain, but when once the skin is cut through, most healthy tissues are almost insensitive to pain. They become tender, however, when inflamed.

The gut and other hollow organs are insensitive to cutting or burning (stimuli to which they are not normally exposed), but very painful when stretched either by unusually bulky contents or unusually strong contractions of their muscles. There are also receptors in muscles, tendons, and joints. These send impulses to the central nervous system, which inform it of the relative positions and movements of different parts of our body.

Receptors and nerves with this function are called proprioceptive, whilst those whose stimuli come from outside are called exteroceptive. Proprioceptive organs may affect the consciousness. Thus we can tell how much our knee is bent even with our eyes shut, owing to the jointorgans, or how great a weight we are holding, owing to the muscle-organs.

But far more important is the aid they give us without our knowing it, in the co-ordination of muscular movement. If proprioceptive impulses cannot reach the brain from the legs, as happens in a disease of the spinal cord called locomotor ataxy, in which sensation is not lost, the patient cannot co-ordinate the movements or postures of his leg muscles.

In walking he raises his foot too high and brings it down too hard. He cannot stand with his eyes shut. There is no weakness of the muscles, but they cannot be used properly, as the brain gets no information as to what they are doing except through the eyes. The spinal cord consists of a central core of nerve-cells, called the grey matter, surrounded by millions of fibres mostly running lengthways, and called the white matter.

Both include a scaffolding of supporting cells. Between each pair of vertebrae a nerve leaves the spinal canal on each side. It enters the spinal cord by a dorsal and a ventral root. The ventral root fibres go to muscles and glands, and are only traversed by impulses going outwards. The dorsal root consists of fibres carrying impulses from receptor organs to the cord. So if a dorsal root is cut we lose the capacity for feeling with a certain area of the skin, while injury to ventral roots leads to paralysis of muscles. But most nerves contain both sensory and motor fibres, so when a nerve is cut both movement and sensation are lost in the area which it supplies.

The separation of the roots serves to bring all the sensory fibres to one cell-area within the cord, all the motor fibres to another. A nerve's only function is to conduct, but the spinal cord not only conducts impulses to and from the brain with its fibres, but gives rise to reflexes by means of its nerve-cells.

This is shown by what happens when it is divided. If a man breaks his spinal cord in the neck, he dies because his breathing muscles are cut off from the brain, and get no nervous impulses to make them work. If it is broken lower down he may live for some time. He has absolutely no feeling in the parts of his body and no voluntary control over the muscles whose nerve-supply comes from the part of the cord below the break.

But if we examine him six months after the accident we find reflexes occurring in the lower part of his body. If, for instance, we pinch his foot it is drawn upwards without his knowledge or will. If the lower part of the cord is destroyed or the nerves to it cut, all reflexes cease. A great deal has been learnt about nervous activity from the study of spinal reflexes.

They are easily studied on the carcass of a frog whose brain has been destroyed by poking a blunt wire into it from behind. If we irritate its skin its hind leg scratches near the place irritated, but its responses are clumsy, and it does nothing without some fairly violent stimulus. Provided they are in nervous connexion with the brain or spinal cord, the muscles of a limb are never quite flabby. They are mostly in a state of gentle but steady contraction or 'tone', so as to keep the limb in a definite posture.

If then the knee is to be bent, as the flexor (bending) muscles of the thigh contract, its extensor muscles must relax. If they relaxed too little or too slowly there would be a strain and a waste of energy. If they relaxed too quickly or completely the movement would proceed too far, and the kneejoint might be dislocated. Exactly the same applies elsewhere. Almost every muscle in the body, those of the trunk, jaws, and eyes, as well as the limbs, has an antagonist, and arrangements must be made for one to relax as the other contracts.

As there are no inhibitory nerves to striped muscles, this can only be done by inhibiting or switching off the activity of those cells in the central nervous system which are sending impulses to the muscle which has to relax. Figure gives an idea of some of the connexions concerned in a simple spinal reflex. An impulse enters the cord through a fibre in a dorsal root from a pain-spot in the foot.

The fibre divides and its branches end near nerve-cells in the grey matter. One of these cells is represented sending a fibre to a flexor muscle of the knee, another sends a fibre to an extensor. When the pain-spot is stimulated the impulses passing along it cause more nervous impulses to be generated in the cell connected with the flexor muscle, less in that connected with the extensor, so the knee tends to bend, and the foot to be withdrawn. Actually things are far more complicated. Stimulation of a single pain-spot will only cause movement after a long time or never, and, if movement occurs, hundreds of nerve-fibres will be conducting impulses at once.

To get a prompt movement one must stimulate a number of spots or fibres from them at once, as when one treads on a hot coal. Though the type of connexion shown in the figure have actually been observed with the microscope, in most reflexes the excitation has to pass through several neurons before it reaches the cell whose axon is the nerve-fibre to the muscle or other effector.

We must now study the function of the spinal cord in conducting nervous impulses in both directions between the body and brain. In a mixed nerve like the sciatic in the thigh, all sorts of fibres with different functions run together. Some are carrying impulses to the muscles, others from the skin and deep receptors.

As they enter the cord they are sorted out according to which way they conduct, and later on a further sorting process occurs. For example, the impulses which on reaching the brain give rise to sensations of temperature, run up the spinal cord by a different path from those which give rise to sensations of touch.

These paths have been located by several different methods, which have also been applied to the study of the brain itself. First, symptoms are observed in patients, and after their death local injuries of the spinal cord due to splinters of metal or bone, burst blood-vessels, or tumours, are found. When the same symptoms are observed in another patient they can often be relieved by the surgeon owing to the knowledge so gained.

To refuse leave to examine the body in such a case is to condemn some one else to die with those symptoms. Again, after destruction or division of some parts of the nervous system one can observe with the microscope the death and degeneration of groups of nerve-fibres. Now we know that when a fibre is divided, only that part dies which is separated from the cell-body and nucleus of the neuron to which it belongs. So we can discover in which direction the cell-bodies of any bundle of fibres lie. But in the central nervous system the long fibres always conduct nervous impulses away from the nucleus, so we discover the direction in which nervous impulses run in the fibres we have cut.

Finally, we can try the effect on an animal of cutting or stimulating some part of its nervous system. (The lower parts of the system will still work after the animal has been made unconscious by an anaesthetic or by removing its cerebrum). By such methods we can distinguish five main pairs of ascending fibre-tracts in the human spinal cord, besides numerous smaller groups. Two of these go to the cerebellum, and their injury does not affect consciousness, but causes unsatisfactory movements and postures, the brain being without information as to what the muscles are doing. Two of them send impulses only to parts of the brain concerned in consciousness. One serves both purposes. Before we study the functions of the brain it will be convenient to deal with the special sense-organs in the head which communicate with it directly and not through the cord. The organs of the chemical senses, taste and smell, are found in the mouth and nose. They work together, and much of the sensation we commonly regard as taste includes an element of smell. With the eyes and nose tightly shut, taste will not distinguish an onion from an apple.

The tasteorgans mostly lie in the papillae which roughen the upper surface of the tongue. There are four elementary kinds of taste, namely: salt, sweet, sour, and bitter. Other tastes are combinations of these. Each elementary taste has different end-organs.

Thus, we taste sweet things best with the tip of the tongue, bitter with the back. The end-organs of smell are a little patch of about onequarter of a square inch of yellow epithelium at the top of the internal cavity of the nose. The corresponding area in a dog is ten or more square inches, in a large shark 24 square feet. In man, smell is an unimportant, almost vestigial sense, but in the dog and many other animals it is the most important of all.

So the dog's world is mainly a world of smells. But even in man it is the most delicate of the senses. We can smell mercaptan at a dilution of 1 milligram in 20,000,000 litres of air.

As about 1 cubic centimetre at a time is in the olfactory part of the nose, this means that we are affected by one twenty-thousand-millionth of a milligram, whereas the smallest object we can see with the naked eye is about a million times as large. In ordinary breathing most of the air goes past the olfactory cavity. In sniffing, some is sucked into it. No satisfactory classification of smells has yet been made.

TRANSPORT ACROSS CELL MEMBRANES

IMPORTANCE OF CELLS

All cells acquire the molecules and ions they need from their surrounding extracellular fluid (ECF). There is an unceasing traffic of molecules and ions

- In and out of the cell through its plasma membrane
  - Examples: glucose, Na^+, Ca^{2+}
- In eukaryotic cells, there is also transport in and out of membrane-bounded intracellular compartments such as the nucleus, endoplasmic reticulum, and mitochondria.
  - *Examples:* proteins, mRNA, Ca^{2+}, ATP

Relative Concentrations

Molecules and ions move spontaneously down their concentration gradient (*i.e.*, from a region of higher to a region of lower concentration) by diffusion. Molecules and ions can be moved against their concentration gradient, but this process, called active transport, requires the expenditure of energy (usually from ATP).

Lipid Bilayers

The lipid bilayer is permeable to water molecules and a few other small, uncharged, molecules like oxygen (O_2) and carbon dioxide (CO_2). These diffuse freely in and out of the cell. The diffusion of water through the plasma membrane is of such importance to the cell that it is given a special name: osmosis.

Lipid bilayers are not permeable to:

- Ions such as
  - K^+, Na^+, Ca^{2+} (called cations because when subjected to an electric field they migrate towards the cathode [the negatively-charged electrode])
  - Cl^-, HCO_3^- (called anions because they migrate towards the anode [the positively-charged electrode])
- Small hydrophilic molecules like glucose
- Macromolecules like proteins and RNA

This page will examine how ions and small molecules are transported across cell membranes. The transport of macromolecules through membranes is described in Endocytosis.

Solving These Problems

Mechanisms by which cells solve the problem of transporting ions and small molecules across their membranes:

- *Facilitated diffusion:* Transmembrane proteins create a water-filled pore through which ions and some small hydrophilic molecules can pass by diffusion. The channels can be opened (or closed) according to the needs of the cell.
- *Active transport:* Transmembrane proteins, called transporters, use the energy of ATP to force ions or small molecules through the membrane against their concentration gradient.

FACILITATED DIFFUSION OF IONS

Facilitated diffusion of ions takes place through proteins, or assemblies of proteins, embedded in the plasma membrane. These transmembrane proteins form a water-filled channel through which the ion can pass down its concentration gradient.

The transmembrane channels that permit facilitated diffusion can be opened or closed. They are said to be "gated".

Ligand-gated Ion Channels

Many ion channels open or close in response to binding a small signalling molecule or "ligand". Some ion channels are gated by extracellular ligands; some by intracellular ligands. In both cases, the ligand is not the substance that is transported when the channel opens.

External Ligands

External ligands (shown here in green) bind to a site on the extracellular side of the channel.

Examples:

- Acetylcholine (ACh). The binding of the neurotransmitter acetylcholine at certain synapses opens channels that admit Na^+ and initiate a nerve impulseor muscle contraction.
- Gamma amino butyric acid (GABA). Binding of GABA at certain synapses — designated $GABA_A$ — in the central nervous system admits Cl^- ions into the cell and inhibits the creation of a nerve impulse.

Internal Ligands

Internal ligands bind to a site on the channel protein exposed to the cytosol.

Examples:

- "Second messengers", like cyclic AMP (cAMP) and cyclic GMP (cGMP), regulate channels involved in the initiation of impulses in neurons responding to odours and light respectively.
- ATP is needed to open the channel that allows chloride (Cl^-) and bicarbonate (HCO_3^-) ions out of the cell. This channel is defective in patients with cystic fibrosis. Although the energy liberated by the hydrolysis of ATP is needed to open the channel, this is not an example of active transport; the ions diffuse through the open channel following their concentration gradient.

MECHANICALLY-GATED ION CHANNELS

Examples:

- Sound waves bending the cilia-like projections on the hair cells of the inner ear open up ion channels leading to the creation of nerve impulses that the brain interprets as sound.
- Mechanical deformation of the cells of stretch receptors opens ion channels leading to the creation of nerve impulses.

Voltage-gated Ion Channels

In so-called "excitable" cells like neurons and muscle cells, some channels open or close in response to changes in the charge (measured in volts) across the plasma membrane. Example: As an impulse passes down a neuron, the reduction in the voltage opens sodium channels in the adjacent portion of the membrane. This allows the influx of Na^+ into the neuron and thus the continuation of the nerve impulse. Some 7000 sodium ions pass through each channel during the brief period (about 1 millisecond) that it remains open. This was learned by use of the patch clamp technique.

The Patch Clamp Technique

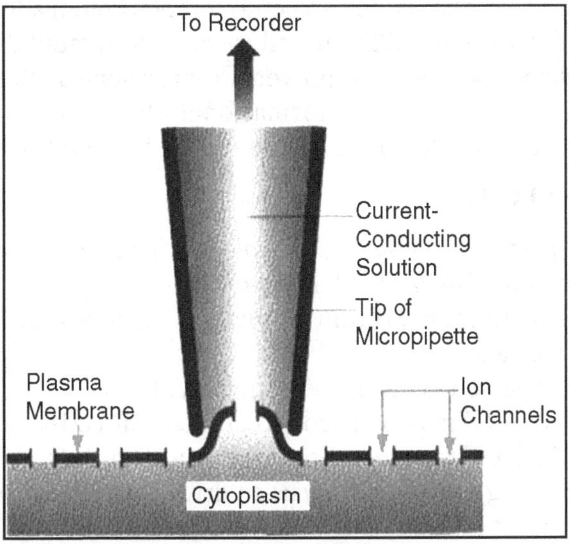

The properties of ion channels can be studied by means of the patch clamp technique.

- A very fine pipette (with an opening of about 0.5 μm) is pressed against the plasma membrane of
- Either an intact cell or
- The plasma membrane can be pulled away from the cell and the preparation placed in a test solution of desired composition.
- Current flow through a single ion channel can then be measured.

Such measurements reveal that each channel is either fully open or fully closed; that is, facilitated diffusion through a single channel is "all-or-none". This technique has provided so much valuable information about ion channels that its inventors, Erwin Neher and Bert Sakmann, were awarded a Nobel Prize in 1991.

FACILITATED DIFFUSION OF MOLECULES

Some small, hydrophilic organic molecules, like sugars, can pass through cell membranes by facilitated diffusion. Once again, the process requires transmembrane proteins.

In some cases, these — like ion channels — form water-filled pores that enable the molecule to pass in (or out) of the membrane following its concentration gradient. Example: Maltoporin. This homotrimer in the outer membrane of E. coli forms pores that allow the disaccharide maltose and a few related molecules to diffuse into the cell.

Another example: The plasma membrane of human red blood cells contain transmembrane proteins that permit the diffusion of glucose from the blood into the cell. Note that in all cases of facilitated diffusion through channels, the channels are selective; that is, the structure of the protein admits only certain types of molecules through. Whether all cases of facilitated diffusion of small molecules use channels is yet to be proven. Perhaps some molecules are passed through the membrane by a conformational change in the shape of the transmembrane protein when it binds the molecule to be transported.

ACTIVE TRANSPORT

Active transport is the pumping of molecules or ions through a membrane against their concentration gradient. It requires:

- A transmembrane protein (usually a complex of them) called a transporter and
- Energy. The source of this energy is ATP.

The energy of ATP may be used directly or indirectly.

- Direct Active Transport. Some transporters bind ATP directly and use the energy of its hydrolysis to drive active transport.
- Indirect Active Transport. Other transporters use the energy already stored in the gradient of a directly-pumped ion. Direct active transport of the ion establishes a concentration gradient. When this is relieved by facilitated diffusion, the energy released can be harnessed to the pumping of some other ion or molecule.

DIRECT ACTIVE TRANSPORT

The Na^+/K^+ ATPase

The cytosol of animal cells contains a concentration of potassium ions (K^+) as much as 20 times higher than that in the extracellular fluid. Conversely, the extracellular fluid contains a concentration of sodium ions (Na^+) as much as 10 times greater than that within the cell.

These concentration gradients are established by the active transport of both ions. And, in fact, the same transporter, called the Na^+/K^+ ATPase, does both jobs. It uses the energy from the hydrolysis of ATP to

- Actively transport 3 Na^+ ions out of the cell
- For each 2 K^+ ions pumped into the cell.

This accomplishes several vital functions:

- It helps establish a net charge across the plasma membrane with the interior of the cell being negatively charged with respect to the exterior. This resting potential prepares nerve and muscle cells for the propagation of action potentials leading to nerve impulses and muscle contraction.
- The accumulation of sodium ions outside of the cell draws water out of the cell and thus enables it to maintain osmotic balance (otherwise it would swell and burst from the inward diffusion of water).

- The gradient of sodium ions is harnessed to provide the energy to run several types of indirect pumps.

The crucial roles of the Na^+/K^+ ATPase are reflected in the fact that almost one-third of all the energy generated by the mitochondria in animal cells is used just to run this pump.

The H^+/K^+ ATPase

The parietal cells of your stomach use this pump to secrete gastric juice. These cells transport protons (H^+) from a concentration of about 4 x 10^{-8} M within the cell to a concentration of about 0.15 M in the gastric juice. Small wonder that parietal cells are stuffed with mitochondria and uses huge amounts of ATP as they carry out this three-million fold concentration of protons.

The Ca^{2+} ATPases

A Ca^{2+} ATPase is located in the plasma membrane of all eukaryotic cells. It uses the energy provided by one molecule of ATP to pump one Ca^{2+} ion out of the cell. The activity of these pumps helps to maintain the ~20,000-fold concentration gradient of Ca^{2+} between the cytosol (~ 100 nM) and the ECF (~20 mM).

In resting skeletal muscle, there is a much higher concentration of calcium ions (Ca^{2+}) in the sarcoplasmic reticulum than in the cytosol. Activation of the muscle fibre allows some of this Ca^{2+} to pass by facilitated diffusion into the cytosol where it triggers contraction.

After contraction, this Ca^{2+} is pumped back into the sarcoplasmic reticulum. This is done by another Ca^{2+} ATPase that uses the energy from each molecule of ATP to pump 2 Ca^{2+} ions.

Pumps 1. – 3. are designated P-type ion transporters because they use the same basic mechanism: a conformational change in the proteins as they are reversibly phosphorylated by ATP. And all three pumps can be made to run backward. That is, if the pumped ions are allowed to diffuse back through the membrane complex, ATP can be synthesised from ADP and inorganic phosphate.

ABC Transporters

ABC ("ATP-Binding Cassette") transporters are transmembrane proteins that

- Expose a ligand-binding domain at one surface and a
- ATP-binding domain at the other surface.

The ligand-binding domain is usually restricted to a single type of molecule. The ATP bound to its domain provides the energy to pump the ligand across the membrane.

The human genome contains 48 genes for ABC transporters. Some examples:

- CFTR — the cystic fibrosis transmembrane conductance regulator
- TAP, the transporter associated with antigen processing.

- The transporter that liver cells use to pump the salts of bile acids out into the bile.
- ABC transporters that pump chemotherapeutic drugs out of cancer cells thus reducing their effectiveness.

ABC transporters must have evolved early in the history of life. The ATP-binding domains in archaea, eubacteria, and eukaryotes all share a homologous structure, the ATP-binding "cassette".

INDIRECT ACTIVE TRANSPORT

Indirect active transport uses the downhill flow of an ion to pump some other molecule or ion against its gradient. The driving ion is usually sodium (Na^+) with its gradient established by the Na^+/K^+ ATPase.

Symport Pumps

In this type of indirect active transport, the driving ion (Na^+) and the pumped molecule pass through the membrane pump in the same direction.

Examples:

- The Na^+/glucose transporter. This transmembrane protein allows sodium ions and glucose to enter the cell together. The sodium ions flow down their concentration gradient while the glucose molecules are pumpedup theirs. Later the sodium is pumped back out of the cell by the Na^+/K^+ ATPase.
- The Na^+/glucose transporter is used to actively transport glucose out of the intestine and also out of the kidney tubules and back into the blood.
- All the amino acids can be actively transported, for example out of the kidney tubules and into the blood, by sodium-driven symport pumps.
- Sodium-driven symport pumps also return neurotransmitters to the presynaptic neuron.
- The Na^+/iodide transporter. This symporter pumps iodide ions into the cells of the thyroid gland (for the manufacture of thyroxine) and also into the cells of the mammary gland (to supply the baby's need for iodide).
- The permease encoded by the lac operon of E. coli that transports lactose into the cell.

Antiport Pumps

In antiport pumps, the driving ion (again, usually sodium) diffuses through the pump in one direction providing the energy for the active transport of some other molecule or ion in the opposite direction.

Example: Ca^{2+} ions are pumped out of cells by sodium-driven antiport pumps. Antiport pumps in the vacuole of some plants harness the outward facilitated diffusion of protons (themselves pumped into the vacuole by a H^+ ATPase)

- To the active inward transport of sodium ions. This sodium/proton antiport pump enables the plant to sequester sodium ions in its vacuole. Transgenic tomato plants that overexpress this sodium/proton antiport pump are able to thrive in saline soils too salty for conventional tomatoes.
- To the active inward transport of nitrate ions (NO_3^-).

SOME INHERITED ION-CHANNEL DISEASES

A growing number of human diseases have been discovered to be caused by inherited mutations in genes encoding channels.

Some examples:

- Chloride-channel diseases
  - Cystic fibrosis;
  - Inherited tendency to kidney stones (caused by a different kind of chloride channel than the one involved in cystic fibrosis).
- Potassium-channel diseases
  - The majority of cases of long QT syndrome, an inherited disorder of the heartbeat;
  - A rare, inherited tendency to epileptic seizures in the newborn;
  - Several types of inherited deafness.
- Sodium-channel diseases
  - Inherited tendency to certain types of muscle spasms;
  - Liddle's syndrome. Inadequate sodium transport out of the kidneys, because of a mutant sodium channel, leads to elevated osmotic pressure of the blood and resulting hypertension (high blood pressure).

Osmosis

- Osmosis is a special term used for the diffusion of water through cell membranes.
- Although water is a polar molecule, it is able to pass through the lipid bilayer of the plasma membrane. Aquaporins — transmembrane proteins that form hydrophilic channels — greatly accelerate the process, but even without these, water is still able to get through.
- Water passes by diffusion from a region of higher to a region of lower concentration. Note that this refers to the concentration of water, NOT the concentration of any solutes present in the water.
- Water is never transported actively; that is, it never moves against its concentration gradient. However, the concentration of water can be altered by the active transport of solutes and in this way the movement of water in and out of the cell can be controlled.

Example: the reabsorption of water from the kidney tubules back into the blood depends on the water following behind the active transport of Na^+.

Hypotonic Solutions

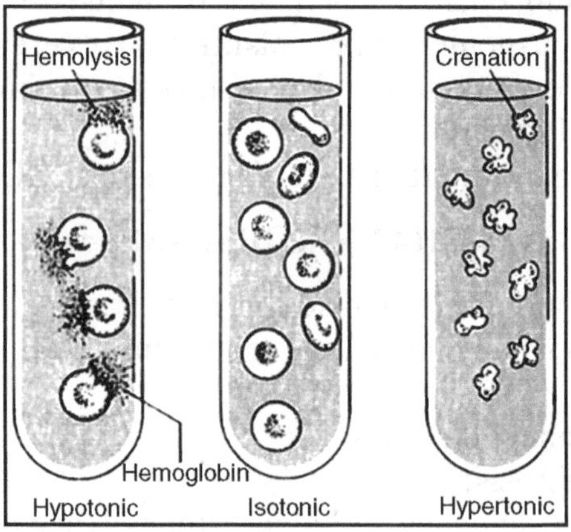

If the concentration of water in the medium surrounding a cell is greater than that of the cytosol, the medium is said to be hypotonic. Water enters the cell by osmosis.

A red blood cell placed in a hypotonic solution (*e.g.*, pure water) bursts immediately ("hemolysis") from the influx of water. Plant cells and bacterial cells avoid bursting in hypotonic surroundings by their strong cell walls. These allow the buildup of turgor within the cell. When the turgor pressure equals the osmotic pressure, osmosis ceases.

Isotonic Solutions

When red blood cells are placed in a 0.9 per cent salt solution, they neither gain nor lose water by osmosis. Such a solution is said to be isotonic. The extracellular fluid (ECF) of mammalian cells is isotonic to their cytoplasm. This balance must be actively maintained because of the large number of organic molecules dissolved in the cytosol but not present in the ECF. These organic molecules exert an osmotic effect that, if not compensated for, would cause the cell to take in so much water that it would swell and might even burst. This fate is avoided by pumping sodium ions out of the cell with the Na^+/ K^+ATPase.

Hypertonic Solutions

If red cells are placed in sea water (about 3 per cent salt), they lose water by osmosis and the cells shrivel up. Sea water is hypertonic to their cytosol. Similarly, if a plant tissue is placed in sea water, the cell contents shrink away from the rigid cell wall. This is called plasmolysis. Sea water is also hypertonic to the ECF of most marine vertebrates. To avoid fatal dehydration, these animals (*e.g.*, bony fishes like the cod) must

- Continuously drink sea water and then
- Desalt it by pumping ions out of their gills by active transport.

Marine birds, which may pass long periods of time away from fresh water, and sea turtles use a similar device. They, too, drink salt water to take care of their water needs and use metabolic energy to desalt it. In the herring gull, shown here, the salt is extracted by two glands in the head and released (in a very concentrated solution — it is saltier than the blood) to the outside through the nostrils. Marine snakes use a similar desalting mechanism.

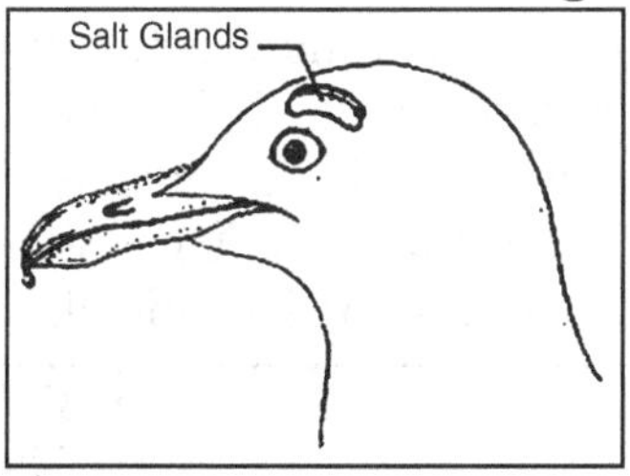

WARM-BLOODED AND COLD-BLOODED

Warm-blooded creatures, like mammals and birds, try to keep the inside of their bodies at a constant temperature. They do this by generating their own heat when they are in a cooler environment, and by cooling themselves when they are in a hotter environment. To generate heat, warm-blooded animals convert the food that they eat into energy. They have to eat a lot of food, compared with cold-blooded animals, to maintain a constant body temperature. Only a small amount of the food that a warm-blooded animal eats is converted into body mass. The rest is used to fuel a constant body temperature.

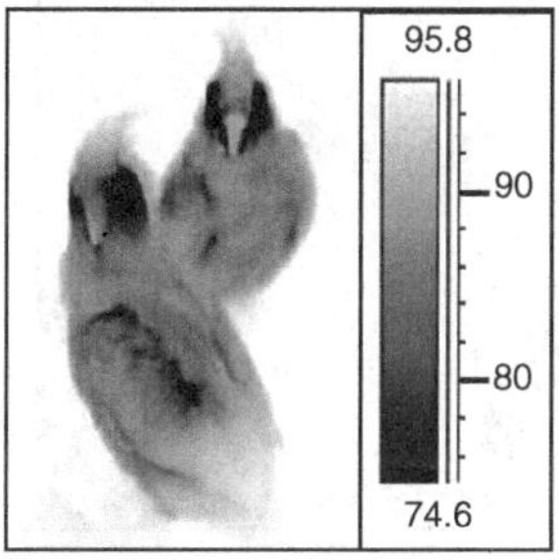

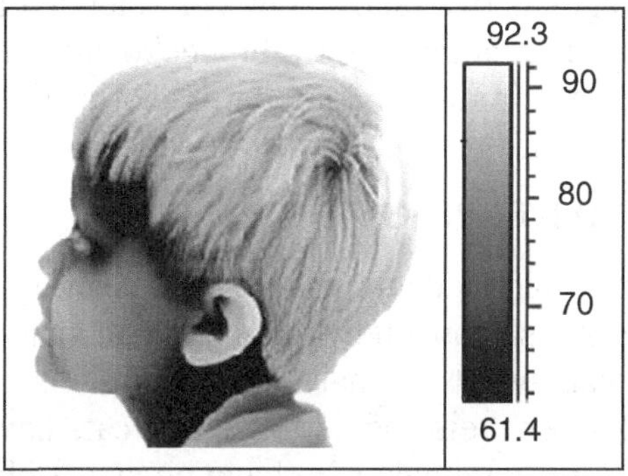

These thermal infrared images of warm-blooded animals, show how birds and mammals maintain body temperatures well above the surrounding, cooler air temperature. Cold-blooded creatures take on the temperature of their surroundings. They are hot when their environment is hot and cold when their environment is cold. In hot environments, cold-blooded animals can have blood that is much warmer than warm-blooded animals.

Cold-blooded animals are much more active in warm environments and are very sluggish in cold environments. This is because their muscle activity depends on chemical reactions which run quickly when it is hot and slowly when it is cold. A cold-blooded animal can convert much more of its food into body mass compared with a warm-blooded animal.

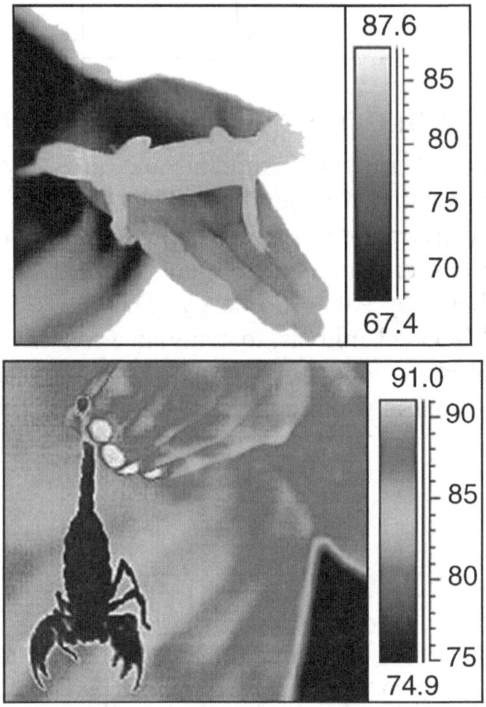

The infrared images above, show how cold-blooded animals take on the temperature of their surroundings. Both the gecko and the scorpion are at the same temperature as the air surrounding them. Notice the difference between these cold-blooded creatures and the warm-blooded humans holding them.

STAYING COOL AND KEEPING WARM

To stay cool, warm-blooded animals sweat or pant to loose heat by water evapouration. They can also cool off by moving into a shaded area or by getting wet. Only mammals can sweat. Primates, such as humans, apes and monkey, have sweat glands all over their bodies. Dogs and cats have sweat glands only on their feet. Whales are mammals who have no sweat glands, but then since they live in the water, they don't really need them. Large mammals can have difficulty cooling down if they get overheated. This is why elephants, for example, have large, thin ears which loose heat quickly. Mammals have hair, fur or blubber, and birds have feathers to help keep them warm. Many mammals have thick coats of fur which keep them warm in winter. They shed much of this fur in the summer to help them cool off and maintain their body temperature. Warm-blooded animals can also shiver to generate more heat when they get too cold. Some warm-blooded animals, especially birds, migrate from colder to warmer regions in the winter.

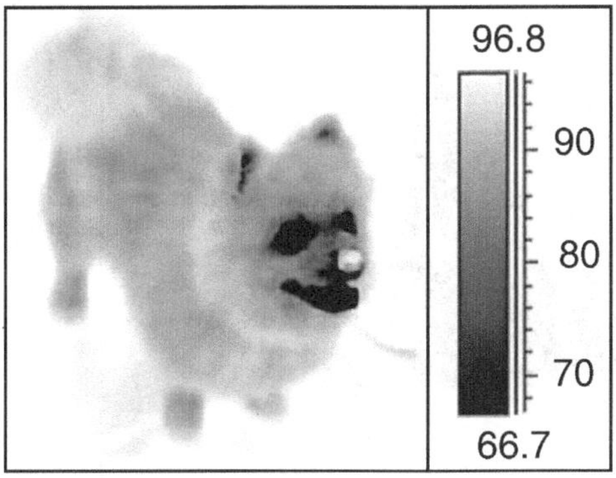

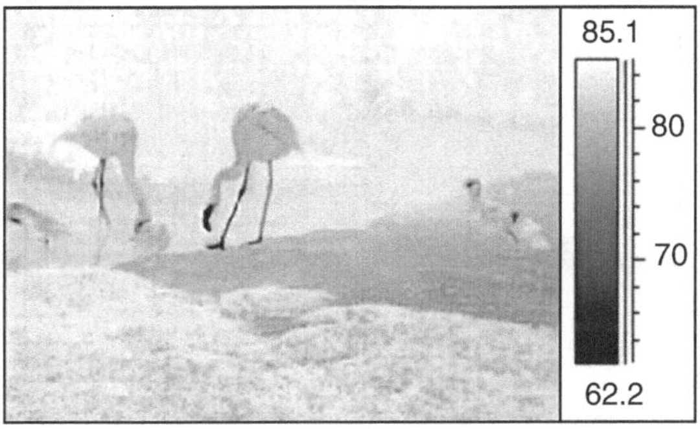

The above infrared images show some ways in which warm-blooded animals try to maintain a constant temperature. The dog in the left image pants when he is too warm. Notice the extra heat radiating from the dog's mouth as he pants. The flamingos in the right image are covered with feathers which help keep these birds warm when it is cool outside. Cold-blooded animals often like to bask in the sun to warm up and increase their metabolism. While basking, reptiles will lie perpendicular to the direction of the sun to maximize the amount of sunlight falling on their skin.

They will also expand their rib cage to increase their surface area and will darken their skin to absorb more heat. When a reptile is too hot, it will lie parallel to the sun's rays, go into a shady area, open its mouth wide, lighten its skin colour or burrow into cool soil. Some cold-blooded animals, such as bees or dragonflies, shiver to stay warm when in a cold environment.

Fish who live in areas where the winters are cold move to deeper waters during the colder months or migrate to warmer waters. Some fish have a special protein in their blood which acts like anti-freeze to help them survive very cold water temperatures. Snakes, lizards, toads, frogs, salamanders and most turtles will hibernate during cool winters. Some insects die when it gets too cold, however others survive by migrating to warmer areas or moving underground. Honeybees stay warm by crowding together and moving their wings to generate heat.

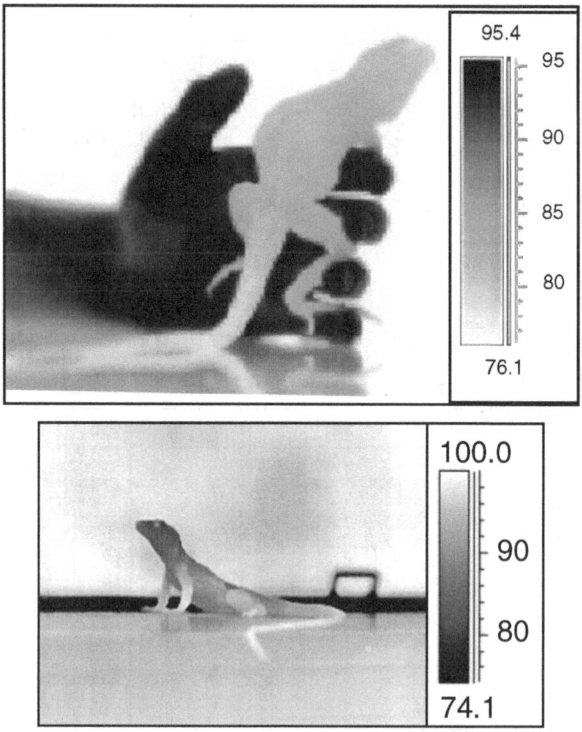

These thermal infrared images of a collard lizard show a cold-blooded animal's body temperature in a cooler and warmer environment. In the image to the left, the lizard is just above room temperature, being warmed by the human hand holding it. To warm up lizards will seek a sunny area and bask in warm sunlight, as in the image to the right.

ADVANTAGES AND DISADVANTAGES

There are many advantages to being warm-blooded. Warm-blooded animals can remain active in cold environments in which cold-blooded animals can hardly move. Warm-blooded animals can live in almost any surface environment on Earth, like in arctic regions or on high mountains where most cold-blooded animals would have difficulty surviving. Warm-blooded animals can remain active, seek food, and defend themselves in a wide range of outdoor temperatures. Cold-blooded animals can only do this when they are warm enough. A cold-blooded animal's level of activity depends upon the temperature of its surroundings.

A reptile, for example, will increase its body temperature before hunting and is better able to escape predators when it is warm. Cold-blooded animals also need to be warm and active to find a mate and reproduce. Being cold-blooded, however, also has its advantages. Cold-blooded animals require much less energy to survive than warm-blooded animals do. Mammals and birds require much more food and energy than do cold-blooded animals of the same weight. This is because in warm-blooded animals, the heat loss from their bodies is proportional to the surface area of their bodies, while the heat created by their bodies is proportional to their mass.

The ratio of a body's surface area to its mass is less the larger the animal is. This means that larger warm-blooded animals can generate more heat than they loose and more easily keep their body temperatures stable. Smaller warm-blooded animals loose heat more quickly. So, it is easier to stay warm by being larger. Warm-blooded animals cannot be too small or else they will loose heat faster than they can produce it.

Being large requires a greater food supply, but for mammals, being small also requires a lot of food to generate more heat. Small mammals need to eat very often to survive because they need more energy to keep a constant body temperature. They also need to eat high energy foods such as fruit, seed, and insects and even other small mammals. Larger mammals can get by with eating lower energy foods or eating less often. In an environment where food is scarce, such as in deserts, reptiles have an advantage.

Since cold-blooded animals do not have to burn a lot of food to maintain a constant body temperature, they are more energy efficient and can survive longer periods without food. Many cold-blooded animals will try to keep their body temperatures as low as possible when food is scarce. Another disadvantage to being warm-blooded is that warm-blooded bodies provide an nice warm environment for viruses, bacteria and parasites to live in. Mammals and birds tend to have more problems with these infections than do reptiles, whose constantly changing body temperatures make life more difficult for these invaders. However, an advantage of this is that mammals and birds have developed a stronger immune system than cold-blooded animals. A reptile's immune system is more efficient when the animals is warmer, however, since bacteria probably grow more slowly in lower temperatures, reptiles sometimes lower their body temperatures when they have an infection.

EXCEPTIONS

Some animals do not fall neatly into the categories of being warm or cold-blooded. Bats, for example, are mammals who cannot maintain a constant body temperature and cool off when they are not active. Echidnas maintain a range of body temperatures which usually lies between 77 and 98.6 degrees Fahrenheit and have difficulty cooling down. Mole Rats are another group of mammals who are unable to regulate their body temperature, however, since they live underground, the temperature of their environment does not change much.

Some warm-blooded animals, such as bears, groundhogs, gophers and bats hibernate during the cold winter. During hibernation these animals live off of stored body fat and can drop their body temperatures by as much as 50 degrees Fahrenheit.

The Hawk Moth is an insect which can raise its body temperature well above the temperature of its surroundings when it is flying because of its huge wing muscles which generate heat when in use. Bees are another example of insects that can raise their body temperatures above that of their environment by moving their wings rapidly to generate heat.

THE ORGANISATION OF ANIMAL BODIES

Living organisms move, feed, respire (burn food to make energy), grow, sense their environment, excrete and reproduce.

These seven characteristics are sometimes summarised by the words "MRS GREN". functions of:

1. Movement
2. Respiration
3. Sensitivity
4. Growth
5. Reproduction
6. Excretion
7. Nutrition

Living organisms are made from cells which are organised into tissues and these are themselves combined to form organs and systems.

Skin cells, muscle cells, skeleton cells and nerve cells, for example. These different types of cells are not just scattered around randomly but similar cells that perform the same function are arranged in groups. These collections of similar cells are known as tissues.

There are four main types of tissues in animals. These are:

1. Epithelial tissues that form linings, coverings and glands,
2. Connective tissues for transport and support
3. Muscle tissues for movement and
4. Nervous tissues for carrying messages.

Epithelial Tissues

Epithelium (plural epithelia) is tissue that covers and lines. It covers an organ or lines a tube or space in the body. There are several different types of epithelium, distinguished by the different shapes of the cells and whether they consist of only a single layer of cells or several layers of cells.

Simple Epithelia – with a Single Layer of Cells

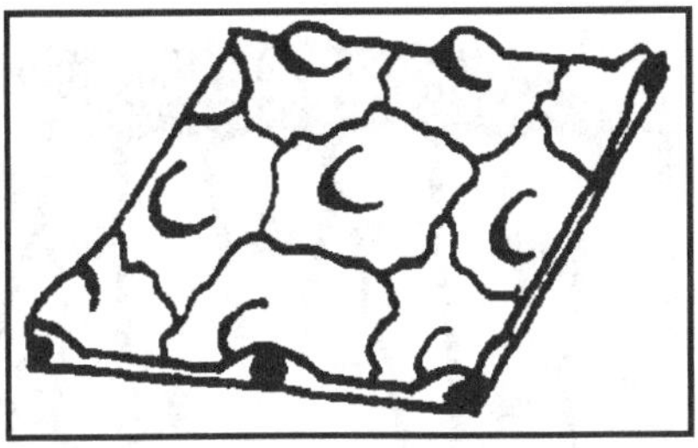

Fig. Squamous Epithelium

Squamous Epithelium

Squamous epithelium consists of a single layer of flattened cells that are shaped rather like 'crazy paving'. It is found lining the heart, blood vessels, lung alveoli and body cavities. Its thinness allows molecules to diffuse across readily.

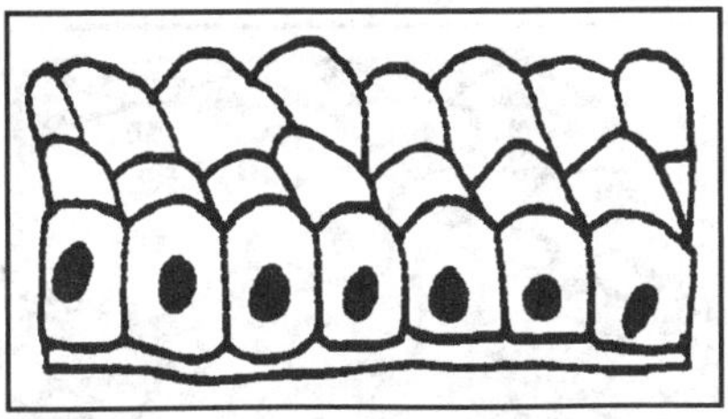

Fig. Cuboidal Epithelium

Cuboidal Epithelium

Cuboidal epithelium consists of a single layer of cube shaped cells. It is rare in the body but is found lining kidney tubules. Molecules pass across it by diffusion, osmosis and active transport.

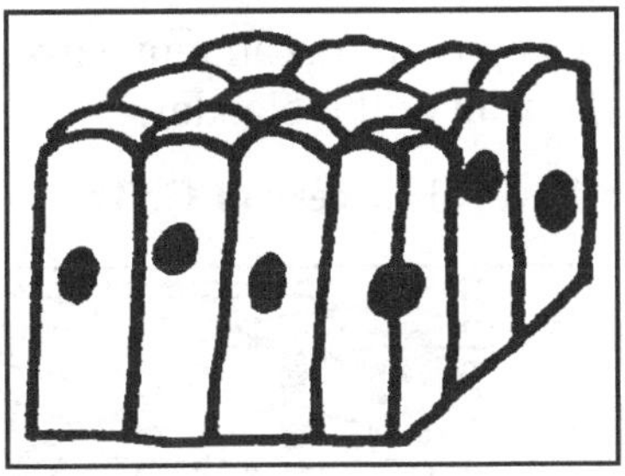

Fig. Columnar Epithelium

Columnar Epithelium

Columnar epithelium consists of column shaped cells. It is found lining the gut from the stomach to the anus. Digested food products move across it into the blood stream.

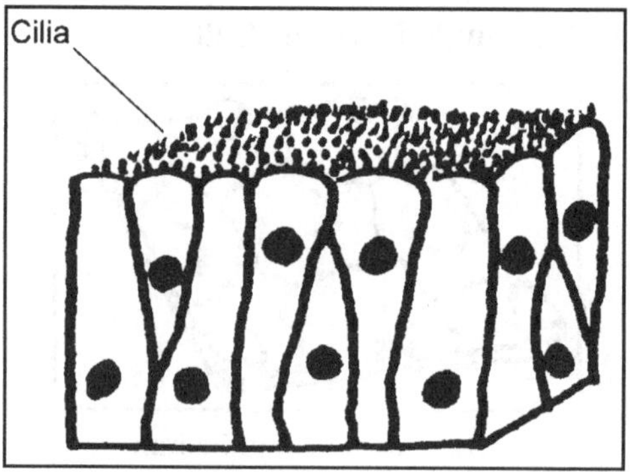

Fig. Columnar Epithelium with Cilia

Columnar Epithelium with Cilia

Columnar epithelium with cilia on the free surface (also known as the apical side of the cell) lines the respiratory tract, fallopian tubes and uterus. The cilia beat rhythmically to transport particles.

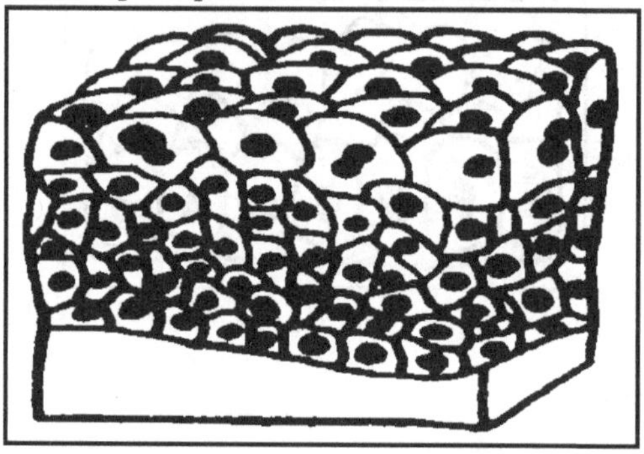

Fig. Transitional Epithelium

Transitional Epithelium–with a Variable Number of Layers

The cells in transitional epithelium can move over one another allowing it to stretch. It is found in the wall of the bladder.

Stratified Epithelia–with Several Layers of Cells

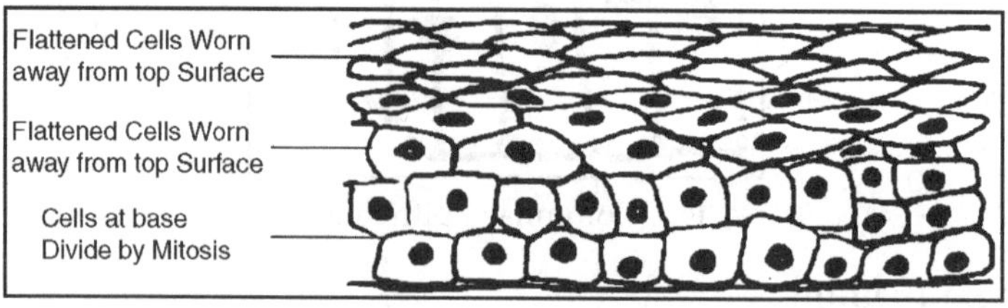
Flattened Cells Worn away from top Surface
Flattened Cells Worn away from top Surface
Cells at base Divide by Mitosis

Fig. Stratified Squamous Epithelium

Epithelia with several layers of cells are found where toughness and resistance to abrasion are needed.

Stratified Squamous Epithelium

Stratified squamous epithelium has many layers of flattened cells. It is found lining the mouth, cervix and vagina. Cells at the base divide and push up the cells above them and cells at the top are worn or pushed off the surface. This type of epithelium protects underlying layers and repairs itself rapidly if damaged.

Keratinised Stratified Squamous Epithelium

Keratinised stratified squamous epithelium has a tough waterproof protein called keratin deposited in the cells. It forms the skin found covering the outer surface of mammals.

Connective Tissues

Blood, bone, tendons, cartilage, fibrous connective tissue and fat (adipose) tissue are all classed as connective tissues. They are tissues that are used for supporting the body or transporting substances around the body. They also consist of three parts: they all have cells suspended in a ground substance or matrix and most have fibres running through it.

Blood

Blood consists of a matrix - plasma, with several types of cells and cell fragments suspended in it. The fibres are only evident in blood that has clotted.

Lymph

Lymph is similar in composition to blood plasma with various types of white blood cell floating in it. It flows in lymphatic vessels.

Connective Tissue 'Proper'

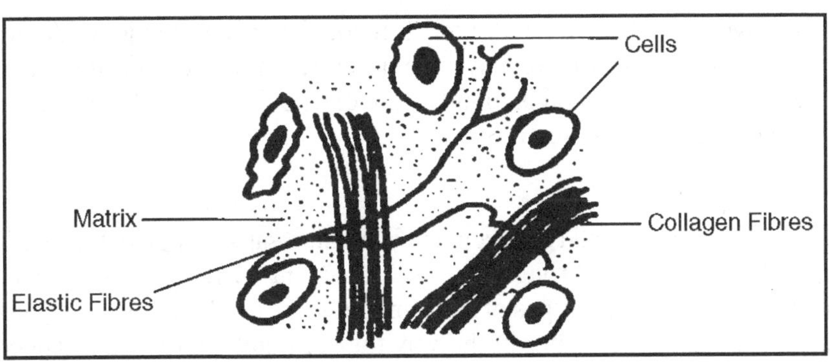

Fig. Loose Connective Tissue

Connective tissue 'proper' consists of a jelly-like matrix with a dense network of collagen and elastic fibres and various cells embedded in it. There are various different forms of 'proper' connective tissue.

Loose Connective Tissue

Loose connective tissue is a sticky whitish substance that fills the spaces between organs. It is found in the dermis of the skin.

Dense Connective Tissue

Dense connective tissue contains lots of thick fibres and is very strong. It forms tendons, ligaments and heart valves and covers bones and organs like the kidney and liver.

Adipose Tissue

Adipose tissue consists of cells filled with fat. It forms the fatty layer under the dermis of the skin, around the kidneys and heart and the yellow marrow of the bones.

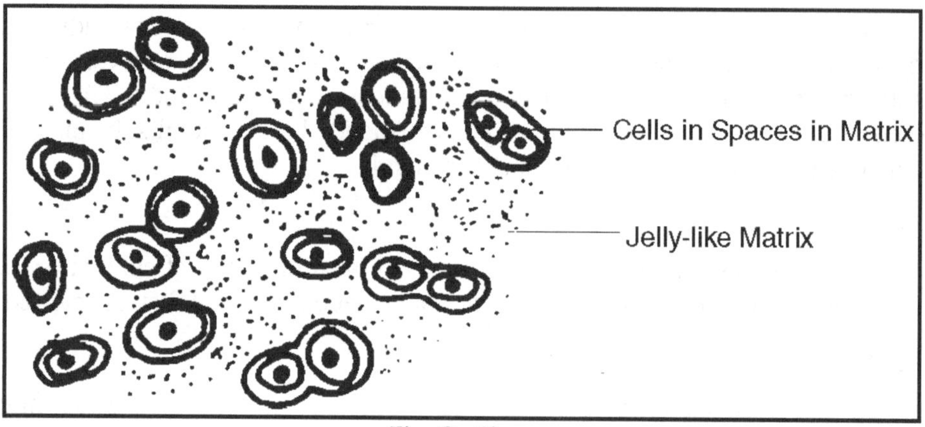

Fig. Cartilage

Cartilage

Cartilage is the 'gristle' of the meat. It consists of a tough jelly-like matrix with cells suspended in it. It may contain collagen and elastic fibres. It is a flexible but tough tissue and is found at the ends of bones, in the nose, ear and trachea and between the vertebrae.

Bone

Bone consists of a solid matrix made of calcium salts that give it its hardness. Collagen fibres running through it give it its strength. Bone cells are found in spaces in the matrix. Two types of bone are found in the skeleton namely spongy and compact bone. They differ in the way the cells and matrix are arranged.

Muscle Tissues

Muscle tissue is composed of cells that contract and move the body. There are three types of muscle tissue:

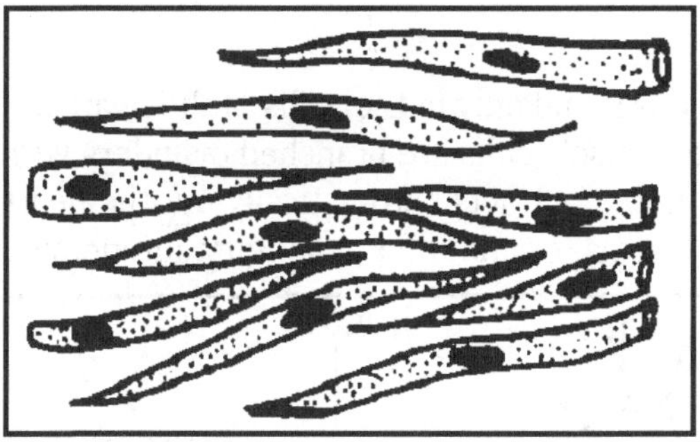

Fig. Smooth Muscle Fibres

Smooth Muscle

Smooth muscle consists of long and slender cells with a central nucleus. It is found in the walls of blood vessels, airways to the lungs and the gut. It changes the size of the blood vessels and helps move food and fluid along. Contraction of smooth muscle fibres occurs without the conscious control of the animal.

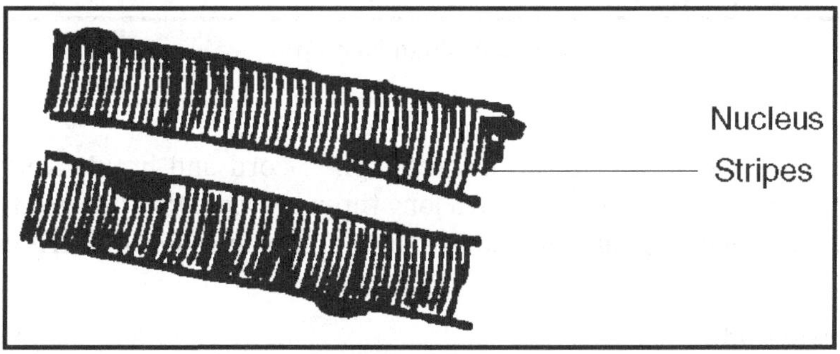

Fig. Skeletal Muscle Fibres

Skeletal Muscle

Skeletal muscle (sometimes called striated, striped or voluntary muscle) has striped fibres with alternating light and dark bands. It is attached to bones and is under the voluntary control of the animal.

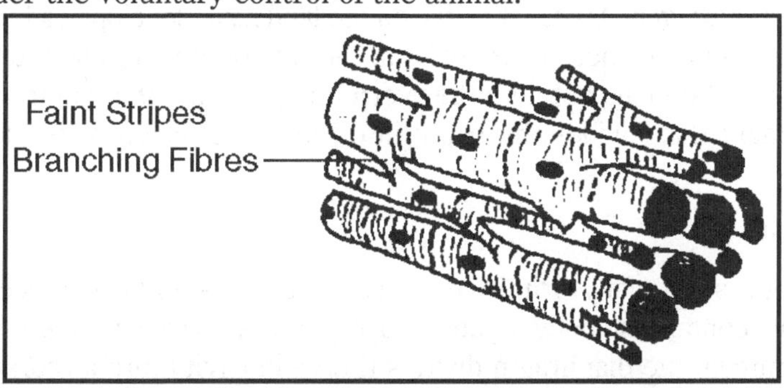

Fig. Cardiac Muscle Fibres

Cardiac Muscle

Cardiac muscle is found only in the walls of the heart where it produces the 'heart beat'. Cardiac muscle cells are branched cylinders with central nuclei and faint stripes. Each fibre contracts automatically but the heart beat as a whole is controlled by the pacemaker and the involuntary autonomic nervous system.

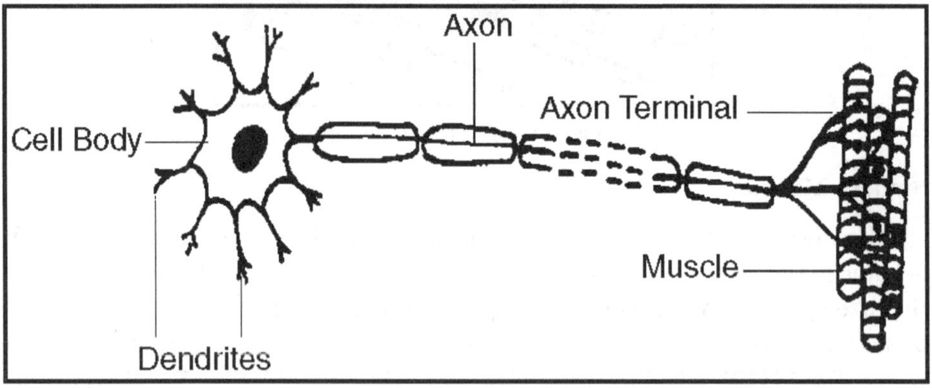

Fig. A Motor Neuron

Nervous Tissues

Nervous tissue forms the nerves, spinal cord and brain. Nerve cells orneurons consist of a cell body and a long thread or axon that carries the nerve impulse. An insulating sheath of fatty material (myelin) usually surrounds the axon.

Vertebrate Bodies

We are so familiar with animals with backbones (*i.e.* vertebrates) that it seems rather unnecessary to point out that the body is divided into three sections. There is a well-defined head that contains the brain, the major sense organs and the mouth, a trunk that contains the other organs and a well-developed tail. Other features of vertebrates may be less apparent.

For instance, vertebrates that live on the land have developed a flexible neck that is absent in fish where it would be in the way of the gills and interfere with streamlining. Mammals but not other vertebrates have a sheet of muscle called the diaphragm that divides the trunk into the chest region or thorax and the abdomen.

Body Cavities

In contrast to many primitive animals, vertebrates have spaces or body cavities that contain the body organs. Most vertebrates have a single body cavity but in mammals the diaphragm divides the main cavity into a thoracic and an abdominal cavity.

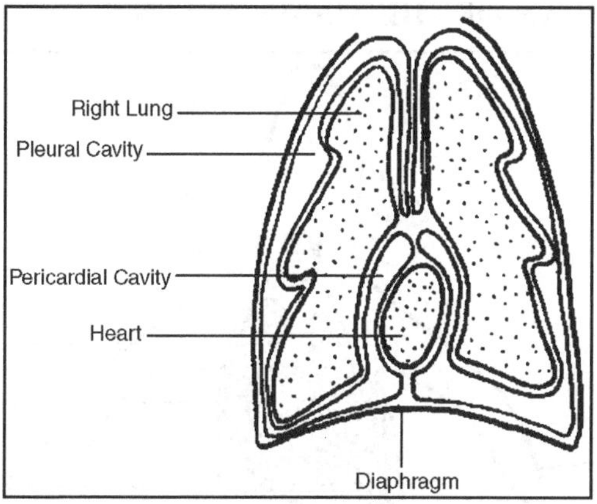

Fig. The Body Cavities

In the thoracic cavity the heart and lungs are surrounded by their own membranes so that cavities are created around the heart - the pericardial cavity, and around the lungs–the pleural cavity.

Organs

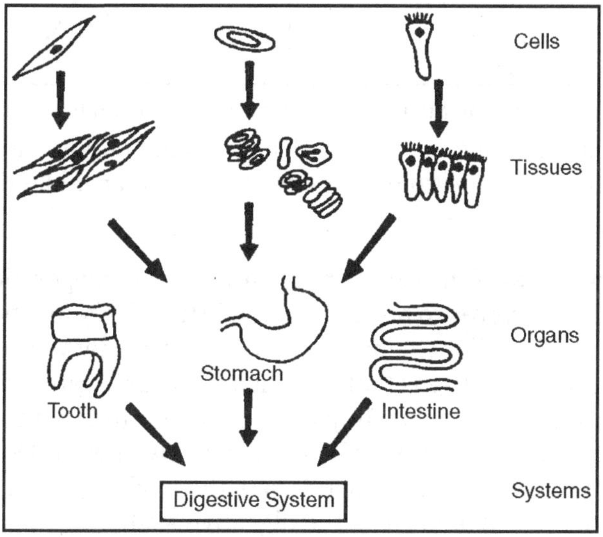

Fig. Cells, Tissues and Organs Forming the Digestive System

Just as the various parts of the cell work together to perform the cell's functions and a large number of similar cells make up a tissue, so many different tissues can "cooperate" to form an organ that performs a particular function. For example, connective tissues, epithelial tissues, muscle tissue and nervous tissue combine to make the organ that we call the stomach. In turn the stomach combines with other organs like the intestines, liver and pancreas to form the digestive system.

GENERALISED PLAN OF THE MAMMALIAN BODY

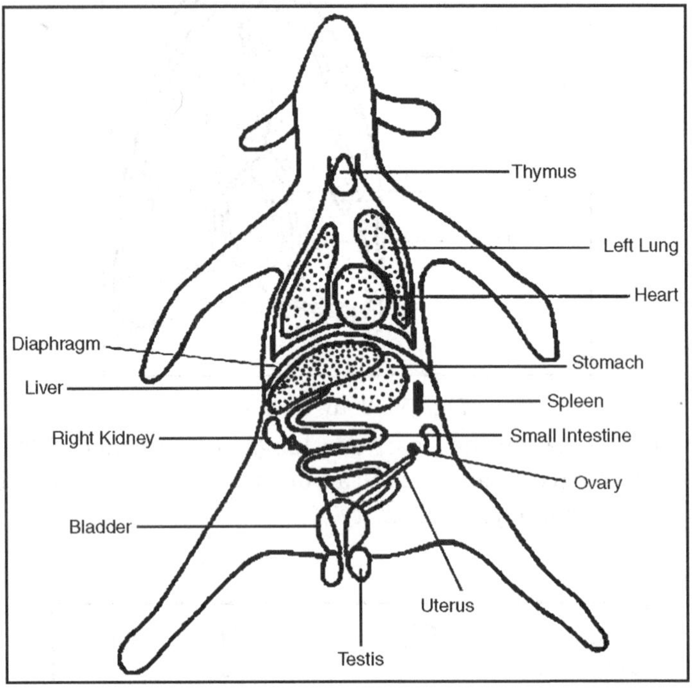

Fig. The Main Organs of the Vertebrate Body

At this point it would be a good idea to make yourself familiar with the major organs and their positions in the body of a mammal like the rabbit.

Body Systems

Organs do not work in isolation but function in cooperation with other organs and body structures to bring about the MRS GREN functions necessary to keep an animal alive. For example the stomach can only work in conjunction with the mouth and oesophagus (gullet). These provide it with the food it breaks down and digests. It then needs to pass the food on to the intestines etc. for further digestion and absorption. The organs involved with the taking of food into the body, the digestion and absorption of the food and elimination of waste products are collectively known as the digestive system.

The 11 Body Systems

- *Skin:* The skin covering the body consists of two layers, the epidermis and dermis. Associated with these layers are hairs, feathers, claws, hoofs, glands and sense organs of the skin.
- *Skeletal System:* This can be divided into the bones of the skeleton and the joints where the bones move over each other.
- *Muscular System:* The muscles, in conjunction with the skeleton and joints, give the body the ability to move.

- *Cardiovascular System:* This is also known as the circulatory system. It consists of the heart, the blood vessels and the blood. It transports substances around the body.
- *Lymphatic System:* This system is responsible for collecting and "cleaning" the fluid that leaks out of the blood vessels. This fluid is then returned to the blood system. The lymphatic system also makes antibodies that protect the body from invasion by bacteria etc. It consists of lymphatic vessels, lymph nodes, the spleen and thymus glands.
- *Respiratory System:* This is the system involved with bringing oxygen in the air into the body and getting rid of carbon dioxide, which is a waste product of processes that occur in the cell. It is made up of the trachea, bronchi, bronchioles, lungs, diaphragm, ribs and muscles that move the ribs in breathing.
- *Digestive System:* This is also known as the gastrointestinal system, alimentary system or gut. It consists of the digestive tube and glands like the liver and pancreas that produce digestive secretions. It is concerned with breaking down the large molecules in foods into smaller ones that can be absorbed into the blood and lymph. Waste material is also eliminated by the digestive system.
- *Urinary System:* This is also known as the renal system. It removes waste products from the blood and is made up of the kidneys, ureters and bladder.
- *Reproductive System:* This is the system that keeps the species going by making new individuals. It is made up of the ovaries, uterus, vagina and fallopian tubes in the female and the testes with associated glands and ducts in the male.
- *Nervous System:* This system coordinates the activities of the body and responses to the environment. It consists of the sense organs (eye, ear, semicircular canals, and organs of taste and smell), the nerves, brain and spinal cord.
- *Endocrine System:* This is the system that produces chemical messengers or hormones. It consists of various endocrine glands (ductless glands) that include the pituitary, adrenal, thyroid and pineal glands as well as the testes and ovary.

Homeostasis

All the body systems, except the reproductive system, are involved with keeping the conditions inside the animal more or less stable. This is called homeostasis. These constant conditions are essential for the survival and proper functioning of the cells, tissues and organs of the body. The skin, for example, has an important role in keeping the temperature of the body constant. The kidneys keep the concentration of salts in the blood within limits and the islets of Langerhans in the pancreas maintain the correct level of glucose in the blood through the hormone insulin. As long as the various body processes remain within normal limits, the body functions properly and is healthy. Once homeostasis is disturbed disease or death may result.

Directional Terms

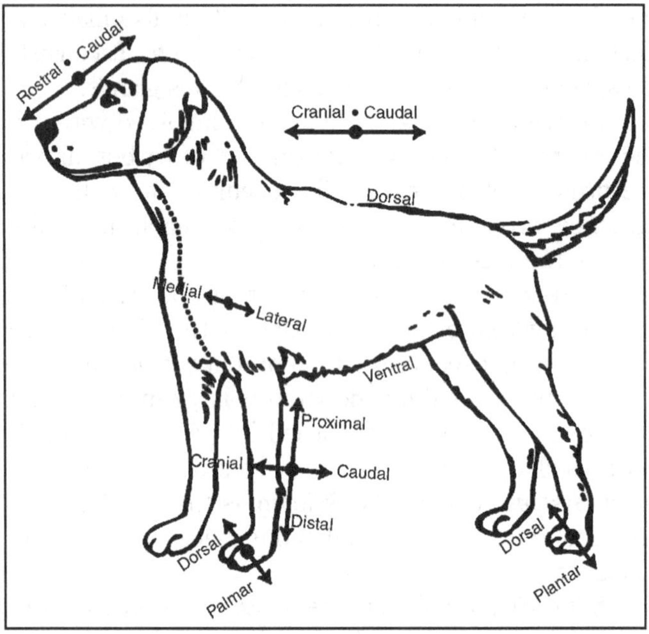

Fig. The Directional Terms Used with Animals

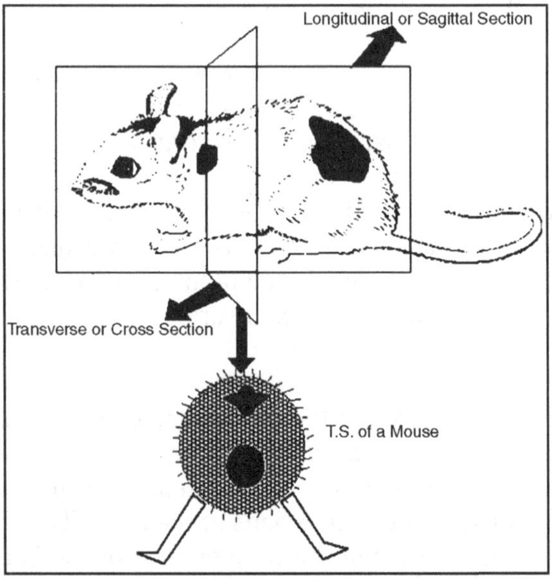

Fig. Transverse and Longitudinal Sections of a Mouse

The systems of the body in the list above will be covered one by one. For each one the structure of the organs involved will be described and the way they function will be explained. In order to describe structures in the body of an animal it is necessary to have a system for describing the position of parts of the body in relation to other parts.

For example it may be necessary to describe the position of the liver in relation to the diaphragm, or the heart in relation to the lungs. Certainly if you work further with animals, in a veterinary clinic for example, it will be necessary to be able to accurately describe the position of an injury. The terms used for this are called directional terms.

The most common directional terms are right and left. However, even these are not completely straightforward especially when looking at diagrams of animals. The convention is to show the left side of the animal or organ on the right side of the page. This is the view you would get looking down on an animal lying on its back during surgery or in a post-mortem. Sometimes it is useful to imagine 'getting inside' the animal (so to speak) to check which side is which.

Term	Definition	Example
Dorsal	Nearer the back of the animal than	The backbone is dorsal to the belly
Ventral	Nearer the belly of the animal than	The breastbone is ventral to the heart
Cranial (or anterior)	Nearer to the skull than	The diaphragm is cranial to the stomach
Caudal (or posterior)	Nearer to the tail than	The ribs are caudal to the neck
Proximal	Closer to the body than (only used for structures on limbs)	The shoulder is proximal to the elbow
Distal	Further from the body than (only used for structures on limbs)	The ankle is distal to the knee
Medial	Nearer to the midline than	The bladder is medial to the hips
Lateral	Further from the midline than	The ribs are lateral to the lungs
Rostral	Towards the muzzle	There are more grey hairs in the rostral part of the head
Palmar	The "walking" surface of the front paw	There is a small cut on the left palmar surface
Plantar	The "walking" surface of the hind paw	The pads are on the plantar side of the foot

Note that we don't use the terms superior and inferior for animals. They are only used to describe the position of structures in the human body (and possibly apes) where the upright posture means some structures are above or superior to others. In order to look at the structure of some of the parts or organs of the body it may be necessary to cut them open or even make thin slices of them that they can be examined under the microscope. The direction and position of slices or sections through an animal's body have their own terminology. If an animal or organ is sliced lengthwise this section is called a longitudinal or sagittal section. This is sometimes abbreviated to LS. If the section is sliced crosswise it is called a transverse or cross section. This is sometimes abbreviated to TS or XS.

4

Animal Experiment

Animal testing, also known as animal experimentation, animal research, and in vivo testing, is the use of non-human animals in experiments. It is estimated that 50 to 100 million vertebrate animals worldwide — from zebrafish to non-human primates — are used annually. Although much larger numbers of invertebrates are used and the use of flies and worms as model organisms is very important, experiments on invertebrates are largely unregulated and not included in statistics. Most animals are euthanized after being used in an experiment. Sources of Labouratory animals vary between countries and species; while most animals are purpose-bred, others may be caught in the wild or supplied by dealers who obtain them from auctions and pounds.

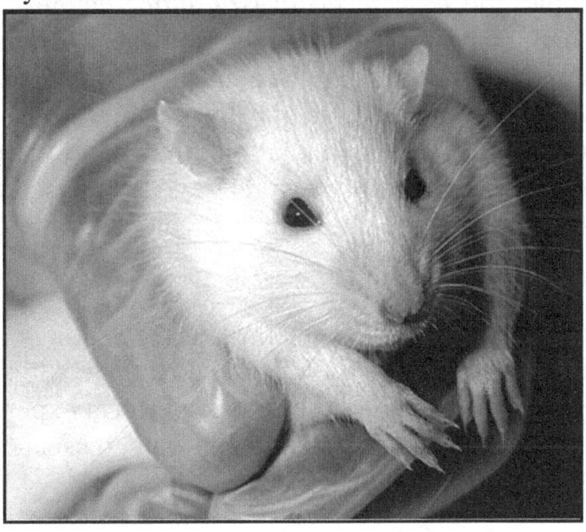

Fig. Animal Testing

The research is conducted inside universities, medical schools, pharmaceutical companies, farms, Defence establishments, and commercial facilities that provide animal-testing services to industry. It includes pure research such as genetics, developmental biology, behavioural studies, as well as applied research such as biomedical research, xenotransplantation, drug testing and toxicology tests, including cosmetics testing. Animals are also used for education, breeding, and Defence research. Supporters of the practice, such as the British Royal Society, argue that virtually every medical achievement in the 20th century relied on the use of animals in some way, with the Institute for Labouratory Animal Research of the U.S. National Academy of Sciences arguing that even sophisticated computers are unable to model interactions between molecules, cells, tissues, organs, organisms, and the environment, making animal research necessary in many areas. Some scientists and animal rights organizations, such as PETA and BUAV, question the legitimacy of it, arguing that it is cruel, poor scientific practice, poorly regulated, that medical progress is being held back by misleading animal models, that some of the tests are outdated, that it cannot reliably predict effects in humans, that the costs outweigh the benefits, or that animals have an intrinsic right not to be used for experimentation. The practice of animal testing is regulated to various extents in different countries.

DEFINITIONS OF ANIMAL EXPERIMENTATION

The terms animal testing, animal experimentation, animal research, *in vivo* testing, and vivisection have similar denotations but different connotations. Literally, "vivisection" means the "cutting up" of a living animal, and historically referred only to experiments that involved the dissection of live animals. The term is occasionally used to refer pejoratively to any experiment using living animals; for example, the *Encyclopaedia Britannica* defines "vivisection" as: "Operation on a living animal for experimental rather than healing purposes; more broadly, all experimentation on live animals", although dictionaries point out that the broader definition is "used only by people who are opposed to such work". The word has a negative connotation, implying torture, suffering, and death. The word "vivisection" is preferred by those opposed to this research, whereas scientists typically use the term "animal experimentation".

HISTORY OF ANIMAL TESTING

The history of animal testing goes back to the writings of the Greeks in the third and fourth centuries BCE, with Aristotle (384-322 BCE) and Erasistratus (304-258 BCE) among the first to perform experiments on living animals. Galen, a physician in second-century Rome, dissected pigs and goats, and is known as the "father of vivisection."

Early Debate

In 1655, physiologist Edmund O'Meara is recorded as saying that "the miserable torture of vivisection places the body in an unnatural state." O'Meara thus expressed one of the chief scientific objections to vivisection: that the pain that the subject endured would interfere with the accuracy of the results. In 1822, the first animal protection law was enacted in the British parliament, followed by the Cruelty to Animals Act (1876), the first law specifically aimed at regulating animal testing. The legislation was promoted by Charles Darwin, who wrote to Ray Lankester in March 1871:

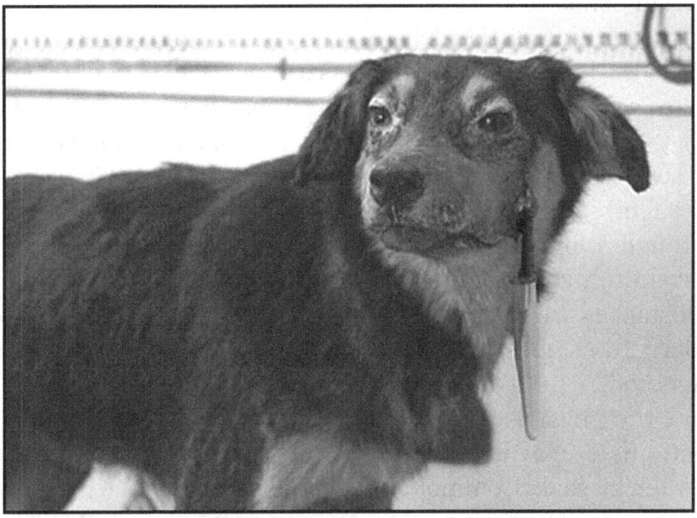

Fig. One of Pavlov's Dogs with a Saliva-catch Container and Tube Surgically Implanted in his Muzzle.

You ask about my opinion on vivisection. I quite agree that it is justifiable for real investigations on physiology; but not for mere damnable and detestable curiosity. It is a subject which makes me sick with horror, so I will not say another word about it, else I shall not sleep to-night."

Opposition to the use of animals in medical research arose in the United States during the 1860s, when Henry Bergh founded the American Society for the Prevention of Cruelty to Animals (ASPCA), with America's first specifically anti-vivisection organization being the American Antivivisection Society (AAVS), founded in 1883.

In the UK, an article in the *Medical Times and Gazette* on April 28, 1877, indicates that anti-vivisectionist campaigners, mainly clergymen, had prepared a number of posters entitled, "This is vivisection," "This is a living dog," and "This is a living rabbit," depicting animals in a poses that they said copied the work of Elias von Cyon in St. Petersburg, though the article says the images differ from the originals. It states that no more than 10 or a dozen men were actively involved in animal testing on living animals in the UK at that time.

Antivivisectionists of the era generally believed the spread of mercy was the great cause of civilization, and vivisection was cruel. However, in the U.S., the antivivisectionists' efforts were defeated in every legislature, overwhelmed by the superior organization and influence of the medical community. The early antivivisectionist movement in the U.S. dwindled greatly in the 1920s, potentially caused by a variety of factors including opposition of the medical community, improvement in medicine through the use of animals, and the tendency of the antivivisectionists to misrepresentation and exaggeration, and their use of inaccurate, vague and outdated references. Overall, this movement had no US legislative success until the passing of the Labouratory Animal Welfare Act, in 1966.

On the other side of the debate, those in Favour of animal testing held that experiments on animals were necessary to advance medical and biological knowledge. Claude Bernard, known as the "prince of vivisectors" and the father of physiology — whose wife, Marie Françoise Martin, founded the first anti-vivisection society in France in 1883 — famously wrote in 1865 that "the science of life is a superb and dazzlingly lighted hall which may be reached only by passing through a long and ghastly kitchen". Arguing that "experiments on animals. are entirely conclusive for the toxicology and hygiene of man.the effects of these substances are the same on man as on animals, save for differences in degree," Bernard established animal experimentation as part of the standard scientific method.

In 1896, the physiologist and physician Dr. Walter B. Cannon said "The antivivisectionists are the second of the two types Theodore Roosevelt described when he said, 'Common sense without conscience may lead to crime, but conscience without common sense may lead to folly, which is the handmaiden of crime.' " These divisions between pro- and anti- animal testing groups first came to public attention during the brown dog affair in the early 1900s, when hundreds of medical students clashed with anti-vivisectionists and police over a memorial to a vivisected dog.

Basic Science Advances

In the 1600s, William Harvey described the movement of blood in mammals. In the 1700s, Antoine Lavoisier, used a guinea pig in a calorimeter to prove that respiration was a form of combustion, and Stephen Hales measured blood pressure in the horse. In the 1780s, Luigi Galvani demonstrated that electricity applied to a dead, dissected, frog's leg muscle caused it to twitch, which led to an appreciation for the relationship between electricity and animation. In the 1880s, Louis Pasteur convincingly demonstrated the germ theory of medicine by giving anthrax to sheep. In the 1890s, Ivan Pavlov famously used dogs to describe classical conditioning.

In 1921 Otto Loewi provided the first strong evidence that neuronal communication with target cells occurred via chemical synapses. He extracted two hearts from frogs and left them beating in an ionic bath. He stimulated the attached Vagus nerve of the first heart, and observed its beating slowed. When the second heart was placed in the ionic bath of the first, it also slowed.

In the 1920s, Edgar Adrian formulated the theory of neural communication that the frequency of action potentials, and not the size of the action potentials, was the basis for communicating the magnitude of the signal. His work was performed in an isolated frog nerve-muscle preparation. Adrian was awarded a Nobel Prize for his work.

In the 1960s David Hubel and Torsten Wiesel demonstrated the macrocolumnar organization of visual areas in cats and monkeys, and provided physiological evidence for the critical period for the development of disparity sensitivity in vision (ie: the main cue for depth perception), and were awarded a Nobel Prize for their work. In 1996 Dolly the sheep was born, the first mammal to be cloned from an adult cell.

MEDICAL ADVANCES

In the 1880s and 1890s, Emil von Behring isolated the diphtheria toxin and demonstrated its effects in guinea pigs. He went on to demonstrate immunity against diphtheria in animals in 1898 by injecting a mix of toxin and antitoxin. This work constituted in part the rationale for awarding von Behring the 1901 Nobel Prize in Physiology and Medicine. Roughly 15 years later, Behring announced such a mix suitable for human immunity which largely banished the diphtheria from the scourges of mankind. The antitoxin is famously commemorated each year in the Iditarod race, which is modeled after the delivery of diphtheria antitoxin to Nome in the 1925 serum run to Nome. The success of the animal studies in producing the diphtheria antitoxin are attributed by some as a cause in the decline of the early 1900s antivivisectionist movement in the USA.

In 1921, Frederick Banting tied up the pancreatic ducts of dogs, and discovered that the isolates of pancreatic secretion could be used to keep dogs with diabetes alive. He followed up these experiments with chemical isolation of insulin in 1922 with John Macleod. These experiments used bovine sources instead of dogs to improve the supply. The first person treated was Leonard Thompson, a 14 year old diabetic who only weighed 65 pounds and was about to slip into a coma and die. After the first dose, the formulation had to be re-worked, a process that took 12 days. The second dose was effective. These two won the Nobel Prize in Physiology or Medicine in 1923 for their discovery of insulin and its treatment of diabetes mellitus. Thompson lived 13 more years taking insulin. Before insulin's clinical use, a diagnosis of diabetes mellitus meant death; Thompson had been diagnosed in 1919.

In the 1943, Selman Waksman's Labouratory discovered streptomycin using a series of screens to find antibacterial substances from the soil. Waksman coined the term antibiotic with regards to these substances. Waksman would win the Nobel Prize in Medicine in 1952 for his discoveries in antibiotics. Corwin Hinshaw and William Feldman took the streptomycin samples and cured tuberculosis in four guinea pigs with it. Hinshaw followed these studies with human trials that provided a dramatic advance in the ability to stop and reverse the progression of tuberculosis. Mortality from tuberculosis in the UK has diminished from the early 20th century due to better hygiene and improved living standards, but from the moment antibiotics were introduced, the fall became much steeper, so that by the 1980s mortality in developed countries was effectively zero. In the 1940s, Jonas Salk used Rhesus monkey cross-contamination studies to isolate the three forms of the polio virus that affected hundreds of thousands yearly. Salk's team created a vaccine against the strains of polio in cell cultures of Rhesus monkey kidney cells. The vaccine was made publicly available in 1955, and reduced the incidence of polio 15-fold in the USA over the following five years.

Albert Sabin made a superior "live" vaccine by passing the polio virus through animal hosts, including monkeys. The vaccine was produced for mass consumption in 1963 and is still in use today. It had virtually eradicated polio in the USA by 1965. It has been estimated that 100,000 Rhesus monkeys were killed in the course of developing the polio vaccines, and 65 doses of vaccine were produced for each monkey.

Also in the 1940s, John Cade tested lithium salts in guinea pigs in a search for pharmaceuticals with anticonvulsant properties. The animals seemed calmer in their mood. He then tested lithium on himself, before using it to treat recurrent mania. The introduction of lithium revolutionized the treatment of manic-depressives by the 1970s. Prior to Cade's animal testing, manic-depressives were treated with lobotomy or electro-convulsive therapy.

In the 1950s the first safer, non-volatile anaesthetic halothane was developed through studies on rodents, rabbits, dogs, cats and monkeys. This paved the way for a whole new generation of modern general anaesthetics - also developed by animal studies - without which modern, complex surgical operations would be virtually impossible.

In 1960, Albert Starr pioneered heart valve replacement surgery in humans after a series of surgical advances in dogs. He received the Lasker Medical Award in 2007 for his efforts, along with Alain Carpentier. In 1968 Carpentier made heart valve replacements from the heart valves of pigs, which are pre-treated with gluteraldehyde to blunt immune response. Over 300,000 people receive heart valve replacements derived from Starr and Carpentier's designs annually. Carpentier said of Starr's initial advances "Before his prosthetic, patients with valvular disease would die".

In the 1970s, leprosy multi-drug antibiotic treatments were refined using leprosy bacteria grown in armadillos, and were then tested in human clinical trials. Today, the nine-banded armadillo is still used to culture the bacteria that causes leprosy, for studies of the proteomics and genomics (the genome was completed in 1998) of the bacteria, for the purposes of improving therapy and developing vaccines. Leprosy is still prevalent in Brazil, Madagascar, Mozambique, Tanzania, India and Nepal, with over 400,000 cases at the beginning of 2004.

The bacteria has not yet been cultured *in vitro* with success necessary to develop drug treatments or vaccines, and mice and armadillos have been the sources of the bacteria for research. The non-human primate models of AIDS, using HIV-2, SHIV, and SIV in macaques, have been used as a complement to ongoing research efforts against the virus. The drug tenofovir has had its efficacy and toxicology evaluated in macaques, and found longterm-highdose treatments had adverse effects not found using shortterm-highdose treatment followed by longterm-lowdose treatment.

This finding in macaques was translated into human dosing regimens. Prophylactic treatment with anti-virals has been evaluated in macaques, because introduction of the virus can only be controlled in an animal model. The finding that prophylaxis can be effective at blocking infection has altered the treatment for occupational exposures, such as needle exposures. Such exposures are now followed rapidly with anti-HIV drugs, and this practice has resulted in measurable transient virus infection similar to the NHP model.

Similarly, the mother-to-fetus transmission, and its fetal prophylaxis with antivirals such as tenofovir and AZT, has been evaluated in controlled testing in macaques not possible in humans, and this knowledge has guided antiviral treatment in pregnant mothers with HIV. "The comparison and correlation of results obtained in monkey and human studies is leading to a growing validation and recognition of the relevance of the animal model. Although each animal model has its limitations, carefully designed drug studies in nonhuman primates can continue to advance our scientific knowledge and guide future clinical trials."

Throughout the twentieth century, research that used live animals has led to many other medical advances and treatments for human diseases, such as: organ transplant techniques and anti-transplant rejection medications, the heart-lung machine, antibiotics like penicillin, and whooping cough vaccine.Presently, animal experimentation continues to be used in research that aims to solve medical problems from Alzheimer's disease, multiple sclerosis spinal cord injury, and many more conditions in which there is no useful *in vitro* model system available.

The earliest references to animal testing are found in the writings of the Greeks in the second and fourth centuries BCE. Aristotle (384-322 BCE) and Erasistratus (304-258 BCE) were among the first to perform experiments on living animals. Galen, a physician in second-century Rome, dissected pigs and goats, and is known as the "father of vivisection."

Animals have been used throughout the history of scientific research. In the 1880s, Louis Pasteur convincingly demonstrated the germ theory of medicine by inducing anthrax in sheep. In the 1890s, Ivan Pavlov famously used dogs to describe classical conditioning. Insulin was first isolated from dogs in 1922, and revolutionized the treatment of diabetes. On November 3, 1957, a Russian dog, Laika, became the first of many animals to orbit the earth. In the 1970s, antibiotic treatments and vaccines for leprosy were developed using armadillos, then given to humans. The ability of humans to change the genetics of animals took a large step forwards in 1974 when Rudolf Jaenisch was able to produce the first transgenic mammal, by integrating DNA from the SV40 virus into the genome of mice. This genetic research progressed rapidly and, in 1996,

Dolly the sheep was born, the first mammal to be cloned from an adult cell. Toxicology testing became important in the 20th century. In the 19th century, laws regulating drugs were more relaxed. For example, in the U.S., the government could only ban a drug after a company had been prosecuted for selling products that harmed customers. However, in response to a tragedy in 1937 where a drug labeled

"Elixir of Sulfanilamide" killed more than 100 people, the U.S. congress passed laws that required safety testing of drugs on animals before they could be marketed. Other countries enacted similar legislation. In the 1960s, in reaction to the Thalidomide tragedy, further laws were passed requiring safety testing on pregnant animals before a drug can be sold. The controversy surrounding animal testing dates back to the 17th century. In 1655, the advocate of Galenic physiology Edmund O'Meara said that "the miserable torture of vivisection places the body in an unnatural state." O'Meara and others argued that animal physiology could be affected by pain during vivisection, rendering results unreliable. There were also objections on an ethical basis, contending that the benefit to humans did not justify the harm to animals.

Early objections to animal testing also came from another angle — many people believed that animals were inferior to humans and so different that results from animals could not be applied to humans.On the other side of the debate, those in Favour of animal testing held that experiments on animals were necessary to advance medical and biological knowledge. Claude Bernard, known as the "prince of vivisectors" and the father of physiology — whose wife, Marie Françoise Martin, founded the first anti-vivisection society in France in 1883 — famously wrote in 1865 that "the science of life is a superb and dazzlingly lighted hall which may be reached only by passing through a long and ghastly kitchen". Arguing that "experiments on animals. are entirely conclusive for the toxicology and hygiene of man.the effects of these substances are the same on man as on animals, save for differences in degree," Bernard established animal experimentation as part of the standard scientific method.

In 1896, the physiologist and physician Dr. Walter B. Cannon said "The antivivisectionists are the second of the two types Theodore Roosevelt described when he said, 'Common sense without conscience may lead to crime, but conscience without common sense may lead to folly, which is the handmaiden of crime.' " These divisions between pro- and anti- animal testing groups first came to public attention during the brown dog affair in the early 1900s, when hundreds of medical students clashed with anti-vivisectionists and police over a memorial to a vivisected dog.

In 1822, the first animal protection law was enacted in the British parliament, followed by the Cruelty to Animals Act (1876), the first law specifically aimed at regulating animal testing. The legislation was promoted by Charles Darwin, who wrote to Ray Lankester in March 1871: "You ask about my opinion on vivisection. I quite agree that it is justifiable for real investigations on physiology; but not for mere damnable and detestable curiosity. It is a subject which makes me sick with horror, so I will not say another word about it, else I shall not sleep to-night."

Opposition to the use of animals in medical research first arose in the United States during the 1860s, when Henry Bergh founded the American Society for the Prevention of Cruelty to Animals (ASPCA), with America's first specifically anti-vivisection organization being the American Antivivisection Society (AAVS), founded in 1883. Antivivisectionists of the era generally believed the spread of mercy was the great cause of civilization, and vivisection was cruel. However, in the USA the antivivisectionists' efforts were defeated in every legislature, overwhelmed by the superior organization and influence of the medical community. Overall, this movement had little legislative success until the passing of the Labouratory Animal Welfare Act, in 1966.

RESEARCH CLASSIFICATION

PURE RESEARCH

Basic or pure research investigates how organisms behave, develop, and function. Those opposed to animal testing object that pure research may have little or no practical purpose, but researchers argue that it may produce unforeseen benefits, rendering the distinction between pure and applied research — research that has a specific practical aim — unclear.

Pure research uses larger numbers and a greater variety of animals than applied research. Fruit flies, nematode worms, mice and rats together account for the vast majority, though small numbers of other species are used, ranging from sea slugs through to armadillos.

Examples of the types of animals and experiments used in basic research include:

- Studies on *embryogenesis* and *developmental biology*. Mutants are created by adding transposons into their genomes, or specific genes are deleted by gene targeting. By studying the changes in development these changes produce, scientists aim to understand both how organisms normally develop, and what can go wrong in this process. These studies are particularly powerful since the basic controls of development, such as the homeobox genes, have similar functions in organisms as diverse as fruit flies and man.
- Experiments into *Behaviour*, to understand how organisms detect and interact with each other and their environment, in which fruit flies, worms, mice, and rats are all widely used. Studies of brain function, such as memory and social Behaviour, often use rats and birds. For some species, Behavioural research is combined with enrichment strategies for animals in captivity because it allows them to engage in a wider range of activities.

- Breeding experiments to study *evolution* and *genetics*. Labouratory mice, flies, fish, and worms are inbred through many generations to create strains with defined characteristics. These provide animals of a known genetic background, an important tool for genetic analyses. Larger mammals are rarely bred specifically for such studies due to their slow rate of reproduction, though some scientists take advantage of inbred domesticated animals, such as dog or cattle breeds, for comparative purposes. Scientists studying how animals evolve use many animal species to see how variations in where and how an organism lives (their niche) produce adaptations in their physiology and morphology. As an example, sticklebacks are now being used to study how many and which types of mutations are selected to produce adaptations in animals' morphology during the evolution of new species.

Applied Research

Applied research aims to solve specific and practical problems. Compared to pure research, which is largely academic in origin, applied research is usually carried out in the pharmaceutical industry, or by universities in commercial partnerships. These may involve the use of animal models of diseases or conditions, which are often discovered or generated by pure research Programmemes. In turn, such applied studies may be an early stage in the drug discovery process. Examples include:

- Genetic modification of animals to study disease. Transgenic animals have specific genes inserted, modified or removed, to mimic specific conditions such as single gene disorders, such as Huntington's disease. Other models mimic complex, multifactorial diseases with genetic components, such as diabetes, or even transgenic mice that carry the same mutations that occur during the development of cancer. These models allow investigations on how and why the disease develops, as well as providing ways to develop and test new treatments. The vast majority of these transgenic models of human disease are lines of mice, the mammalian species in which genetic modification is most efficient. Smaller numbers of other animals are also used, including rats, pigs, sheep, fish, birds, and amphibians.
- Studies on models of naturally occurring disease and condition. Certain domestic and wild animals have a natural propensity or predisposition for certain conditions that are also found in humans. Cats are used as a model to develop immunodeficiency virus vaccines and to study leukemia because their natural predisposition to FIV and Feline leukemia virus. Certain breeds of dog suffer from narcolepsy making them the major model used to study the human condition. Armadillos and humans are among only a few animal species that naturally suffer

from leprosy; as the bacteria responsible for this disease cannot yet be grown in culture, armadillos are the primary source of bacilli used in leprosy vaccines.

- Studies on induced animal models of human diseases. Here, an animal is treated so that it develops pathology and symptoms that resemble a human disease. Examples include restricting blood flow to the brain to induce stroke, or giving neurotoxins that cause damage similar to that seen in Parkinson's disease. Such studies can be difficult to interpret, and it is argued that they are not always comparable to human diseases. For example, although such models are now widely used to study Parkinson's disease, the British anti-vivisection interest group BUAV argues that these models only superficially resemble the disease symptoms, without the same time course or cellular pathology. In contrast, scientists assessing the usefulness of animal models of Parkinson's disease, as well as the medical research charity *The Parkinson's Appeal*, state that these models were invaluable and that they led to improved surgical treatments such as pallidotomy, new drug treatments such as levodopa, and later deep brain stimulation.

XENOTRANSPLANTATION

Xenotransplantation research involves transplanting tissues, or organs from one species to another, as a way to overcome the shortage of human organs for use in organ transplants. Current research involves using primates as the recipients of organs from pigs that have been genetically-modified to reduce the primates' immune response against the pig tissue. Although transplant rejection remains a problem, recent clinical trials that involved implanting pig insulin-secreting cells into diabetics did reduce these people's need for insulin.

The British Home Office released figures in 1999 showing that 270 monkeys had been used in xenotransplantation research in Britain during the previous four years. Documents leaked from Huntingdon Life Sciences to *The Observer* in 2003 showed, between 1994 and 2000, wild baboons were imported to the UK from Africa to be used in experiments that involved grafting pigs' hearts and kidneys onto the primates' necks, abdomens, and chests. *The Observer* reports that some baboons died after suffering strokes, vomiting, diarrhea, and paralysis, while others died *en route* to the UK. The experiments were conducted by Imutran Ltd, a subsidiary of Novartis Pharma AG in conjunction with Cambridge University and Huntingdon Life Sciences. Novartis told the newspaper that developing new cures for humans invariably means experimenting on live animals.

The newspaper also wrote that researchers were deliberately underestimating the suffering in order to obtain licences. A report from Imutran said: "The Home Office will attempt to get the kidney transplants classified as 'moderate,' ensuring that it is easier for Imutran to receive a licence and ignoring the 'severe' nature of these Programmemes."

TOXICOLOGY TESTING AND SAFETY TESTING OF ANIMAL

Toxicology testing, also known as safety testing, is conducted by pharmaceutical companies testing drugs, or by contract animal testing facilities, such as Huntingdon Life Sciences, on behalf of a wide variety of customers. According to 2005 EU figures, around one million animals are used every year in Europe in toxicology tests; which are about 10 per cent of all procedures. According to *Nature*, 5,000 animals are used for each chemical being tested, with 12,000 needed to test pesticides. The tests are conducted without anesthesia, because interactions between drugs can affect how animals detoxify chemicals, and may interfere with the results.

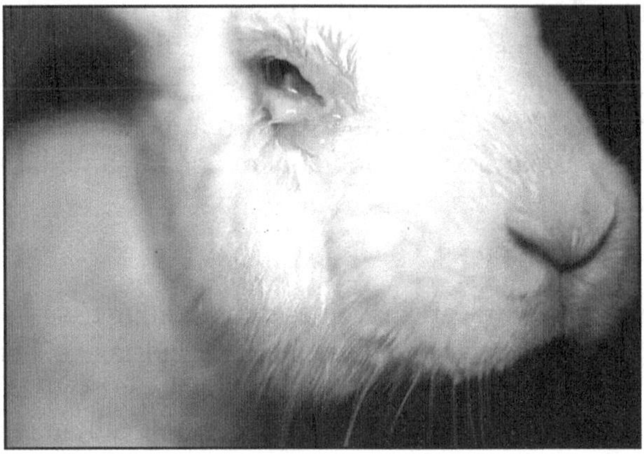

Fig. A Rabbit During a Draize Test.

Toxicology tests are used to examine finished products such as pesticides, medications, food additives, packing materials, and air freshener, or their chemical ingredients. Most tests involve testing ingredients rather than finished products, but according to BUAV, manufacturers believe these tests overestimate the toxic effects of substances; they therefore repeat the tests using their finished products to obtain a less toxic label.

The substances are applied to the skin or dripped into the eyes; injected intravenously, intramuscularly, or subcutaneously; inhaled either by placing a mask over the animals and restraining them, or by placing them in an inhalation chamber; or administered orally, through a tube into the stomach, or simply in the animal's food. Doses may be given once, repeated regularly for many months, or for the lifespan of the animal.

There are several different types of acute toxicity tests. The LD50 ("Lethal Dose 50 per cent") test is used to evaluate the toxicity of a substance by determining the dose required to kill 50 per cent of the test animal population. This test was removed from OECD international guidelines in 2002, replaced by methods such as the fixed dose procedure, which use fewer animals and cause less suffering. *Nature* writes that, as of 2005, "the LD50 acute toxicity test. still accounts for one-third of all animal [toxicity] tests worldwide." Irritancy is usually measured using the Draize test, where a test substance is applied to an animal's eyes or skin, usually an albino rabbit. For Draize eye testing, the recommended protocol involves observing the effects of the substance at intervals and grading any damage or irritation, but that the test should be halted and the animal killed if it shows "continuing signs of severe pain or distress". The Humane Society of the United States writes that the procedure can cause redness, ulceration, hemorrhaging, cloudiness, or even blindness. This test has also been criticized by scientists for being cruel and inaccurate, subjective, over-sensitive, and failing to reflect human exposures in the real world. Although no accepted *in vitro* alternatives exist, a modified form of the Draize test called the *low volume eye test* may reduce suffering and provide more realistic results, but it has not yet replaced the original test.

The most stringent tests are reserved for drugs and foodstuffs. For these, a number of tests are performed, lasting less than a month (acute), one to three months (subchronic), and more than three months (chronic) to test general toxicity (damage to organs), eye and skin irritancy, mutagenicity, carcinogenicity, teratogenicity, and reproductive problems. The cost of the full complement of tests is several million dollars per substance and it may take three or four years to complete.

These toxicity tests provide, in the words of a 2006 United States National Academy of Sciences report, "critical information for assessing hazard and risk potential". However, as *Nature* reported, most animal tests either over- or underestimate risk, or do not reflect toxicity in humans particularly well, with false positive results being a particular problem. This variability stems from using the effects of high doses of chemicals in small numbers of Labouratory animals to try to predict the effects of low doses in large numbers of humans. Although relationships do exist, opinion is divided on how to use data on one species to predict the exact level of risk in another.

COSMETICS TESTING

Cosmetics testing on animals is particularly controversial. Such tests, which are still conducted in the U.S., involve general toxicity, eye and skin irritancy, phototoxicity (toxicity triggered by ultraviolet light) and mutagenicity.

Cosmetics testing is banned in the Netherlands, Belgium, and the UK, and in 2002, after 13 years of discussion, the European Union (EU) agreed to phase in a near-total ban on the sale of animal-tested cosmetics throughout the EU from 2009, and to ban all cosmetics-related animal testing. France, which is home to the world's largest cosmetics company, L'Oreal, has protested the proposed ban by lodging a case at the European Court of Justice in Luxembourg, asking that the ban be quashed. The ban is also opposed by the European

Federation for Cosmetics Ingredients, which represents 70 companies in Switzerland, Belgium, France, Germany and Italy.

DRUG TESTING

Before the early 20th century, laws regulating drugs were lax. Nowadays all new pharmaceuticals undergo rigorous animal testing before being licensed for human use. Tests on pharmaceutical products involve:

- *Metabolic tests*, investigating pharmacokinetics - how drugs are absorbed, metabolized and excreted by the body when introduced orally, intravenously, intraperitoneally, intramuscularly, or transdermally.
- *Toxicology tests*, which gauge acute, sub-acute, and chronic toxicity. Acute toxicity is studied by using a rising dose until signs of toxicity become apparent. Current European legislation demands that "acute toxicity tests must be carried out in two or more mammalian species" covering "at least two different routes of administration". Sub-acute toxicity is where the drug is given to the animals for four to six weeks in doses below the level at which it causes rapid poisoning, in order to discover if any toxic drug metabolites build up over time. Testing for chronic toxicity can last up to two years and, in the European Union, is required to involve two species of mammals, one of which must be non-rodent.
- *Efficacy studies*, which test whether experimental drugs work by inducing the appropriate illness in animals. The drug is then administered in a double-blind controlled trial, which allows researchers to determine the effect of the drug and the dose-response curve.
- Specific tests on *reproductive function*, *embryonic toxicity*, or *carcinogenic potential* can all be required by law, depending on the result of other studies and the type of drug being tested.

Education, Breeding, and Defence

Animals are also used for education and training; are bred for use in Labouratories; and are used by the military to develop weapons, vaccines, battlefield surgical techniques, and defensive clothing. For example, in 2008 the United States Defence Advanced Research Projects Agency used live pigs to study the effects of improvised explosive device explosions on internal organs, especially the brain.

There are efforts in many countries to find alternatives to using animals in education. Horst Spielmann, German director of the Central Office for Collecting and Assessing Alternatives to Animal Experimentation, while describing Germany's progress in this area, told German broadcaster ARD in 2005: "Using animals in teaching curricula is already superfluous. In many countries, one can become a doctor, vet or biologist without ever having performed an experiment on an animal."

ETHICS

The ethical questions raised by performing experiments on animals are subject to much debate, and viewpoints have shifted significantly over the 20th century. There remain strong disagreements about which animal testing procedures are useful for which purposes, as well as disagreements over which ethical principles apply, and to which species of animals. The dominant ethical position, worldwide, is that achievement of scientific and medical goals using animal testing is desirable, provided that animal suffering and use is minimized. The British government has additionally required that the cost to animals in an experiment be weighed against the gain in knowledge.

A wide range of minority viewpoints exist as well. The view that animals have moral rights (animal rights) is a philosophical position proposed by Tom Regan, who argues that animals are beings with beliefs, desires and self-consciousness. Such beings are seen as having inherent value and thus possessing rights. Regan still sees clear ethical differences between killing animals and killing humans, and argues that to save human lives it is permissible to kill animals.

However, some such as Bernard Rollin have taken his position further and argue that any benefits to human beings cannot outweigh animal suffering, and that human beings have no moral right to use an individual animal in ways that do not benefit that individual. Another prominent position is articulated by Peter Singer, who sees no convincing reason to include a being's species in considerations of whether their suffering is important in utilitarian moral considerations.

Although these arguments have not been widely accepted, in response to these concerns some governments such as the Netherlands and New Zealand have outlawed invasive experiments on certain classes of non-human primates, particularly the great apes.

Some medical schools and agencies in China, Japan, and South Korea have built cenotaphs for killed animals. In Japan there are also annual memorial services (*Ireisai* pa—my) for animals sacrificed at medical school.

PROMINENT CASES

In 1997, People for the Ethical Treatment of Animals (PETA) filmed staff inside Huntingdon Life Sciences (HLS) in the UK, Europe's largest animal-testing facility, hitting puppies, shouting at them, and simulating sex acts while taking blood samples. The employees were dismissed and prosecuted, and HLS's licence to perform animal experiments was revoked for six months. The broadcast of the undercover footage on British television in 1997 triggered the formation of Stop Huntingdon Animal Cruelty, an international campaign to close

HLS, which has been criticized for its sometimes violent tactics. In February 1997 a team at the Roslin Institute in Scotland announced the birth of Dolly the sheep, a ewe that had been cloned from tissue taken from another adult sheep. Dolly was produced through nuclear transfer to an unfertilised oocyte, and was the only lamb that survived from 277 attempts at this technique. Dolly appeared to be a normal sheep, living for six years and giving birth to several lambs, but was euthanized in 2003 after contracting a progressive lung disease. Although the production of Dolly was a scientific breakthrough, it was controversial, since it showed that not only could cloned animals be produced for use in farming, but also that it would now be, in principle, possible to clone a human being.

Covance

In 2004, German journalist Friedrich Mülln shot undercover footage of staff in Covance, Münster, Europe's largest primate-testing Centre, making monkeys dance in time to blaring pop music, handling them roughly, and screaming at them. The monkeys were kept isolated in small wire cages with little or no natural light, no environmental enrichment, and high noise levels from staff shouting and playing the radio (video). Primatologist Dr. Jane Goodall described the living conditions of the monkeys as "horrendous." Primatologist Stephen Brend told BUAV that using monkeys in such a stressed state is "bad science," and trying to extrapolate useful data in such circumstances an "untenable proposition." Covance obtained a restraining order preventing Mülln from performing any further undercover research against the company for three years, and required him and PETA to turn over the material they obtained from Covance. PETA is further prevented from attempting to infiltrate Covance for five years.

The British Union for the Abolition of Vivisection (BUAV) raised concerns about primate experiments at the University of Cambridge in 2002. In a series of court cases, the BUAV alleged that monkeys had undergone surgery to induce a stroke, and were left alone after the procedure for 15 hours overnight. Researchers had trained the monkeys to perform certain tasks before inflicting brain damage and re-testing them. The monkeys were only given food and water for two hours a day, to encourage them to perform the tasks. The judge hearing BUAV's application for a judicial review rejected the allegation that the Home Secretary had been negligent in granting the university a license. The British government's chief inspector of animals conducted a review of the facilities and experiments. It concluded the veterinary input at Cambridge was "exemplary"; the facility "seems adequately staffed"; and the animals afforded "appropriate standards of accommodation and care."

One of the cases of alleged abuse involved Britches, a macaque monkey born in 1985 at the University of California, Riverside, removed from its mother at birth, and left alone with its eyelids sewn shut, and a sonar sensor on its head, as part of an experiment to test sensory substitution devices for blind people. 260 animals, including Britches, were stolen from the Labouratories at the University of California, Riverside in a raid by the Animal Liberation Front. The university alleged that damage to the monkey's eyelids, caused by the sutures according to the ALF, had in fact been caused by an ALF veterinarian, and that the sonar device had been removed and re-attached by the activists. The ALF reported that Britches was later transferred to a sanctuary in Mexico. University officials reported that hundreds of thousands of dollars of damage was done by the theft, and by smashing Labouratory equipment, and years of medical research were lost.

COLUMBIA UNIVERSITY

CNN reported in October 2003 that a post-doctoral "whistleblowing" veterinarian at Columbia University approached the university's Institutional Animal Care and Use Committee about experiments being carried out by an assistant professor of neurosurgery, E. Sander Connolly. Connolly was allegedly causing strokes in baboons by removing their left eyeballs and using the eye sockets to reach a critical blood vessel to their brains. A clamp was placed on the blood vessel until the stroke was induced, after which Connolly would try to treat the condition with an experimental drug. In a letter to the National Institute of Health, PETA cited the case of a baboon they said was unable to sit up or eat, and remained slouched over in its cage, before dying two days later. An investigation by the United States Department of Agriculture found the experiments did not violate federal guidelines. Connolly abandoned the research saying he felt under attack after receiving a threatening e-mail, but continued to believe his experiments were humane and potentially valuable.

THREATS TO RESEARCHERS

In 2006, a primate researcher at the University of California, Los Angeles (UCLA) shut down the experiments in his lab after threats from animal rights activists. The researcher had received a grant to use 30 macaque monkeys for vision experiments; each monkey was anesthetized for a single physiological experiment lasting up to 120 hours, and then euthanized. The researcher's name, phone number, and address were posted on the website of the Primate Freedom Project. Demonstrations were held in front of his home. A Molotov cocktail was placed on the porch of what was believed to be the home of another UCLA primate researcher; instead, it was accidentally left on the porch of an elderly woman unrelated to the university.

The Animal Liberation Front claimed responsibility for the attack. As a result of the campaign, the researcher sent an email to the Primate Freedom Project stating "you win," and "please don't bother my family anymore." In another incident at UCLA in June 2007, the Animal Liberation Brigade placed a bomb under the car of a UCLA children's ophthalmologist who experiments on cats and rhesus monkeys; the bomb had a faulty fuse and did not detonate. UCLA is now refusing Freedom of Information Act requests for animal medical records.

These attacks, as well as similar incidents that caused the Southern Poverty Law Centre to declare in 2002 that the animal rights movement had "clearly taken a turn toward the more extreme," this prompted the US government to pass the Animal Enterprise Terrorism Act and the UK government to add the offense of "Intimidation of persons connected with animal research organisation" to the Serious Organised Crime and Police Act 2005. Such legislation, and the arrest and imprisonment of extremists may have decreased the incidence of attacks.

ALTERNATIVES TO ANIMAL TESTING

Scientists and governments state that animal testing should cause as little suffering to animals as possible, and that animal tests should only be performed where necessary. The "three Rs" are guiding principles for the use of animals in research in most countries:

- Reduction refers to methods that enable researchers to obtain comparable levels of information from fewer animals, or to obtain more information from the same number of animals.
- Replacement refers to the preferred use of non-animal methods over animal methods whenever it is possible to achieve the same scientific aim.
- Refinement refers to methods that alleviate or minimize potential pain, suffering or distress, and enhance animal welfare for the animals still used.

Although such principles have been welcomed as a step forwards by some animal welfare groups, they have also been criticized as both outdated by current research, and of little practical effect in improving animal welfare.

5

Scientific Researches in Animal Biotechnology

Animal biotechnology is an area of scientific research that is under constant evolution. Although no genetically modified (GM) animal is currently on the market, the United States Food and Drug Administration (FDA) is looking into the authorization of a fast-growth transgenic salmon. Some countries are worried about the imminent availability of such animals on the market, given the many diverse uncertainties, and have asked the Food and Agriculture Organization of the United Nations (FAO) and the Codex Alimentarius to determine risks associated with genetically modified organisms and to draw up procedures of analysis and international standards for derived products. The Codex Alimentarius Commission was created in 1963 by FAO and the World Health Organization (WHO) to establish food standards, guidelines and other normative texts, under the Joint FAO/WHO Food Standards Programme.

The basic aims of this programme are to protect consumer health, to promote fair trade in food and to coordinate food standardization by governmental and non-governmental organizations. At its twenty-third session, the Codex Alimentarius Commission set up the Intergovernmental Task Force on Foods Derived from Biotechnology to draw up science-based standards, regulations and recommendations for foods derived from biotechnology and for novel characteristics of foods introduced by biotechnology. FAO and WHO hold regular consultations of scientific experts to discuss the safety and nutritional value of genetically modified food in support of the work of the Task Force. These consultations seek to provide FAO, WHO and their member countries with scientific advice on the safety and nutritional value of foods derived from biotechnology, on the basis of existing scientific data and research carried out by national authorities, FAO, WHO, and other relevant international organizations or forums. They serve to transmit the advisory opinions of experts, who are independent of the Commission, to specialized committees and task forces. Strategies to assess the safety and nutritional value of foods derived from biotechnology are examined on the basis of increasing public concerns and the outcomes of the many tests carried out to date.

Recommendations are also made on the priorities of further research into the safety and nutritional value of foods derived from biotechnology.

It was in this context that I was tasked with carrying out a literature survey in preparation for an expert consultation to be held in 2003/2004 on the subject of foods derived from genetically modified animals. This meant collating recent information on animal biotechnology (including insects) and on the status of GM animals and derived foods, with a special focus on food safety. However, while highlighting safety, the report necessarily had to consider the broader implications of environment, ethics and animal welfare. This survey is based on many (mostly recent) documents and reports, but draws especially upon a report on animal biotechnology, which I believe anyone interested in the topic should read, that was compiled in 2002 by several American scientific committees on behalf of the US Food and Drug Administration. In 2020, the world's population could amount to 8 billion people, with 6.7 billion living in the developing countries.

A problem of food security would thus co-exist with the already manifest problem of soil erosion and resource depletion, notably fishery resources. Biotechnology is championed as a solution to the anticipated food deficit, but also holds promise for crop and animal production, human and animal health, and animal welfare. What do we mean by biotechnology? There are several definitions, but the most frequent refers simply to organisms whose genetic material has been modified by a means that cannot be achieved by conventional breeding techniques. The Codex definitions adopted by the Cartagena Protocol on Biosafety are as follows. A living modified organism (LMO) is understood as any living organism that possesses a novel combination of genetic material obtained through modern biotechnology. "Modern biotechnology" is understood as the application of in vitro nucleic acid techniques, including the recombination of deoxyribonucleic acid and the direct introduction of nucleic acids into cells or organelles, or the fusion of cells beyond the taxonomic family, that overcomes natural physiological reproductive or recombination barriers and that are not techniques used in traditional breeding and selection.

More simply, the term GMO applies to any biological entity capable of producing or transferring genetic material, this having been modified in a manner that is not effected naturally by propagation and/or by natural recombination. Since they were first domesticated, animals have been bred by humans for chosen properties and traits, initially by human selection, and subsequently with the assistance of genetic engineering. The purpose of applying biotechnology to animals is essentially to increase their productivity and yield, to improve their resistance to disease and parasites, and to improve the nutritional and technological qualities of foods derived from these transgenic animals. Related techniques can also be used to control human and animal disease. The first deals with the many forms of animal biotechnology and directly resulting problems, which are listed in detail. There is then a chapter on the specific case of transgenic animals to protect human health. While the term biotechnology encompasses many techniques, notably techniques applied to animal production, the focus here is on everything related to genetic engineering and cloning. Genetically modified animals thus include animals resulting from any form of cloning, animals that have been genetically modified to produce meat and other products for human consumption, and animals that have been genetically modified for purposes of human health. Biotechnology has opened up wide possibilities in many fields: from agriculture to pharmaceuticals. It has also raised increasing concern, with sometimes fierce debate on GM animals involving scientists, food producers, consumers, public interest groups, especially environmental groups, national authorities and decision-makers. The second part of the report looks at environmental concerns, dwelling briefly on transgenic insects, and highlights concerns about animal health and welfare. The third part looks at concerns about the safety of transgenic animals and derived products. These are closely allied to current with public fears and a complex interplay of political, economic, scientific and social considerations.

TECHNICAL PROBLEMS RELATING TO GERMLINE MODIFICATION

EXPRESSION OF RANDOMLY INSERTED GENES

Controlling the expression of the introduced gene seems impossible, as the gene needs to be expressed in the appropriate tissue, at the correct time and at an adequate level. In practice, the transgene either fails to express itself or else expresses itself in a variable and inappropriate manner. These problems arise from the limited understanding and difficult control of the complex system of regulation of transcription (promoters, regulatory elements, etc.). Expression of the inserted gene is influenced by many control elements located around the integration site. As a result, the transgene is often unexpressed or, more rarely, expressed abnormally, which of course reduces the efficiency of these techniques. The methylation of certain nucleotides also seems to be linked to the absence of expression of certain genes. Methylation is a very important regulatory mechanism in somatic cells. The absence of specific (unknown) signals to regulate the intervention of this mechanism would appear to prevent the expression of the transgene. Appropriate vectors permitting the insertion of the transgene and the regulatory process are currently under development, in particular certain lentiviruses, such as FIV or BIV, that would appear to have the appropriate properties.

Surplus Animals

The problem with these techniques is that many animals fail to present the anticipated properties, do not possess the transgene or display major genetic abnormalities. Also, several animal generations are required to evaluate the stability and effects of the transgene. Failure is high, so these techniques are now turning increasingly towards the culture of modified and selected cells followed by nuclear transfer to create the desired animals, thus reducing "surplus" transgenic animal numbers.

Uniqueness of Transgenic Animals

One characteristic of GM animals is their considerable variability, which is linked to:

- The number of transgene sequences contained in the cells;
- The variable transgene insertion site(s) and consequences (unique phenotype);
- The level of expression of the transgene;
- The variability of abnormalities and their frequency.

A direct consequence is the extreme difficulty of assessing the risks that are associated with these individuals.

PROBLEMS LINKED TO GERMLINE MANIPULATION

Unexpected Genetic Side Effects

Traditional outcrossings, like the different kinds of mutation (for example, deletion, duplication, insertion, inversion, translocation, transposons, and even aneuploids and polyploids), often cause the involuntary suppression or modified expression of certain genes. If detected, such abnormalities are generally rejected. Depending on the location of the chromosomes into which the modified genes have been integrated, these undesired effects can also occur with genetic engineering.

The insertion of a transgene into a functional gene can cause genetic modification and varying degrees of dysfunction. The insertion of a transgene into a silent gene could activate the expression of that gene. Mammals possess a large proportion of noncoding genome sequences, which lessens the risk of modification/inactivation of genes associated with insertion of the transgene. However, the problem remains, and abnormalities of expression of genes situated near the integration site have been observed.

Certain consequences are highlighted in the literature and need to be evaluated:

- Abnormalities of immune system (suppression of certain immune mechanisms, sensitivity to disease, abnormal expression of genes and induction of immunity tolerance);
- Alterations to physiological mechanisms, fertility, foetal development, etc. We can also add:
- The passage of pathogens across interspecies barriers;
- The activation of latent viruses.

Gene interaction is too complex to fully appreciate the possible biological consequences of inserting a foreign gene into a genome. Assessing this phenomenon is further complicated by the fact that gene expression is also partly determined by environmental factors and inevitably depends on the genetic make-up of the host.

UNFORESEEN CONSEQUENCES OF MODIFICATION

Consequences such as changed characteristics of food absorption, fertility and sexual maturity are discussed. The introduction of the growth hormone gene into fish increases their nutritional needs and changes their metabolic and physiological parameters. Behavioural abnormalities are also reported, such as increased aggressiveness among transgenic mice, and the disappearance of maternal behaviour or avoidance of risk among certain transgenic fish. The abnormalities noted among transgenic fish can be transmitted to their offspring. The insertion of a gene encoding human cell-surface proteins into pigs for xenotransplantation could render these animals susceptible to human diseases, as has been observed with mice, increasing their risk of illness and helping propagate certain human diseases. The possibility that pig viruses could become virulent for human cells also represents a high risk.

GENE MARKERS

Markers are generally inserted into vectors along with the transgene, in order to select the cells that possess the desired transgene. It could for example be a sequence encoding resistance to an antibiotic. While some researchers consider these markers harmless, others point out that these DNA sequences can provoke side effects in both the transgenic animal (acquisition of antibiotic resistance in host bacteria) and the consumer (allergenicity). Although the likelihood of side effects is probably low, it would seem impossible to disprove such a possibility.

UNDESIRED INSERTS

Additional sequences unrelated to the specific transgene but contained in the vector construct can be introduced into target cells. Such sequences are difficult to detect and remove. In particular, retroviruses are produced by cells possessing a large number of endogenous viruses and viral DNA sequences. The accidental introduction of these sequences when inserting the transgene is therefore possible, and genetic side effects can be foreseen. There could also be a recombination of different sequences leading to the generation of novel infectious viruses.

CREATION OF NEW PATHOGENS

Such transgenic animals and derived products could be the source of new diseases or more virulent modified pathogens. The risk is accentuated by the limitations of methods of analysis and detection of new unforeseen pathogens. The gene for antibiotic resistance used as a marker could pose a problem if integrated into the genome of a virulent pathogen. Retroviruses used as vectors can combine with endogenous or exogenous viruses and generate a more virulent virus. The insertion of regulatory sequences or new genes into a viral genome could thus modify the pathogenecity of a micro-organism.

MOBILIZATION OF THE TRANSGENE/ HORIZONTAL TRANSFER OF THE TRANSGENE

Using viruses as vectors carries the risk of transmitting the transgene to other individuals, which would be possible if the viral vector were related to a virus pathogenic to the targeted species. The two viruses could combine to form a virus that could spread the transgene among the animal population. The transgene could also be mobilized through the endogenous retroviruses that normally replicate at low level in the host organism. Similarly, the presence of moveable transposons in the genome of transgenic animals could facilitate the mobility of the inserted transgene, notably its horizontal transfer. The possibility of transgenes transferring horizontally is however disputed.

PROBLEMS RELATED TO CLONING

The two cloning techniques differ according to the type of nuclear donor cell, which can be a (differentiated) somatic cell or an (undifferentiated) germline cell. The somatic cell nuclear transfer technique differs from the latter in two essential respects: the length of the inserted chromosome telomeres which is shorter because of the absence of telomerase but restored among transgenic animals, and the level of DNA methylation of somatic cells. The inappropriate level of methylation and the inability to correct the level are thought to cause developmental abnormalities in embryos produced with this technique. The conditions needed for the reprogramming of the inserted nucleus are disputed. Although nuclear reprogramming is currently a problem, the clear progress made in recent years suggests that it is not insurmountable.

Efficiency of Techniques

The somatic cell nuclear transfer technique is not very efficient. High prenatal mortality and abnormal development, perinatal mortality and abnormal placentation among cattle and sheep have been observed, as have respiratory distress, lethargy, cardiomyopathy, pulmonary hypertension and problems of regulation of insulin levels or hypoglycaemia. These problems would appear to stem from the methods and media of embryonic cell culture, the nuclear transfer method or a combination of the two. A reprogramming of inserted genes during fertilization and early embryo development have been observed.

Reduction of the Gene Pool

Cloning could significantly reduce the gene pool. However, it could also help maintain certain character traits or foster genetic diversity where seemly impossible (sterility, etc.). A reduction in genetic diversity prevents future enhancement of species and homogeneity within animal species could mean greater susceptibility to disease.

GENERAL PRINCIPLES OF RISK ANALYSIS

Risk analysis has three elements: risk assessment, risk management and risk communication. The first two are most important as concerns risk analysis applied to the environment.

In risk assessment, the risk has two components:

1. A potential hazard
2. The likelihood of that event taking place.

Thus the risk is the *potential hazard* x *the probability of exposure*.

Risk assessment is a process based on scientific data and involving the following stages:

- Hazard identification;
- Hazard characterization;
- Exposure assessment;
- Risk characterization.

Potential hazards and the likelihood of their occurrence are studied in this manner and models are built to predict risk. Risk management, which is distinct from risk assessment, consists of examining policy alternatives with all interested parties, bearing in mind risk assessment and other factors relevant to protection of consumer health and promotion of fair trade, while, where needed, determining appropriate prevention and control options.

An environmental hazard is not so easy to quantify as a health hazard, and concerns a public good rather than a private good (health). When an appropriate risk management strategy is applied to environmental problems and not to safety problems, the problem must first be set out, as must the objectives and values that will serve to seek a solution.

All options are then examined to cover the maximum number of solutions, for weighing the advantages and drawbacks of a vast range of possible solutions helps get all parties involved. Risk communication is the interactive exchange of information and ideas between risk assessors, risk managers, consumers, industry, academia and other interested parties of the risk analysis process. The exchange of information concerns factors linked to the risk, as well as the ways in which the risk is perceived, and includes a presentation of the conclusions of the risk assessment and a justification for the risk management decisions.

Risk assessment relating to the environment is a complex undertaking because it is very difficult to identify and quantify all the potential risks of releasing GM animals into the environment. The risk analysis procedure needs to be adapted and the animals need to be classified according to their capacity for dispersal in the environment.

Proposed stages are:

- Identification of potential harms;
- Identification of hazards that could cause these harms;
- Definition of what exposure means for gm animals and likelihood of exposure;
- Estimation of likelihood of risk;
- Classification of risks according to their priorities.

As not all potential risks can be identified, the process of risk analysis needs to be ongoing to take account of new information as it arises.

CLASSIFICATION OF TRANSGENIC ANIMALS ACCORDING TO RISK TO THE ENVIRONMENT

The harm can be partly envisaged: perturbation to ecosystems, reduction or even elimination of wild populations, etc. The hazard is the transgenic animal itself, whose presence in an environment can have direct and indirect consequences for natural ecosystems through the action of various factors.

The risk is not so much that the animal finds itself in the environment but that it finds itself there AND establishes itself. It is therefore a matter of studying the impact of the establishment of transgenic animals on the wild populations.

The establishment of a GM animal and thus of the transgene in the environment depends on three factors: its capacity for survival and breeding (which itself depends on five factors: viability of juveniles and adults, age at sexual maturity, fecundity, fertility and reproductive success); capacity of escape and dispersal; and the characteristics of the receiving community.

A reduced community of wild animals will be under greater threat from the introduction of transgenic animals than a large community that will be able to withstand the impact of the transgene.

If a transgenic animal is better adapted to environmental conditions than its wild peers, it will establish itself among the wild population, which it might in fact replace. If not, the transgenic animal will disappear. If the fitness of the transgenic animal is the same as that of the wild animal, they might be able to coexist.

Fitness can be determined prospectively or retrospectively.The prospective method studies four factors: heightened adaptability to environmental conditions, traits and characteristics of the GM animal, capacity to produce novel products and animal's aptitude to escape.

HEIGHTENED ADAPTABILITY TO ENVIRONMENTAL CONDITIONS

Heightened adaptability to environmental conditions, such as capacity to resist cold or disease, enables GM animals to establish themselves in an environment or to colonize ecosystems in which their wild counterparts cannot survive.

Enhanced Existing Traits

Enhanced traits often relate to rate of growth, feed efficiency or production performance (*e.g.* milk or eggs). An enhanced trait can sometimes be countered by physiological imbalance or increased food requirement, as has been observed among some transgenic farm animals. Genetic enhancement by means of genetic engineering differs from enhancement through the traditional selective breeding of animals with interesting traits, in the sense that the characteristics associated with the interesting trait do not follow the same evolutionary path.

A transgenic animal can have a vascular or skeletal system that is completely unsuited to its improved rate of growth, which produces a developmental imbalance of physiological systems and renders the animal less fit for survival. Transgenic animals developed for production and breeding often present an altered characteristic that counterbalances the impact of the improvement and therefore represent a low risk of establishment in the environment.

However, in some cases the improved trait could outweigh the altered characteristic; for example, it has been noted among certain transgenic fish that a 25% increase in size boosted their reproductive success by 400% as compared to the norm.

Such success benefits the transgenic animal and rapidly disseminates the transgene among the wild population, even if the transgene reduces the lifespan of the transgenic animal. In such a case, the aggregate impact favours the establishment of the transgenic animal in the environment, an advantage that is further accentuated if the conspecific wild population is small. Fragile wild communities could be reduced or even disappear.

PRODUCTION OF NOVEL PRODUCTS

Transgenic animals producing more proteins and pharmaceutical substances in their milk, urine, or any biological by-product, have only limited capability of establishment in the environment, because they have not acquired any special advantage in fitness and their added functionality in fact requires higher energy expenditure which makes them less competitive with their wild conspecifics. Such transgenic animals therefore only represent a low risk for the environment.

PRODUCTION OF ANIMALS OR ANIMAL PRODUCTS FOR HUMAN HEALTH

Companion animals genetically engineered to reduce allergenicity and animals modified for xenotransplantation only present a low risk of establishment in the environment. Their fitness remains unchanged or perhaps compromised. Transgenic insects modified to control the spread of a vector-borne human disease such as malaria are meant to establish themselves in the environment.

GENETICALLY MODIFIED ANIMALS

ALLERGENICITY AND HYPERSENSIBILITY

Most food allergens are proteic, well known and identified. As regards the safety of new proteins in foods derived from transgenic animals, the possibility that a new protein could cause an allergic reaction among certain individuals needs to be assessed.

FAO has published an approach for assessing the potential allergenicity of new proteins extracted from foods derived from transgenic animals, using the decision tree reproduced in Figure.

If the new protein is produced from a transgene that is known to have allergenic potential, or if the animoacid sequence is similar to that of a known allergenic protein, then the allergenic potential of the new protein can be tested with the serum of individuals with known food allergies.

The problem arises for proteins with unknown allergenic potential which cannot be easily assessed, as there is no existing human immunoserum. The problem is further compounded when the new protein derives from an existing protein that has no known allergenic potential.

Thus, assessing the potential allergenicity of a protein from a transgene remains one of the major difficulties in the overall safety assessment of transgenic foods. Assessment of allergenicity requires an understanding of several factors, including the source of the transgene protein, its level of expression, its chemical and physical properties, and its similarities to any known allergen.

All these factors have to be considered together to have an idea of the potential allergenicity of the new protein. The absence of appropriate and effective methods of analysis is a major problem, as is the feasibility of performing adequate assessments for an increasing number of transgenic products.

In this connection, WHO and FAO are working on the development of a standardized protocol for the assessment of allergenicity. The animal model for allergenicity tests of products derived from transgenic animals is recognized as effective.

In vivo allergenicity tests among humans would be the best option but raises ethical problems. Post-market surveillance of a product is also advocated, but modalities for doing this are difficult to determine.

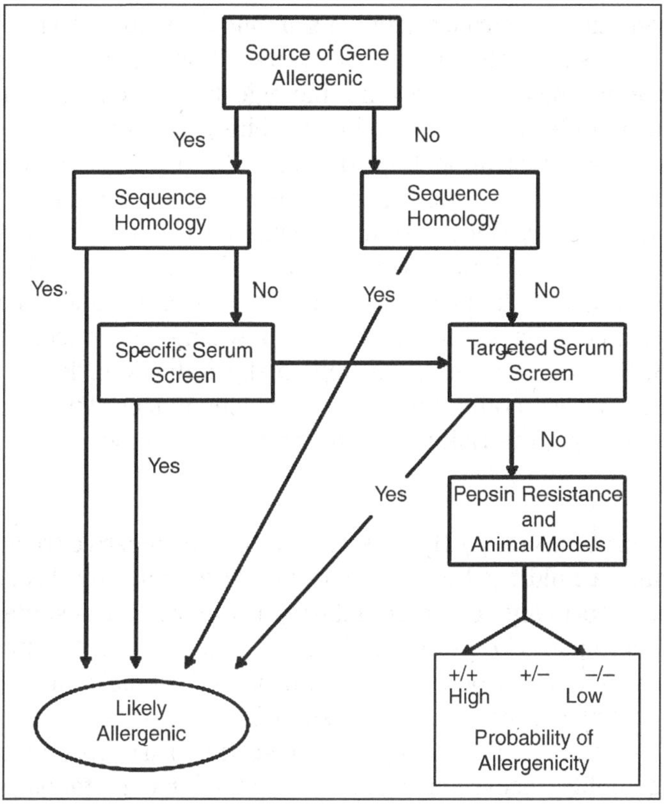

Fig. FAO/WHO 2001, Decision Tree to Assess the Potential Allergenicity of Foods Derived from Biotechnology.

Other Bioactive Compounds

Some transgenic animals are designed to express biopharmaceuticals. That these products could retain their bioactivity in the organism after consumption of the food is a safety concern. All proteins and polypeptides are normally broken down in the digestive tract, thus destroying their bioactivity. Only small peptides pass the barrier of the digestive epithelium. The problem remains, however, for people whose digestive epithelium has been compromised by disease or injury. Similarly, the digestive epithelium of young children is permeable to proteins for a period of a few weeks to a few months, during which these proteins could enter the bloodstream.

This poses a real problem for bioactive peptides contained the milk. The peptides or proteins could have a negative impact on the digestive system. The production of bactericidal proteins in milk to reduce cattle susceptibility to mastitis from *Staphylococcus aureus* or to control bacterial disease in fish could upset the bacteriological equilibrium of the intestinal flora of consumers.

It could also lead to pathogens resistant to these antimicrobials. Many transgenic fish express a growth hormone gene, which is usually of fish origin.

Can this growth hormone cause problems among consumers? The FDA reports that studies have shown that non-human growth hormones, whether of bovine, ovine, porcine or whale origin, are not biologically active among humans. Nor are digested peptide fragments or insulin-like growth factors I secreted in response to GH administration. Moreover, the IGF-I is destroyed by heat along with the active growth hormones. In the (unlikely, given their age) case of young children being fed transgenic fish or milk containing GH, this would be destroyed during heating. The problem however remains for individuals whose digestive tract has been impaired by disease, digestive ulcer or age and which therefore absorbs proteins that have not been broken down and introduces them into the organism. So the risk varies according to the individual. For a susceptible individual, the hazard could have severe consequences, while for a healthy individual of any age, the risk is thought to be low to moderate.

Toxicity

Because proteins are partly broken down in the digestive tract, their direct toxicity is only a mild food safety concern. Moreover, any direct toxicity of proteins would normally be detected during pre-market assessment. The risk is therefore minimal. The problem arises in connection with unintended and unanticipated effects of products derived from GM animals, linked not only to the proteins that are directly expressed by a transgene but also to any unintended by-products. For example, the insertion of a transgene could disturb a specific metabolic process and cause the expression of metabolites with some toxicity. What we need to know is whether there are effective methods of analysis and screening that can detect a toxic substance or a change in metabolism that introduces toxicity. Whole foods can have a tiny concentration of proteins expressed by a transgene or arising as a by-product of the transgene. Such toxicity can be very difficult to detect given the sensitivity limits imposed by laboratory animal numbers, the small quantities of substances tested in whole foods, and the possibility that any negative effect will seldom occur.

Methods include:

- Analysis of the structural/functional relationship of the substance and of its physical and chemical properties and comparison with existing databases of toxic agents to see if the molecule has similarities with a known toxic agent.
- *In vitro method:* Testing the stability of molecules under different conditions or the ability of the molecule to act on other molecules with specific functions. Few *in vitro* tests have been validated and extrapolated *in vivo* as this is difficult, for the method is still fraught with uncertainties.
- *Animal model*: The best indicator of possible toxicity. However, extrapolation remains uncertain, hence the use of safety factors. This model serves to determine acute, subchronic or chronic toxicity. The

problem is that the dietary regime needs to be balanced if parallel side effects are not to be caused (high possibility of bias). A precise diet, specific doses and clear protocols are required.

Institutions, Scientific Expertise and International Standards

International agencies have been charged with establishing international standards for GMOs and derived products. Codex is developing principles for risk analysis applied to foods from GMOs. The first principle is to have a pre-market assessment involving case-by-case study of the direct and indirect consequences of inserting a new gene (toxicity, allergenicity, properties of compounds, stability of genome, nutritional effects and other impacts). Codex principles are however for reference only and not binding.

Evaluation of Safety of Foods Derived from Genetically Modified Animals

As concerns examination of the safety of GM foods, the risks associated with genetic engineering are the involuntary modification of the host genetic substance, which can induce changes in food components, including the toxic substances.

Evaluation of the safety of GM foods should therefore include the following procedures:

- Identification of the organism that has been modified and of the source organism(s) of the inserted gene(s). The origin and nature of all the genetic elements that have been introduced into the modified organism need to be identified, including the structural and regulatory sequences and all other parts of the vector sequences. The possibility of horizontal transfer of genes and related consequences also needs to be studied. If the transfer of genes resistant to antibiotics is intended, the possible health implications of concentrations of micro-organisms in the human digestive tract or other parts of the body need to be considered.
- Identification of primary and secondary genetic products, including a description of the characteristics of the inserted gene. Identification of hazards requires an understanding of the expressed inserted genes, the characteristics, concentration and location of expressed food products and the consequences of expression. For each protein resulting from genetic modification, the factors taken into account include possible toxicity and allergenicity from exposure to the expressed protein.
- Evaluation of the safety of new substances anticipated in the foods (*i.e.* proteins, glucides and lipids).
- Assessment of unanticipated effects on the composition of foods, including assessment of changes in the concentration of nutritive or toxic substances occurring naturally, identification of anti-nutritional

factor compounds significantly altered in GM foods and assessment of the safety of compounds showing significant modified concentration.
- Evaluation of any toxin produced directly by modification.
- Evaluation of type of treated food, assuming normal manufacturing procedures.
- Evaluation of food consumption patterns, including identification of potential human population consuming GM foods and probable consumption levels, and evaluation of possible consequences if the consumption of modified foods differs from that of equivalent traditional foods.
- Assessment of allergenicity of new foods.

Current approaches to assessing the toxicity of specific proteins are based on internationally approved, acute or chronic testing on laboratory rodents or on fast-growth domesticated species, such as chickens. However, no repeated dose testing with GM foods or food products has yet been published. As regards allergenicity, most scientists now base their evaluations on a decision tree that has been designed to evaluate the potential allergenicity of foods from GM plants, in the light of current knowledge of what is defined as an allergen and how to better identify an allergen.

Concept of Substantial Equivalence

The OECD's principal contribution to the evaluation of safety of foods from genetically modified animals has been its publication *Safety evaluation of foods derived by modern biotechnology: concepts and principles*. According to this report, the most practical way of determining the relative safety of a new food product is to determine whether it is substantially equivalent to its conventional counterpart, where this exists.

This concept was initially applied to organisms of terrestrial origin but, with certain qualifications, was then also applied to products of aquatic biotechnology. Substantial equivalence recognizes that the purpose of evaluation is not to guarantee absolute safety, but to determine whether the transgenic food presents more risks than its conventional counterpart, should this exist. It is generally agreed that such evaluation requires an integrated, specific and gradual approach.

The factors taken into consideration when a transgenic food is compared to its conventional counterpart are (as detailed in the previous chapter on the evaluation of safety of foods derived from transgenic animals):
- Its identity, source and composition; its characteristics in relation to the "natural" product;
- The effects of processing and cooking;
- The processing stage, the dna itself and the products of protein expression of the introduced dna; its nutritional qualities;
- The effects on its function;

- Its potential toxicity and allergenicity, as well as possible secondary effects;
- Consumption of the transgenic food and the nutritional impact of its introduction.

Interactions between environmental factors and animal genotype also need to be taken into account. These variations can influence the phenotype and composition of the modified animal and need to be studied during the evaluation of equivalence. If the food derived from a GMO is judged to be substantially equivalent to its conventional counterpart, it is then considered to present the same level of risk. Otherwise, further tests are needed. Confirmation of substantial equivalence does not mean that the product of a genetically modified animal is identical to the conventional product. Comparison does not take all elements into account and substantial equivalence only provides assurance that the appropriate components of safety of the product will be present in equivalent quantities.

As the comparative approach links the composition of new foods to existing products with a history of safe use, the consequences of introducing new foods into a diet can be foreseen. The concept means that all similarities between foods from genetically modified animals and conventional foods can be judged to be safe. Differences noted during comparison are subject to further meticulous examination which includes the testing of traditional nutritive elements and toxicological or immunological testing or long-term studies, depending on the differences noted. Foods from transgenetic animals might not have any conventional equivalent or the differences between these foods and their conventional equivalents may not be sufficiently characteristic. The history of safe use of the conventional product could not therefore be used to assess the safety of the new food under study.

Substantial equivalence cannot be used to determine the safety of foods for which there is no comparator. However, that a novel food does not bear much resemblance to its counterpart does not necessarily make it dangerous. Its safety needs to be determined by using traditional food safety approaches, with supplementary testing on the consequences of modification.

Post-Approval Monitoring of Foods Derived from Transgenic Animals

It is widely accepted that foods and food products need to be thoroughly evaluated before being placed on the market, if consumers, animal health and the environment are to be protected. If the assessment raises safety concerns, the product will not be approved for commercial release. Some countries therefore fail to see any scientific justification for the post-approval monitoring of these products. Other countries, on the other hand, see the monitoring of possible negative or positive impacts of novel foods as a logical follow-up to the initial science-based risk assessment. They argue that post-approval monitoring should be mandatory to consolidate the initial pre-market risk assessment, which was based on the then state of scientific knowledge. This could apply to any pre-market assessment. It is recognized that it is sometimes difficult to draw clear conclusions from epidemiological studies, especially when applied to food compounds. Post-approval monitoring is advocated as the only feasible way of demonstrating the absence of possible long-term or unexpected consequences of consuming a novel food. Implementing this strategy is not easy, however.

SCIENCE, INSTITUTIONS, SOCIETY AND POLICIES

Problems Linked to Scientific Uncertainties

There are many scientific uncertainties relating to animal biotechnology. Current understanding is considered to be inexact, uncertain and insufficient as regards technique, methodology and epistemology. There are too many factors, variables and interactions to accurately assess the level of risk. These interactions are not always known or understood. Genetic engineering has unexpected secondary consequences and the aggregate impact of these consequences on intended transgene impact cannot be anticipated. Similarly, genes have pleiotropic effects that are impossible to foresee. It is therefore clearly impossible to envisage all the potential risks. Some of these may not be identified and therefore not studied. On the other hand, analysis of a non-existent risk is a waste of time and resources, and can result in unnecessary costly management measures. In addition, estimating potential risk by using inherently biased methodology must necessarily lead to error. Regulatory bodies make their decisions on the basis of science-based risk assessment.

Scientific uncertainties should therefore be priority research areas in both the private and the public sector. A process of consultation with all stakeholders is required to establish agreed and validated risk assessment protocols and to share results and experiences. There are at least four direct consequences of existing scientific uncertainties: application of the precautionary principle in certain national regulations; extreme precaution in risk analysis; stated need for post-approval monitoring of transgenic animals; and the need for further research.

Policy Context, National and International Agencies

Animal biotechnology raises a number of policy problems. Which standards apply to biotechnology products? A major problem is that the risks concern a variety of areas: human and animal health, animal welfare and the environment. How can these different areas be integrated into the decision-making and regulatory process? The welfare of transgenic animals is usually covered by legislation on animal welfare in general. Is specific regulation on the welfare of transgenic animals required? Another problem is the absence of regulation on transgenic insects.

There is clear need to clarify the scope and limits of different regulatory and control agencies, and national and international organizations as regards the different areas that affected by biotechnology. Should their remit be extended beyond public health and environment to include social and economic aspects, given that these are also relevant? Many different agencies are involved: those responsible for the environment (field releases and trials), food and human health, imports and exports, and animal protection and health. It is important to define individual responsibilities, legitimacy and role. Transgenic animals and derived food products are governed by regulation on novel foods (Novel Food Regulation introduced in 1997 by the European Commission) in Europe and (Novel Food Regulation part of the Food and Drugs Act of October 1999) in Canada. For Canada, the concept of novel food includes any food from plants, animals or micro-organisms that has been genetically modified in such a way that new traits have emerged, or are no longer observed, or are observed at unusual levels. In Canada, protocols are drawn up by Health Canada to assess the safety of novel food. In the USA, the US Federal Drug and Cosmetics Act has been amended to include GM food.

To summarize, approaches differ in many respects:

- *Basic legislation*: Some countries (Canada, USA) have incorporated GMO legislation into existing legislation; others (Australia, Japan) have issued specific legislation for biotechnology, resulting in a mass of sometimes extremely complex regulations.
- *Transparency of decision-making*: Some countries do not consider public opinion (Canada) and only provide a summary of information once a decision has been made, without prior notification. Conversely, others announce their intentions, consult public opinion and issue reports that summarize positions and decisions (EU, USA).
- *Approach to risk assessment and in particular to the principle of precaution*: Some countries seek to eliminate all risk and only decide once every aspect has been assessed; others decide on the basis of existing rather than potential risks.
- *Conceptual approach*: For some, the risk to be assessed concerns the product (Canada), while for others it concerns biotechnology in general (Japan, EU, Australia)
- *Independence of decision-making*: Are all links between governments, scientists, industry and expert committees legitimate? In the USA, there is sometimes a close link between decision-makers and assessors.

Good practices often advocated include greater transparency and public involvement, standardized risk assessment concepts, uniform understanding of the principle of substantial equivalence, and distinction between technique and product. According to the British Better Regulation Task Force, regulation should be transparent, accessible, targeted, complete and proportionate to cost and risk.

Convergence of Policy, Science, Ethics and Public Opinion

Concerns that are not science-based should not guide scientific examination. However, such concerns do inherently influence the scientists' mindset, the way they address questions to policy-makers and their presentation of scientific response to public health and environmental concerns. At the same time, government agencies are influenced in their priorities and decisions by the issues raised by public opinion.

Public Perception of Transgenic Animals and Derived Products

The Consumers' Perspective

Recent events regarding the application of modern biotechnology to animals and food production have received considerable attention and raised serious public concern. The introduction of new characteristics into food that differ significantly from those of traditional foods could accentuate these concerns in the future. It therefore seems necessary to keep the public informed of safety assessment procedures applied to novel foods. Another difficulty is the differing consumer needs and expectations in the world regarding food quantity and quality, and the differing nutritional values and cultures. These factors need to be taken into account when examining food production, trade and recent events such as crop enhancement and functional foods. Food safety is a universal concern of consumers who need reassurance that marketed transgenic products have been properly tested for deficiencies and checked for safety. The five eurobarometers conducted in the European Union since 1991 (the last in 2002) give a certain idea of how the European public perceives GMOs.

In many countries this perception is in fact increasingly negative, with concerns relating to:

- The unexpected effects and consequences of gmos on human health and environment;
- The potential irreversibility of negative effects;
- The ethical acceptability of gmos;
- The usefulness of gmos;
- Animal welfare;
- Relational imbalances between producers, farmers and consumers;
- The equality of peoples in the face of biotechnology.

There is a clear distinction in the way GMOs are perceived according to their intended application. On the one hand, we have biomedical applications which are considered useful, morally acceptable and are encouraged, while, on the other, we have agrifood applications which are considered redundant and hazardous to society. Public reaction varies according to familiarity and preoccupation with the subject. However, some observers report a difference between what the public says and what the public does or is. People *think as citizens and not as consumers*. The perception of risk differs between the experts and the public. The way the experts estimate risk does not appear to coincide with the public's perception of risk. There appears to be a lack of trust in regulatory bodies and scientific experts, which in part explains the increasing consultation of public opinion, the greater emphasis on transparency and the release of public information. Assessors have identified three categories of public opinion: unconditional supporters, those who accept the risks and opponents.

Acceptance of GMOs is conditioned by four factors: material values, optimism, confidence and preoccupation with issues linked to GMOs and derived products. Survey responses vary according to connotations underlying related terms, such as "genetic" and "biotechnology", so depend directly on the social and scientific climate at the time of the survey. Consumers believe they have a right to be informed on the products they purchase. However, the question of whether the labelling of transgenic foods is the most appropriate and realistic way of enabling consumers to make enlightened choices is a matter of fierce debate in many countries. The Codex Alimentarius Commission is currently examining this issue.

Several governments have adopted policies and procedures on GMO labelling, and significant differences exist. Provisions for labelling from production to consumption can pose insurmountable problems for countries with limited capacity but anxious to enter international markets. Public opinion in the USA appears to be less animated, and opinions seem stronger on genetically modified animals than on genetically modified crops. The American people appear to be aware of and encourage the potential benefits of biotechnology, with one survey revealing that 62% believe biotechnology will produce additional benefits over the next five years. Such benefits include improved quality, taste and diversity of food, improved human health and nutrition, reduced use of pesticides and insecticides, lower food costs and improved yields. The current use of GM crops does not seem to be a problem for the US population. Do they feel the same way about GM animals? Survey data reveal inadequate methodology, with the use of closed questions and an interpretation of results that needs to be shorn of the deep-seated mental prejudices of both assessors and the public. Questionnaires often focus on GM plants, while it might be illuminating to distinguish between GM plants and GM animals to gauge the level of public concern about genetically modified animals.

Communication between the Public, Assessors and Decision-makers

The OECD countries and intergovernmental organizations are seeking new ways of sharing their experience. They are seeking to boost the dissemination of information and real consumer understanding of the safety issue. Some countries have adopted measures for the public exchange of information on the safety assessment of GM foods. The public are invited to comment on the reports and proceedings of safety assessment bodies. Some regulatory bodies actively consult the public on food safety and regulations. Some make all information supporting an application available to the public, except confidential commercial information. The Internet is increasingly used to inform the public of safety assessment and approval procedures, and is a good source of information on approved foods and food products.

Some countries are looking into the possibility of using the Internet to make application details accessible to the widest possible audience, in order to make the assessment process as transparent and understood as possible. The OECD's on-line BioTrack site is a useful source of information on regulations in member countries, with information on ministries and agencies, and details of laws, regulations and guidelines. It also has two important databases: one on products that have been marketed; the other on GM field tests carried out in OECD countries. Other approaches adopted with huge success in selected countries include the appointment of consumer representatives to safety assessment committees. Consensus conferences have also been attempted with varying degrees of success.

Ethical Considerations

Up until now, the idea of food products from transgenic animals has not been well received by consumers. Surveys have constantly shown that the public is better disposed towards transgenic plants than transgenic animals. There is greater reluctance towards trials involving animals and changes in animal make-up and therefore broader possible implications. Various cultures and religions limit or forbid the consumption of certain foods of animal origin. The public seems however to be more disposed to consume by ingestion or injection pharmaceutical products derived from transgenic animals. Various ethical issues have been raised.

Distribution of Benefits

One preoccupation is the possible impact of biotechnology on agricultural structure, especially the potential elimination of small livestock farms in the face of the cost of producing transgenic animals. People are worried about the impact of a dismantled agricultural society on the environment, sustainable agriculture and quality of life. The public points to the concentration of production and its direct consequences on markets and consumers, and is wary of the dependence of livestock farmers and food producers on multinationals. There is mental conflict between the law of the market and the traditions, cultural identities and needs of society.

Nutrition and Food Safety

There seems to be general consensus among scientists that the consumption of food derived from transgenic animals is no more hazardous than the consumption of conventional products. However, the public thinks differently. Some people refer to specific diets based on cultural or religious considerations. For example, the consumption of an animal or a food from a transgenic animal that contains proteins or genes of animals whose consumption is forbidden by culture or religion could pose a problem. Another point often stressed is the social divide from different levels of access to biotechnology in developing and developed countries.

Respect for Life and the Unnatural Nature of GMOs

Some people do not believe that technical and economic pressures justify the commercialization of life and the patenting of living organisms. Overstepping of the species barrier and the large-scale industrial production of genetic animals are seen as contrary to nature. This argument is frequently refuted by biologists who stress that the continuous natural evolution or the human selection of animal genotypes has favoured certain genes and eliminated others. Finally, biotechnology and conventional livestock practices might seem to pose similar problems, in that both seek maximized productivity and both cause animal dysfunctioning and welfare and health problems. However, such problems seem to be magnified (some would say disproportionately) in the context of biotechnology.

Animal biotechnology is a recent science and therefore difficult to view in the light of experience. Many uncertainties and many doubts exist. Information currently available will have to be constantly updated with data and results of analyses and trials of transgenic animals and derived food products, so that techniques, regulations and public opinion can evolve and adapt; so that doubts can be clarified and problems resolved; and so that agreed protocols of analysis and international standards can be determined. Given the rapid progress being made and the prospects of animal biotechnology, it is almost certain that improved techniques will boost benefits. However, the trade-off between risk, cost and benefit will always have to be examined. Ongoing oversight, greater transparency of results from scientific trials, greater transparency of regulatory and decision-making processes and closer cooperation among all stakeholders are required for the safety evaluation of products derived from transgenic animals.

METHODS FOR MAKING TRANSGENIC ANIMALS

Transgenic animals are usually made by cloning the transgene of interest (for example human insulin) then inserting that gene into the genome of a newly fertilized egg. The egg is then cultured to the blastocyst stage and implanted into to uterus of a surrogate mother.

One method of inserting foreign DNA into an egg is microinjecting it into the male pronucleus. The male pronucleus is used because it is larger than the female pronucleus. Eggs are matured using hormones to increase ovulation in a group of animals. Then the eggs are harvested and injected with hundreds of copies of the desired DNA using a micropipette.

If the procedure is a success, the animal produced will have altered DNA throughout every cell in its body. But because of the randomness of this procedure, in some cases the DNA doesn't integrate or only some of the cells have the new DNA sequence. When this occurs the resulting animal is a "mosaic animal", not all the cells contain the transgene DNA sequence. The offspring of these particular animals will sometimes carry the gene and sometimes not. A major benefit of making transgenic animals using microinjection is that it can be used on a wide variety of animals.

A second technique for making a transgenic animal uses embryonic stem cells or ES cells to introduce the new DNA sequence. ES cells are cells that regenerate and differentiate into other cells. They are undifferentiated cells that have the potential to differentiate into any type of cell, somatic cells or germ line cells, so if the transgene can be inserted into an ES cell, the cell can then be used to create the transgenic animal. These cells become very useful when it is important to target gene sequences to specific sites in the genome because ES cells can be incorporated into a blastocyst and differentiate normally or be grown *in vitro*.

The process of making a transgenic animal using ES cells starts by obtaining ES cells from the blastocyst of donor mice. The cells are taken from an embryo that has not yet been implanted in the uterine wall. The fertilized embryos are collected from female mice a few days after fertilization or the mice are given steroids that prevent implantation while embryonic cell division occurs. The embryos are harvested and cultured using an embryonic fibroblast feeder layer that produces leukemia inhibitory factor. This factor will help reduce the differentiation of the cells. The inner cell mass of the harvested embryos dissociates from Trophoblast cells. This allow the ES cells from the inner cell mass to be selected individually for undifferentiated morphology, indicating their likely pluripotency, then they are allowed to grow and multiply. The DNA is introduced into the ES cells by microinjection, viruses, chemicals, or electroporation. Electroporation is a process that uses a pulse of high voltage to make cell membranes permeable and allow the introduction of new DNA. The electric charge is passed through a plate with DNA layered on top of cells. The negative charge of DNA caused by its phosphate residues is attracted to positive electrodes. Once the DNA is absorbed in the cell, the DNA moves into the cytoplasm and integrates into the cellular DNA.

The cells become ES cell lines that can be evaluated for their potential as gene targeting tools or used in studies of cellular differentiation. If the transgene successfully incorporated, the ES cells can be injected into a blastocyst, and the embryo implanted as before to make the transgenic animal. A gene targeting process is used to introduce the desired DNA sequence into ES cells. In gene targeting, a piece of DNA that carries the transgene or DNA sequence of interest is introduced into the ES cells of a mouse by electroporation. Inside the ES cell the DNA sequence can insert directly in the intact genome at a specific region. ES cells that successfully incorporate the sequence are added to an embryo in its early stages.

This is done by either injecting the ES cells in an embryo or culturing them with it.

Effects on neighbouring is implanted in a surrogate mother. When the chimeric mouse is born the colour is usually different from that of the host because the gene for the coat colour is often chosen to be from the ES cells genetic makeup and not the host. This is an easy way to confirm the success of the procedure. The chimera then carries the new gene in its germ line and can be selectively bred to establish the gene permanently in a new mouse.

Another method for inserting the foreign DNA into the ES cells is to use viruses. A retroviruse can be modified so that it carries a desired DNA sequence in its DNA. The disease causing genes are removed from the virus so disease is not introduced to the transgenic animal. The virus can infect the ES cells with a specific gene but does not infect all of the ES cells with the retroviral DNA. Germ line cells need to be infected for the procedure to be successful.

A third method used to deliver the new DNA into the ES cells is DNA microinjection. This is done by microinjection of the DNA sequence into the ES cells in the blatocyst of the host animal. This process produces a mosaic animal that does not always carry the transgene in its germ line. The process is often repeated to gain more transgenic animals. A versatile approach to enhance the delivery of non-viral DNA involves complexation with cationic polymers, which can be designed to overcome the barriers to effective gene transfer. DNA is packaged into a polymetric or scaffolding. Liposomes are usually used to fuse to the ES cell membrane and insert the DNA. Polylysine and plasmid DNA can also be used to make an attraction between biotin and avidin. A mixture of the biotin-modified and unmodified cationic polymers are electrostatically complexed with non-viral DNA and tethered to a substrate containing non-glycosylated avidin. The cells that were used, HEK293T and NIH/3T3, grew along the surface, then were directly exposed to the tethered complexes and are easily transformed. Transfection is a function of the surface DNA quantities and the number of tethers in the complex.

This process has shown to be much more efficient than traditional bulk delivery. The success rate for these methods of creating transgenic animals that can birth animals containing the transgene is very low. If the genetic manipulation does not cause an abortion, the result is a first generation of animals that need to be tested for the expression of the transgene.Depending on the technique used, the first generation may result in chimeras, and various tissues need to be tested for transgene insertion. When the transgene has integrated into the germ cells, the so-called germ line chimeras are then inbred for 10 to 20 generations until homozygous transgenic animals are obtained and the transgene is present in every cell. At this stage, embryos carrying the transgene can be frozen and stored for subsequent implantation. Assays Used for Screening Transgenic Animals There are several ways of testing the effectiveness of the transgenic method used to determine whether the transgene incorporated into the various tissues of the animal. Foreign DNA can be detected in the genome of a transgenic animal using either a Southern assay, or PCR.

One of the more reliable tests is the "Southern Blot" test. A Southern blot is a method of identifying a specific DNA band on an agarose gel electrophoresis by marking specific DNA sequences (Answers.com). This technique uses a restriction enzyme to split DNA at specific locations, and then the fragmented DNA is put through an agarose gel. An electric current is run through the agarose gel. DNA moves towards the positive electrodes because it is negatively charged. The size of the DNA affects how far it migrates through the gel, the smaller DNA fragments have an easier time migrating through the gel, so those fragments move the farthest on the gel.

The pattern of DNA in the gel is then blotted to a membrane that retains the pattern, but allows hybridization to a probe to illuminate a specific gene (like the transgene). The DNA from the animal is compared with the position of the DNA of the transgenic DNA. If the sample contains the transgene, the transgenic DNA was successfully integrated into the animal's cell. A Western Blot is another way to determine if an animal's tissue is expressing the transgene, *i.e.* is making the transgenic protein.

This method takes into account that transgenic animals are engineered to produce specific protein. These proteins can be detected in a similar way as the DNA in the southern blot. In the western blot, whole cell extracts containing protein are electrophoresed to separate the proteins by size, and then blotted. Lighter proteins will travel further. The protein is then blotted to membrane made of nitrocellulose and a specific protein is visualized among the bands present using an antibody solution. The antibody recognizes and attaches to the transgenic protein, allowing its detection. If the protein that the antibody binds to is present in the sample the antibody will bind to it and it will create a dark spot in the gel.

An Enzyme Linked Immunosorbent Assay or ELISA is another technique used for screening transgenic animals. It is used to measure the levels of antibodies found in the transgenic animal's serums, blood and urine. Animals produce antibodies when substances are introduced which are foreign to the body. An antigen or protein is added to a plastic well to which it attaches. The serum of the animal is then added and if the animal is positive for the antibodies to the protein, they will bind to the proteins. Antigens attached to an enzyme are then added to the mixture and they will bind the antibodies. The enzymes react with a chromogen substrate to produce a colour. If the colour changes then the animal is positive for the antibodies against the transgenic protein. The type of transgenic animal to be made is a very important question. There are several factors that need to be taken into account when deciding what animals need to be used. Disease models are usually mice since they have a short gestation time which allows more data to be obtained. Transpharmers are usually cows, sheep, or goats since they produce large quantities of milk containing the product. It is important to look at the gestation time, number of progeny, and amount of milk per year of the animal depending on what it is to be used for. Transgenic animals are very useful and help scientists gain a better understanding of animal and human biological function.

METHODS TO CONTROL GENE EXPRESSION

USE OF LONG GENOMIC DNA FRAGMENT

The majority of DNA in somatic cells of animals is methylated on the C of CpG motifs. This results in the specific inactivation of the corresponding genes. Mammalian genomes contain about 25,000 genes and only 2,000 are active in somatic cells. About 1,000 genes, known as housekeeping genes, are active in all cell types whereas the other 1,000 genes are specifically active in given cell types to support their differentiated state. During gametogenesis and the early embryo development, DNA is heavily demethylated to blunt the gene expression programme of gonad cells from which gametes derive. After embryo implantation, DNA is progressively and selectively methylated to define which gene in the different cell types will have to be active or not in foetuses, newborns and adults.

The mechanisms which control this programme of the gene expression are only partly known. It implies the contribution of multiple DNA regulatory sequences, some of them being located far upstream or downstream of the genes. The low expression of many transgenes containing only the transcribed regions with a promoter, proximal enhancers, at least one intron and a transcription terminator, has revealed that remote regulatory regions must be involved in the control of gene expression. In a limited but significant number of cases, using long genomic DNA regions (up to 200 kb) surrounding the gene of interest greatly increases the proportion of active transgenes and also often the level of their expression.

Interestingly and expectedly, association of classical plasmid expression vectors with long DNA fragments markedly enhances the functioning of the transgenes. This point is examplified by a milk protein gene, the WAP (whey acidic protein gene) gene. A 30 kb genomic fragment containing the pig WAP gene expressed the WAP gene in transgenic mice very poorly whereas fragments of 80 kb or 145 kb allowed a high expression of the gene, although not as a function of the integrated copy number and at various levels according to species. Interestingly, coding sequences added after the WAP gene promoter in the 145 kb BAC (bacterial artificial chromosome) were expressed at a much higher level than when they were under the dependency of the only WAP gene promoter.

SPECIFIC INHIBITION OF GENE EXPRESSION

Transgenesis is mostly used to add foreign genetic information into an animal. Inactivating a gene in an animal is also essential, particularly for the identification of the function of the gene. Indeed, inactivating a gene may have a much stronger impact than adding a gene to an animal and thus reveal the function of the gene. A gene is usually activated to eliminate the corresponding protein in the animal. This can be achieved by different techniques and at different levels of the protein synthesis process.

AT THE GENE LEVEL

The gene knockout is currently performed early in development and this event is irreversible. Experimenters may wish to prevent the expression of a gene reversibly, in a given cell type only and at chosen periods of the animal's life. Available methods make the gene knockout possible in a given cell type at a chosen moment. This technique, which has been used successfully for more than one decade, leads to an irreversible inactivation of the gene.

AT THE MRNA LEVEL

It is possible to inhibit a mRNA specifically by adding to the cells short synthetic oligonucleotides, having a sequence complementary to that of the targeted mRNA. These oligonucleotides contain some analogues of natural deoxyribonucleotides to enhance their stability *in vivo*. The binding of the oligonucleotides to the corresponding mRNA induces a degradation of the mRNA. This tool is currently used to inhibit the expression of genes in cultured cells. Oligonucleotides are also administered to patients to tentatively inhibit viral genes in order to block infections. This approach has met limited success so far.

Another possibility to inhibit a mRNA consists of introducing in a cell an anti-sense RNA generated by the transcription of the non-coding strand of the gene. The anti-sense RNA forms a double strand RNA with the mRNA which cannot be translated anymore. In practise, this method is rarely efficient, as the mRNA and the anti-sense RNA each form multiple short double strands with their own sequences. These RNA are also more or less associated with proteins. These two events prevent the easy formation of a double strand mRNA-anti-sense RNA. Hence, anti-sense RNAs meet success at most when a single region strand of the anti-sense is complementary to a single strand region of the targeted mRNA.

Ribozymes are short RNAs capable of cleaving a complementary RNA. This natural mechanism does not imply the contribution of proteins as ribozymes possess an intrinsic RNase activity. The use of ribozymes has proved disappointing in practise as, like antisense RNAs, they do not easily reach their target RNA sequence.

The discovery of interfering RNA one decade ago has profoundly improved the situation. It was unexpectedly found that a long double strand RNA can induce the degradation of a RNA having a complementary structure. Soon after, it was shown that the long double strand RNAs are randomly cut into 19–21 nucleotide fragments known as siRNA (small interfering RNA). One of the two strands of the siRNA is kept and targeted to a mRNA having a complementary sequence. This induces the degradation of the mRNA. It was also demonstrated that synthetic siRNAs transfected into cells had an RNAi effect. Soon after, the use of promoters directed by RNA polymerase III could synthesize siRNAs. In practise, a synthetic gene, containing the targeted 19–21 nucleotide sequence, followed a short random sequence and by the targeted sequence in the opposite orientation is linked to a promoter acting with RNA polymerase III (usually U6 or H1 gene promoters).

The RNAs synthesized by such vectors form a 19–21 nucleotide double strand RNA separated by a loop containing the random sequence. These RNAs known as shRNAs (short hairpin RNA) are processed in cells to generate active siRNAs. The recent discovery of the role of microRNAs has increased the possibility to use interfering RNAs. Indeed, microRNAs (miRNAs) are present in all eukaryotic cells. They are encoded by short genes expressed under the control of RNA polymerase II promoters.

The primary products of these genes are 135 nucleotides RNAs which are processed and transferred to the cytoplasm where they are transformed into siRNAs. The mature miRNAs which are fully complementary to the targeted mRNA induce a degradation of this mRNA. The miRNAs, which are only partially complementary to the targeted mRNA and which recognize a sequence located in the 3'UTR (3'untranslated region) of the mRNA, inhibit translation of this mRNA without inducing its degradation.

A mammalian genome contains several hundreds of miRNA genes. Their function is essential as they control the expression of a large proportion of the genes by modulating translation of the mRNAs. On the contrary, the siRNAs described above appear more as a defence mechanism degrading exogenous double strand RNAs (*e.g.* some viral RNAs) as well as badly shaped cellular RNAs. The possibility to generate transgenic animals expressing siRNAs preventing specifically the expression of a gene by degrading the corresponding mRNA or inhibiting its translation has opened avenues for the control of gene expression *in vivo*. This approach has met brilliant success in plants.

A rapidly increasing number of transgenic plants expressing genes coding for siRNAs resistant to pathogens or having a metabolic pathway specifically blocked are available. The application of the siRNA approach is not so easy in animals for several reasons. Long double strand RNAs induce interferons and some unspecific immune reactions and they cannot be easily used. The siRNAs are auto-amplified in plants in lower invertebrates but not in vertebrates. Moreover, the reliable expression of transgenes coding for siRNAs is more difficult in animals than in plants, as promoters directed by RNA polymerase III are generally poorly active in transgenic animals unless they are inserted into lentiviral vectors or associated with vectors directed by RNA polymerase II. It remains that the use of RNA polymerase II promoters to direct the synthesis of siRNAs offers unprecedented possibilities for experimenters and biotechnologists to modulate specific gene expression in a potent and subtle manner.

AT THE PROTEIN LEVEL

In most cases, the expression of a gene is achieved to suppress or inactivate the corresponding protein in cells or whole living organisms. This goal can be reached directly using different techniques. One of them consists of expressing a gene coding for an antibody specifically recognizing and inactivating the targeted protein. This kind of antibodies, known as intrabodies, must not be secreted and can even be targeted to some cell compartments to reach the intracellular proteins.

Another possibility relies on the overexpression of a gene coding for an inactive analogue of the targeted protein. The protein encoded by the gene can suppress or greatly attenuate the activity of the protein of interest by playing the role of a decoy.

This was exemplified more than one decade ago. A gene coding for an inactive analogue of an insulin receptor still capable of binding the hormone allowed the generation of transgenic mice that were no more sensitive to insulin and thus suffering from type II diabetes. This strategy is currently used in nature. This is namely the case for some hormone receptors and transcription factors which exist under different forms synthesized in the same cells in a controlled manner.

CONTROL OF TRANSGENE EXPRESSION BY EXOGENOUS FACTORS

All the vectors described above and used to express transgenes contain promoters which are naturally active in the cells of the transgenic animals. This implies that the transgenes are regulated by the natural inducers of the host genes. In some cases, artificial promoters containing natural or mutated regulatory elements associated in a non natural manner are used to direct transgene expression. Transgene expressed under the direction of injected oestrogens is one example among many others. This approach is fundamentally limited. The oestrogenic inducers will stimulate or inhibit not only the transgene but a number of host genes, leading to complex and unknown side effects in the animals.

To circumvent these problems, artificial promoters, containing regulatory elements from both animal genes and bacterial genes, have been designed. The resulting promoters are active in animal cells but controlled by substances active in bacteria but not in animals. The most popular system is based on the use of the bacterial tetracycline repressor gene. In practise, the transgene becomes reversibly activated only when tetracycline is administered to the animals. A number of similar systems are available and currently used in transgenic animals with good success. These tools virtually offer the possibility to express a transgene precisely in a given cell type and at a given moment.

DELETION OF TRANSGENES OR GENOMIC DNA REGIONS

Deletion of genomic DNA regions is required in some circumstances. Conventional homologous recombination makes gene deletion, known as knockout, possible. Another possibility consists of using the Cre-LoxP or Flp-FRT sytems.

A LoxP sequence must first be added on both ends of the fragment to delete. The presence of the Cre recombinase will then recombine the two LoxP sites leading to a deletion of the DNA fragment located between the LoxP regions. The Cre recombinase may be synthesized by the corresponding gene under the direction of a cell specific promoter. The Cre recombinase will be present and the deletion of the DNA fragment will take place only in the cells in which the promoter is active.

This process can be controlled by still more sophisticated tools. The promoter directing the Cre gene expression can be under the dependency of tetracycline. The deletion of the DNA fragment will then occur only in the chosen cell type and at the chosen moment. Another level of control can be obtained by using an engineered Cre recombinase which becomes reversibly active in the presence of an oestrogen analogue, 4-hydroxy tamoxifen.

This offers the advantage of having the active Cre recombinase for short periods of time. This prevents the non-specific action of the Cre recombinase which can recognize cryptic sites in the host genome and induce illegitimate recombinations damaging the integrity of the host DNA. The Cre-LoxP approach may be implemented to withdraw a given gene or a regulatory region from a genome.

In the first case, the operation is known as conditional knockout. The same technique may also be used to activate a gene conditionally. In this case, a DNA sequence having an inhibitory action on transcription and bordered by two LoxP sequences may be added between the promoter of a gene and its transcription start site.

The gene will remain silent until the inhibitory sequence is deleted by the action of the Cre recombinase. Another application of this tool is the elimination of marker genes. This is the case when pluripotent cells or the cloning techniques are implemented.

The marker genes and selection genes are not required for the action of the transgene. Their presence in the animals may have no effects, yet their elimination has been recommended by FAO/WHO and Codex Alimentarius.

CURRENT CONTEXT OF GENETICALLY ENGINEERED ANIMALS

Genetic engineering technology has numerous applications involving companion, wild, and farm animals, and animal models used in scientific research. The majority of genetically engineered animals are still in the research phase, rather than actually in use for their intended applications, or commercially available.

COMPANION ANIMALS

By inserting genes from sea anemone and jellyfish, zebrafish have been genetically engineered to express fluorescent proteins — hence the commonly termed "GloFish." GloFish began to be marketed in the United States in 2003 as ornamental pet fish; however, their sale sparked controversial ethical debates in California — the only US state to prohibit the sale of GloFish as pets. In addition to the insertion of foreign genes, gene knock-out techniques are also being used to create designer companion animals.

For example, in the creation of hypoallergenic cats some companies use genetic engineering techniques to remove the gene that codes for the major cat allergen.

Companion species have also been derived by cloning. The first cloned cat, "CC," was created in 2002. At the time, the ability to clone mammals was a coveted prize, and after just a few years scientists created the first cloned dog, "Snuppy".

With the exception of a couple of isolated cases, the genetically engineered pet industry is yet to move forward. However, it remains feasible that genetically engineered pets could become part of day-to-day life for practicing veterinarians, and there is evidence that clients have started to enquire about genetic engineering services, in particular the cloning of deceased pets.

WILD ANIMALS

The primary application of genetic engineering to wild species involves cloning. This technology could be applied to either extinct or endangered species; for example, there have been plans to clone the extinct thylacine and the woolly mammoth.

Holt et al point out that, "As many conservationists are still suspicious of reproductive technologies, it is unlikely that cloning techniques would be easily accepted. Individuals involved in field conservation often harbour suspicions that hi-tech approaches, backed by high profile publicity would divert funding away from their own efforts

." However, cloning may prove to be an important tool to be used alongside other forms of assisted reproduction to help retain genetic diversity in small populations of endangered species.

FARM ANIMALS

As reviewed by Laible, there is "an assorted range of agricultural livestock applications [for genetic engineering] aimed at improving animal productivity; food quality and disease resistance; and environmental sustainability." Productivity of farm animal species can be increased using genetic engineering. Examples include transgenic pigs and sheep that have been genetically altered to express higher levels of growth hormone.

Genetically engineered farm animals can be created to enhance food quality. For example, pigs have been genetically engineered to express the Ä12 fatty acid desaturase gene (from spinach) for higher levels of omega-3, and goats have been genetically engineered to express human lysozyme in their milk. Such advances may add to the nutritional value of animal-based products.

Farm species may be genetically engineered to create disease-resistant animals. Specific examples include conferring immunity to offspring via antibody expression in the milk of the mother; disruption of the virus entry mechanism (which is applicable to diseases such as pseudorabies); resistance to prion diseases; parasite control (especially in sheep); and mastitis resistance (particularly in cattle).

Genetic engineering has also been applied with the aim of reducing agricultural pollution. The best-known example is the Enviropig; a pig that is genetically engineered to produce an enzyme that breaks down dietary phosphorus (phytase), thus limiting the amount of phosphorus released in its manure.

Despite resistance to the commercialization of genetically engineered animals for food production, primarily due to lack of support from the public, a recent debate over genetically engineered AquAdvantage Atlantic salmon may result in these animals being introduced into commercial production.

Effort has also been made to generate genetically engineered farm species such as cows, goats, and sheep that express medically important proteins in their milk. According to Dyck et al, "transgenic animal bioreactors represent a powerful tool to address the growing need for therapeutic recombinant proteins."

In 2006, ATryn® became the first therapeutic protein produced by genetically engineered animals to be approved by the Food and Drug Administration (FDA) of the United States. This product is used as a prophylactic treatment for patients that have hereditary antithrombin deficiency and are undergoing surgical procedures.

RESEARCH ANIMALS

Biomedical applications of genetically engineered animals are numerous, and include understanding of gene function, modeling of human disease to either understand disease mechanisms or to aid drug development, and xenotransplantation. Through the addition, removal, or alteration of genes, scientists can pinpoint what a gene does by observing the biological systems that are affected. While some genetic alterations have no obvious effect, others may produce different phenotypes that can be used by researchers to understand the function of the affected genes.

Genetic engineering has enabled the creation of human disease models that were previously unavailable. Animal models of human disease are valuable resources for understanding how and why a particular disease develops, and what can be done to halt or reverse the process.

As a result, efforts have focused on developing new genetically engineered animal models of conditions such as Alzheimer's disease, amyotrophic lateral sclerosis (ALS), Parkinson's disease, and cancer. However, as Wells (13) points out: "these [genetically engineered animal] models do not always accurately reflect the human condition, and care must be taken to understand the limitation of such models."

The use of genetically engineered animals has also become routine within the pharmaceutical industry, for drug discovery, drug development, and risk assessment.

As discussed by Rudmann and Durham: "Transgenic and knock out mouse models are extremely useful in drug discovery, especially when defining potential therapeutic targets for modifying immune and inflammatory responses...Specific areas for which [genetically engineered animal models] may be useful are in screening for drug induced immunotoxicity, genotoxicity, and carcinogenicity, and in understanding toxicity related drug metabolizing enzyme systems."

Perhaps the most controversial use of genetically engineered animals in science is to develop the basic research on xenotrans-plantation — that is, the transplant of cells, tissues, or whole organs from animal donors into human recipients.

In relation to organ transplants, scientists have developed a genetically engineered pig with the aim of reducing rejection of pig organs by human recipients. This particular application of genetic engineering is currently at the basic research stage, but it shows great promise in alleviating the long waiting lists for organ transplants, as the number of people needing transplants currently far outweighs the number of donated organs.

However, as a direct result of public consultation, a moratorium is currently in place preventing pig organ transplantation from entering a clinical trial phase until the public is assured that the potential disease transfer from pigs to humans can be satisfactorily managed. According to Health Canada, "xenotransplantation is currently not prohibited in Canada. However, the live cells and organs from animal sources are considered to be therapeutic products (drugs or medical devices)...No clinical trial involving xenotransplantation has yet been approved by Health Canada".

ETHICAL ISSUES OF GENETIC ENGINEERING

Ethical issues, including concerns for animal welfare, can arise at all stages in the generation and life span of an individual genetically engineered animal. The following sections detail some of the issues that have arisen during the peer-driven guidelines development process and associated impact analysis consultations carried out by the CCAC. The CCAC works to an accepted ethic of animal use in science, which includes the principles of the Three Rs (Reduction of animal numbers, Refinement of practices and husbandry to minimize pain and distress, and Replacement of animals with non-animal alternatives wherever possible).

Together the Three Rs aim to minimize any pain and distress experienced by the animals used, and as such, they are considered the principles of humane experimental technique. However, despite the steps taken to minimize pain and distress, there is evidence of public concerns that go beyond the Three Rs and animal welfare regarding the creation and use of genetically engineered animals.

6

Blood Components of Animal

Whole blood is collected from a donor animal for blood transfusion purposes into a blood bag containing citrate phosphate dextrose as the anticoagulant. Donor animals should be selected with care and strict attention should be paid to the blood collection technique to maintain sterility at all times.

Once the blood has been collected, it can be kept and used in its natural state or can be converted into a variety of components. These blood components are packed red blood cells, platelet-rich plasma, platelet concentrates, fresh plasma, fresh frozen plasma, frozen plasma, cryoprecipitate and cryosupernant.

Double, triple and quadruple blood bags (a single whole blood collection bag with various satellite bags) are used for producing and separating components within a sterile closed environment. Blood component production is highly desirable for several reasons, including maximization of the yield of products from a single blood donation and ability to use the optimal products (in high concentrations) for specific diseases (thus minimizing the amount of unnecessary foreign material the recipient animal is exposed to). The most commonly available blood components are whole blood, packed red blood cells, fresh frozen plasma and cryoprecipitate.

Some definitions may be useful for understanding blood components:

- *Whole blood:* This is blood collected directly from a donor animal into a blood transfusion bag containing citrate-phosphate-dextrose with (CPDA-1) or without adenine (CPD) as an anticoagulant. In general, for dogs, a 500 ml transfusion bag is used (which contains approximately 63 ml of anticoagulant, obtaining approximately 450 ml blood from the donor dog).

  Whole blood can be used immediately or stored at 4 C for future transfusion or separation into blood components. Additives can be used to improve red cell storage viability.
- *Packed red blood cells:* These are a concentrated source of red blood cells that remain in a small amount of plasma upon removal of supernatant plasma after centrifugation of the blood transfusion bag containing whole blood.

Packed cells are an excellent source of red blood cells for anemic animals that need the additional oxygen-carrying capacity these cells provide.

Packed red cells can be used immediately or stored at 4°C. They need dilution in sterile isotonic solution prior to infusion (due to the high hematocrit, packed cells without dilution are very thick and flow sluggishly through infusion lines). The current standard for red cell storage is that there should be about 75 per cent posttransfusion viability after storage, that is at least 75 per cent of the transfused red cells must remain in the recipient's circulation 24 hours after transfusion. The posttransfusion viability of canine red cells collected into CPDA-1 is 20 days.

Additives have been developed that can be added in a sterile fashion (they are attached to the original transfusion bag as a satellite bag) to packed red cells (or whole blood bags) to optimise red cell storage viability. These additives usually contain dextrose and adenine for red cell energy metabolism and mannitol, which decreases red cell lysis. Several additives have been evaluated with canine red blood cells. Both Nutricel and Adsol increase the posttransfusion viability of stored canine red cells to 35 and 37 days, respectively.

- *Platelet-rich plasma (PRP):* Platelet-rich plasma is produced by separating plasma from red blood cells (within 6 hours of whole blood collection) using a slow spin to prevent pelleting of the platelets. Platelet-rich plasma is useful for the treatment of disorders of platelet number and function but must be infused within 8 to 12 hours (maintained at room temperature) due to platelet instability (which limits its use).
- *Platelet concentrates:* Platelet concentrates are produced by separating most of the plasma from platelet-rich plasma. Platelet concentrates are used similarly to platelet-rich plasma.
- *Platelet-poor plasma (PPP):* Platelet-poor plasma is produced by separating plasma from red blood cells using a high spin to pellet platelets with the red cells. This is the starting point for production of most blood components. Separation of platelets is desirable because they provide an additional source of foreign antigens and micro-aggregation can cause transfusion reactions. Approximately 200 to 400 ml of plasma are obtained from each whole blood transfusion bag. One unit of plasma is defined as that obtained from a single whole blood transfusion bag.
- *Fresh plasma:* This is platelet-poor plasma that is separated from red cells and infused within 6 hours of blood collection (with the blood bag being maintained at 4°C until separation).

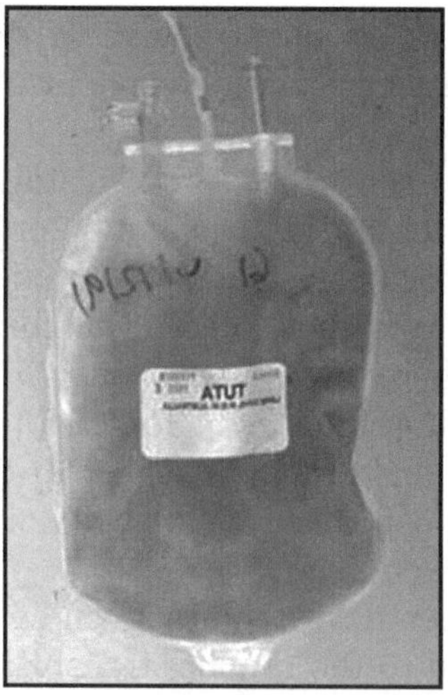

- *Fresh frozen plasma (FFP):* This is platelet-poor plasma that is separated from red cells within 6 hours of blood collection and frozen in a dedicated freezer (at or below –20°C). Fresh frozen plasma and fresh plasma contain all coagulation factors and plasma proteins (such as albumin).
  Fresh frozen plasma is stable for 1 year if maintained in a dedicated freezer (one that does not undergo freeze-thaw cycles like household freezers) at or below –20 C.
  One unit of FFP is defined as that obtained from a single whole blood transfusion bag (approximately 250 ml).
- *Cryoprecipitate (CPP):* Cryoprecipitate is a concentrated source of von Willebrand factor, fibrinogen, factor VIII and fibronectin. It is produced by slow-thawing (at 4°C) fresh frozen plasma, followed by centrifugation at 4°C. Cryoprecipitable proteins (those mentioned above) precipitate at this temperature and are maintained in a very small amount of remaining plasma (approximately 1/10 of the starting volume of FFP, or about 20 to 30 ml). Cryoprecipitate is stable for 1 year from the date of collection of the whole blood for transfusion purposes (not the date of preparation of the product) if maintained at or below–20 C in a dedicated freezer. One unit of cryoprecipitate is defined as that obtained from a single FFP bag (approximately 250 mL plasma).
- *Cryosupernant (Cryosuper):* Cryosupernant is the remaining plasma after removal of the pelleted cryoprecipitate. This is a source of all coagulation and plasma proteins, except for factor VIII, fibrinogen, von Willebrand factor and fibronectin. Cryosupernant is stable for 5 years if stored in a dedicated freezer at or below –20°C.
- *Frozen plasma:* Frozen plasma has several sources. It can be plasma

that is separated and frozen longer than 6 hours after whole blood collection. It can be fresh plasma that is not used within 6 hours of collection and then frozen. It can be fresh frozen plasma maintained for longer than 1 year in a dedicated freezer. Frozen plasma lacks certain coagulation factors which are quite unstable.

BLOOD OF ANIMALS

When Animal Blood is used in cooking: for example, in thesausagesknown as blackpuddings, the addition of several aromaticspicesis necessary so as to overcome its alkaline flatness, and lack of savour. "Blood," says Dr. Thudicum, "is not capable of giving a savoury extract (to gravy), although the blood of each species of eatable animal has its particular, and distinctive flavour; that of the ox, and cow being remarkably redolent of musk." But among civilized nations the pig is the only animal of which the Blood furnishes a distinct article of food; mixed withfat, and spices, whilst enclosed in prepared intestines, this pig's blood is made into black puddings.

Chemically the Blood of animals contains a considerable quantity of iron, besides albumin, fibrin, hydrogen, some traces of prussicacid, and some empyreumaticoil. The serum, or thin part of the Blood, includes sulphur. Experimentally it turns out that the blood of snails, which is colourless, contains as much iron as that of the ox, or calf, this fact going to prove that the red colour of animal Blood is not due, as is generally supposed, to the presence of iron in that fluid. The saline constituents of Blood are phosphates of lime, and magnesium, with chlorides, sulphates, and phosphates of potash and soda.

In Pickwick, Mr. Roker, the coarse turnkey at the Fleet Prison for debt, when showing Mr. Pickwick what were to be his wretched quarters there, turned fiercely round on him whilst he was mildly expostulating, and uttered in an excited fashion "certain unpleasant invocations concerning his own eyes, limbs, and circulating fluids".

Pliny tells us that the Blood of animals (and, indeed, human Blood as well) was administered in his time for curative purposes; so likewise the Blood of the ox is in medicinal vogue today in certain parts of the Western Hemisphere. This is because of the well-ascertained fact that iron, particularly its organicsalt (haemoglobin) as found in Blood, forms one of the most important constituents. It may be thus supplied from the pig in the culinary form of black puddings; as likewise from the ox, or sheep, if so desired. Among the Boers in South Africa dog's Blood is an established remedy for convulsions, and fits.

It is of modern discovery that in health the humanliverhas to receive a comparatively large allowance of iron, for carrying on the vital processes of combustion and oxidation, as its special functions. This iron is best obtained from the food, and not through any form of physics.

We know that many animals, especially beasts of prey, derive their needful supply of iron exclusively from meat containing a large proportion of Blood, which is rich in organic iron. Towards overcoming the natural repugnance of a patient to drinking animal Blood for acquiring its iron remedially, some skilful foreign chemists have produced this essential product of late in a compact form, which they term "Sanguinal," as a brownish red powder consisting (as is asserted) of pure crystallised haemoglobin, with the mineral Blood constituents, and of muscle albumin. Hypothetically it is fair to suppose that in this way the red corpuscles of a bloodless patient may be beneficially augmented.

Pepys observed about a Mr. Andrews who was dining with him, "What an odd, strange fancy he hath to raw meat, that he eats it with no pleasure unless the Blood run about his chops," which it did now by a leg of mutton that was not above half-boiled; but "it seems at home all his meat is dressed so, beefand all".

Practical experiments have shown that metallic iron, in whatever form it is administered medicinally, can be recovered from the excretions, absolutely undiminished in quantity, so that evidently no particle thereof is assimilated into the system.

Nevertheless, the machinery of red Blood-making is undoubtedly started afresh by giving iron, whether in food, or in physic (much more problematically). In 1902 Professor Bunge read an important paper on "Iron in Medicine" before the German Medical Congress.

He advocated an increased attention to foods containing iron, as a substitute for its administration in drug-form. "Spinach," said he, "is richer in iron than yolk of egg, and yolk of egg than beef; milk is almost devoid of iron; and, as if to provide against this defect, the Blood of the infant mammal is more plentifully endowed with the essential ingredients than that of adults, thus showing that nature is always self-provident.

" Garden spinach (one of the "Goosefoot" order), than which no better blood-purifier grows amongst vegetables, contains iron as one of its most abundant salts; hence it is a valuable food for bloodless persons; moreover, in both salinity, and digestibility it leads the kitchen greens, its amount of salts being 2 per cent, whereby it helps to furnish red colouring matter (haemoglobin) for the blood.

In the fruit world even the apple does not afford so much iron as this vegetable, neither does the strawberry. Spinach insists on having a rich soil in which to grow, out of which it extracts a large proportion of saline matters.

Its full green juice abounds in chlorophyll, insomuch that the spinach may be cooked entirely in its own fluids, and in the steam which will arise from them.

This brilliant green principle of colour, elaborated from the yellow and blue rays of the sunlight, is peculiarly salubrious. Evelyn (Acetaria) has said, "Spinach being boil'd to a pulp, and without other water than its own moisture, is a most excellent condiment for almost all sorts of boil'd flesh, and may accompany a sick man's diet. 'Tis laxative and emollient, and therefore profitable for the aged". Savoy, a nutritious, and wholesome companion of spinach, contains the greatest amount of vegetable oil of all this class of kitchen plants; and spinach runs the luxuriant Savoy very close in its complement of bland oil-salts, which render the juices nourishing. Quite half a pint of spinach-oil might be expressed from a hundred pounds of the vegetable, and sometimes more than this from the same quantity of Savoy.

BLOOD CIRCULATION SYSTEM OF ANIMAL

The circulatory system is the continuous system of tubes through which the blood is pumped around the body. It supplies the tissues with their requirements and removes waste products. In mammals and birds the blood circulates through two separate systems - the first from the heart to the lungs and back to the heart again (the pulmonary circulation) and the second from the heart to the head and body and back again.

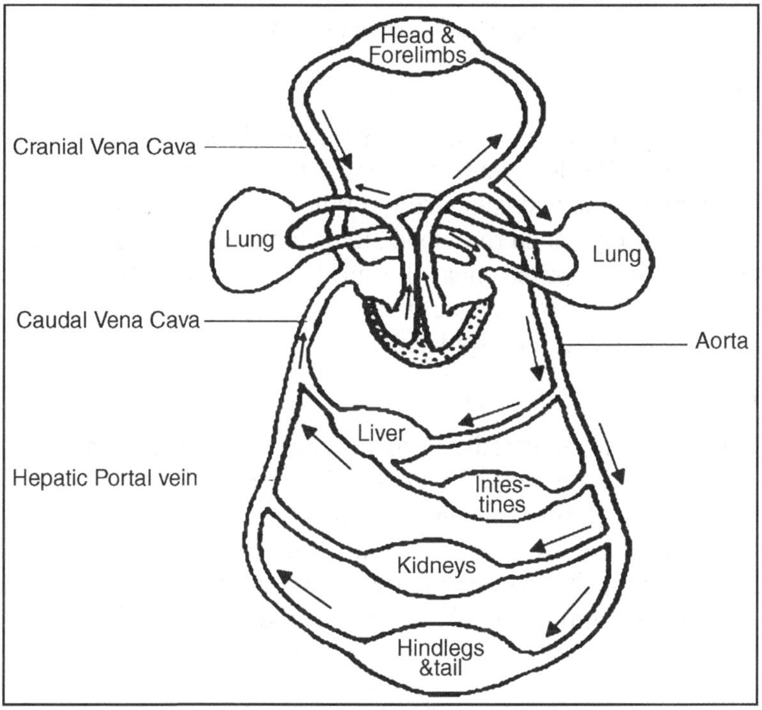

Fig. The Mammalian Circulatory System

The tubes through which the blood flows are the arteries, capillaries and veins. The heart pumps blood into arteries that carry it away from the heart. The arteries divide into very thin vessels called capillaries that form a network between the cells of the body. The capillaries then join up again to make veins that return the blood to the heart.

Arteries

Arteries carry blood away from the heart. They have thick elastic walls that stretch and can withstand the surges of high pressure blood caused by the heartbeat. The arteries divide into smaller vessels called arterioles. The hole down the centre of the artery is called the lumen. There are three layers of tissue in the walls of an artery. It is lined with squamous epithelial cells. The middle layer is the thickest layer. It made of elastic fibres and smooth muscle to make it stretchy. The outer fibrous layer protects the artery. The pulse is only felt in arteries.

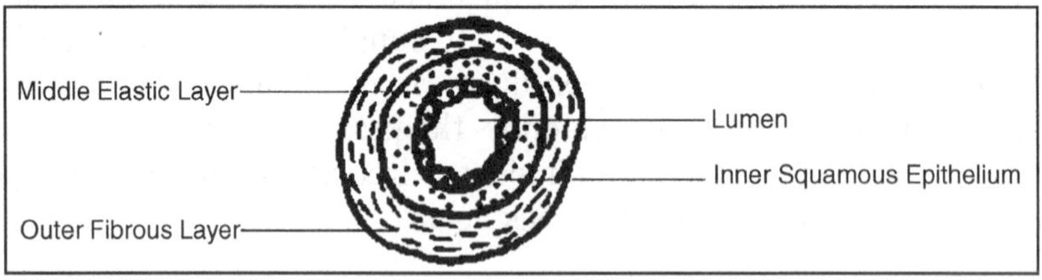

Fig. Cross Section of an Artery

The Pulse

The pulse is the spurt of high pressure blood that passes along the aorta and arteries when the left ventricle contracts. As the pulse of blood passes along an artery the elastic walls stretch. When the pulse has passed the walls contract and this helps push the blood along. The pulse is easily felt at certain places where an artery passes near the surface of the body. It is strongest near the heart and becomes weaker as it travels away from the heart. The pulse disappears altogether in the capillaries.

Capillaries

Arterioles divide repeatedly to form a network penetrating between the cells of all tissues of the body. These small vessels are called capillaries. The walls are only one cell thick and some capillaries are so narrow that red blood cells have to fold up to pass through them. Capillaries form networks in tissues called capillary beds. The capillary networks in capillary beds are so dense that no living cell is far from its supply of oxygen and food.

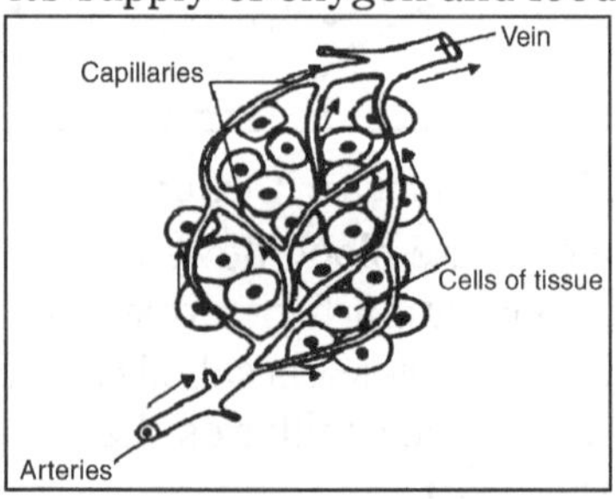

Fig. A Capillary Bed

The Formation of Tissue Fluid and Lymph

The thin walls of capillaries allow water, some white blood cells and many dissolved substances to diffuse through them. These form a clear fluid called tissue fluid (or extracellular fluid orinterstitial fluid) that surrounds the cells of the tissues. The tissue fluid allows oxygen and nutrients to pass from the blood to the cells and carbon dioxide and other waste products to be removed from the tissues.

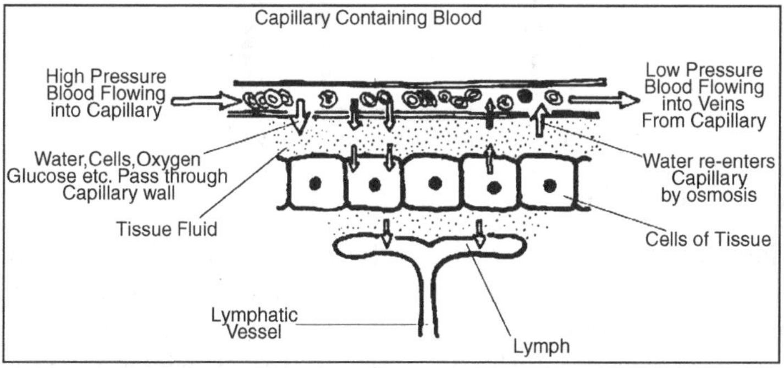

Fig. The Formation of Tissue Fluid and Lymph from Blood

Some tissue fluid finds its way back into the capillaries and some of it flows into the blind-ended lymphatic vessels that form a network in the tissues. Once the tissue fluid has entered the lymphatics it is called lymph although its composition remains the same. The lymph vessels have walls that are even thinner than the capillaries. This means that molecules and particles that are larger than those that can pass into the blood stream *e.g.* cancer cells and bacteria can enter the lymphatic system. These are then filtered out as the lymph passes through lymph nodes.

Veins

Capillaries unite to form larger vessels called venules that join to form veins. Veins return blood to the heart and since blood that flows in veins has already passed through the fine capillaries, it flows slowly with no pulse and at low pressure. For this reason veins have thinner walls than arteries although there have the same three layers in them as arteries. As there is no pulse in veins, the blood is squeezed along them by the contraction of the skeletal muscles that lay alongside them. Veins also have valves in them that prevent blood flowing backwards.

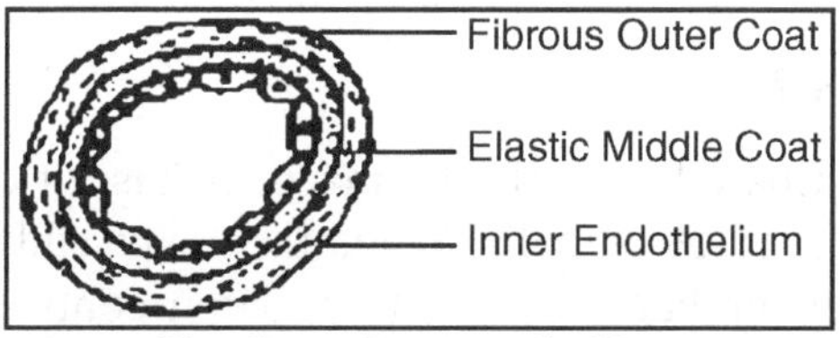

Fig. Cross Section of a Vein

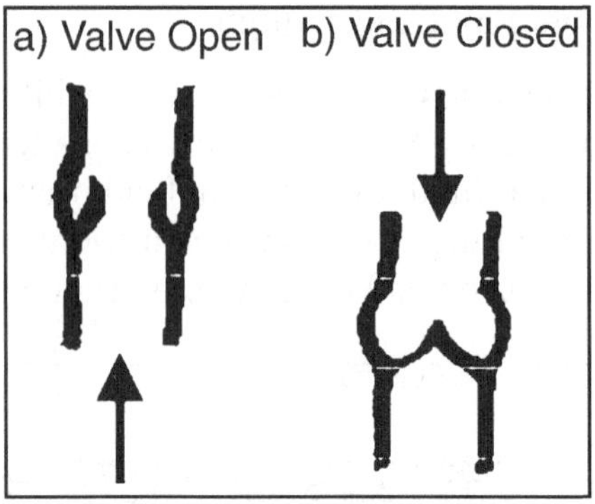

Fig. a) and b) Valves in a Vein

Regulation of Blood Flow

The flow of blood along arteries, arterioles and capillaries is not constant but can be controlled depending upon the requirements of the body. For example more blood is directed to the skeletal muscles, brain or digestive system when they are active. Regulation of the blood flow to the arterioles of the skin is also important in controlling body temperature. The size of the vessels is adjusted by the contraction or relaxation of smooth muscle fibres in their walls.

Oedema and Fluid Loss

Oedema is the swelling of the tissues due to the accumulation of tissue fluid. This may occur because the tissue fluid is prevented from returning to the bloodstream and accumulates in the tissues. This may be caused by physical inactivity (*e.g.* long car or plane trips in humans) or because of imbalances in the proteins in the blood. This is what causes the "pot-belly" of the malnourished child or worm-infested puppy.

Loss of body fluid can be caused not only by drinking insufficient liquid but also through diarrhea and vomiting or sudden loss of blood due to haemorrhage. The effect is to reduce the volume of the blood which decreases the blood pressure. This could be dangerous because the supply of adequate blood to the brain depends upon maintaining the blood pressure at a constant level. To compensate for the loss of fluid various mechanisms come into play. First of all the blood vessels contract in order to try and maintain the pressure. Then, since the loss of fluid tends to make the blood more concentrated and increases its osmotic pressure, fluid is drawn into the blood from the tissues by osmosis.

The Spleen of Stomach

The spleen is situated near the stomach. It has a rich blood supply and acts as a reservoir of red blood cells. When there is a sudden loss of blood, as happens when a haemorrhage occurs, the spleen contracts to release large numbers of red blood cells into the circulation. The spleen also destroys old red cells and makes new lymphocytes but it is not an essential organ because its removal in adult life seems to cause few problems. In the foetus, the spleen makes both red and white cells.

Important Blood Vessels of the Systemic (Body) Circulation

Blood is pumped out into the body via the main artery, the aorta. This takes the blood to the head, the limbs and all the body organs. After passing through a network of fine capillaries, the blood is returned to the heart in the largest vein, the vena cava. Arteries and veins to and from many organs often run alongside each other and have the same name *e.g.* the renal artery and vein serve the kidney, the femoral artery and vein serve the hind limbs and the subclavian artery and vein serve the forelimbs. However, blood to the head passes along the carotid artery and returns to the cranial vena cava via the jugular vein.

One variation on this arrangement is found in the blood vessels that serve the digestive tract. A variety of arteries take blood from the aorta to the intestines but blood from the intestines is carried by the hepatic portal vein to the liver where the digested food can be processed. This vessel is unlike others in that it transports blood from one organ to another rather than to or from the heart like arteries or veins.

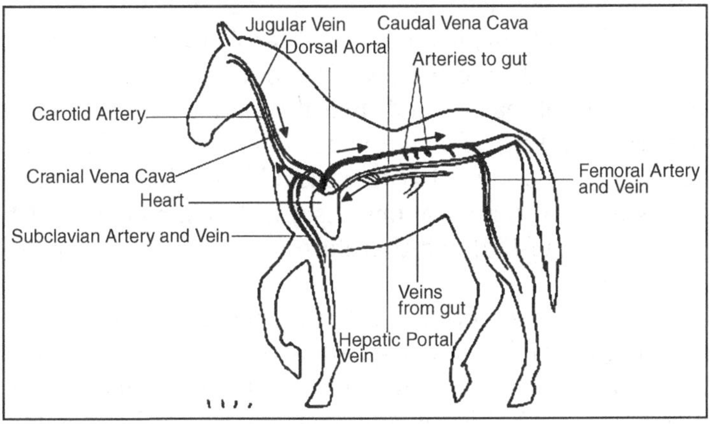

Fig. The Main Arteries and Veins of the Horse

Blood Pressure

The blood pressure is the pressure of the blood against the walls of the main arteries. The pressure is highest as the pulse produced by the contraction of the left ventricle passes along the artery. This is known as the systolic pressure. Pressure is much lower between pulses. This is known as the diastolic pressure. Blood pressure is measured in millimetres of mercury. A blood pressure that is higher than expected is known as hypertension while a pressure lower than expected is known as hypotension.

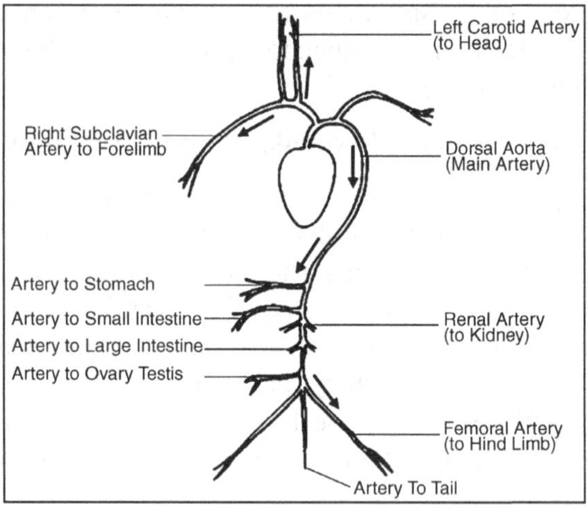

Fig. The Main Arteries of the Body

BLOOD COAGULATION AND ANTI COAGULANTS

ANTICOAGULANTS

Heparin is the prototypical anticoagulant. It was discovered in the liver of dogs in 1916 and was purified in the 1930s. It requires a plasma factor called antithrombin for its anticoagulant action. Heparin can be purified from the tissues of different animals. It cannot be given orally. It is widely used in medical practice for a number of reasons and clinical situations. It is commonly used to keep IV lines from clotting off, and it is used in a number of clinical situations where either a clot has occurred or there is a high risk of a clot occurring and causing serious medical complications. Its effect is immediate but has a short duration of activity (half-life) and therefore is most often given continuously through an IV line.

Alternatively, it is sometimes given as subcutaneous (under the skin) injections on a regular and frequent schedule (such as every four to six hours). The most feared side effects of heparin are bleeding and *heparin induced thrombocytopenia* (H.I.T.) Heparin administration must be monitored closely by means of a test called the P.T.T. (partial thromboplastin time). Other side effects of heparin include osteoporosis (with long term use), allergic reactions and elevation of liver enzymes. Warfarin is the dominant oral anticoagulant in the United States. It is derived from dicumarol, which is found in moldy sweet clover and caused an epidemic of cattle deaths in the early 1920s before the cause was discovered. In the 1930s it was discovered that vitamin K is necessary to prevent bleeding, and dicumarol and related compounds such as warfarin are known to work by inhibiting coagulation factors that require vitamin K (but this fact was not discovered until the 1970s). Warfarin received approval in the 1950s for clinical use.

Side effects of warfarin include paradoxically increased clotting activity for the first 24 to 36 hours of treatment, allergic reaction, drug interactions and severe skin reaction (necrosis) that may be associated with other conditions. The anticoagulation effect of warfarin is delayed for several days before becoming apparent. Therefore, heparin is often started in the hospital until the warfarin effect occurs.

Low Molecular Weight Heparins are stripped down versions of conventional (sometimes also called unfractionated.) heparin. Low molecular weight heparin molecules are about one third the size of unfractionated heparin, but contain the key five sugar sequence (pentasaccharide) that is responsible for the anticoagulant activity. Low molecular weight heparins can be given subcutaneously in a fixed dose and do not require monitoring. They can be used at home.

Fondaparinux is the most stripped down version of heparin. It consists of the five sugar sequence (pentasaccharide) that gives unfractionated heparin its anticoagulant activity. It is manufactured synthetically. Bivalirudin is another synthetic anticoagulant. It is derived from the anti-clotting substance found in leeches.

New Types of Oral Anticoagulants

The ideal anticoagulant drug would be one with a wide therapeutic index, oral administration, once a day administration, easy reversibility and availability of an effective antidote, short half life, lack of need for laboratory monitoring and reasonable cost.

While unfractionated heparin, low molecular weight heparins and warfarin in their own respects fulfil some of the above characteristics, none of them are by any means ideal and they all fall far short of fulfilling all of the above criteria.

- *Direct thrombin inhibitors (DTI): dabigatran* (Pradaxa-Boehringer Ingelheim) is a DTI that has been shown to be as effective and safe as enoxaparin (Lovenox) in reducing VTE after orthopedic surgery. As the name implies, it works by directly inhibiting the thombin molecule in the coagulation cascade. It does not require an intermediate molecule to be effective. It received approval in Europe for use after orthopedic operations to prevent blood clots from occurring.
- *Factor Xa inhibitors:* These drugs work by inhibiting the molecule Factor Xa in the coagulation cascade. Rivaroxaban (Xarelto-Bayer) has received approval in Canada and the EU for prevention of VTE in patients undergoing elective total hip or total knee replacement surgery. Apixaban failed to meet pre-specified criteria of non-inferiority in a study comparing it to enoxaparin in post-op patients but was numerically very similar in efficacy and statistically superior in terms of bleeding complications.

WHAT IS COAGULATION

Coagulation is the series of events that result in the formation of a clot. In the body, coagulation occurs after any injury to a blood vessel or tissue, in order to stop bleeding. Coagulation involves the interaction of cells lining the injured blood vessel (*endothelial cells*), Specialised blood cells called *platelets* that form a plug in the region of the damaged blood vessel, and circulating *coagulation factors*.

What are Coagulation Factors

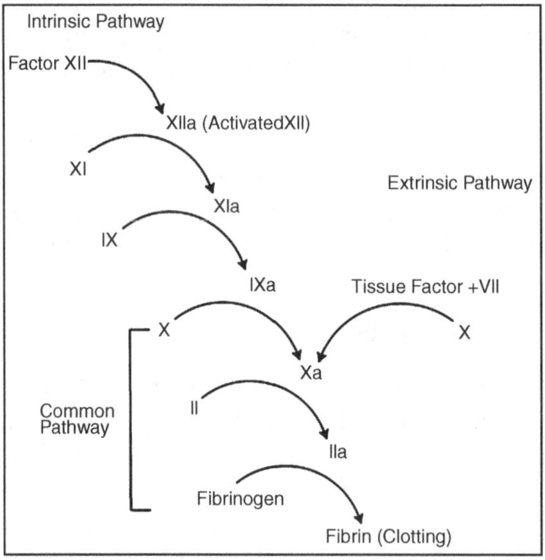

Coagulation factors are substances that are made in the liver and circulate in the blood stream. They become 'activated' when blood vessel or tissue injury occurs, and in co-operation with platelets, produce a clot at the site of injury. There are thirteen different coagulation factors. These factors are activated in a specific sequence, following two different pathways or sequences (the intrinsic and extrinsic pathways), and a final common pathway. In the body, there is interaction between the intrinsic and extrinsic coagulation pathways. In the laboratory, the activity of the coagulation factors comprising these pathways is measured separately.

When are Coagulation Tests Performed

Coagulation tests may be undertaken for a variety of reasons. Some breeds of dogs are known to have a higher incidence of clotting factor deficiencies and with these breeds, coagulation tests may be used for 'screening purposes' prior to diagnostic or surgical procedures. "Some breeds of dogs are known to have a higher incidence of clotting factor deficiencies..." If an animal experiences episodes of bleeding for an unknown reason, evaluation of clotting function should be undertaken. Severe liver disease may lead to problems with blood clotting because the liver is the site of production of coagulation factors.

Are there any screening tests that can be used in the veterinary clinic to evaluate coagulation?

Yes. The most commonly performed test is the evaluation of platelet numbers. Platelets are blood components that are involved in the formation of platelet 'plugs' at the site of blood vessel injury. Platelets not only provide the initial 'patch' at injured sites, they also form a framework that allows coagulation factors to accumulate at the injured site and subsequently form a more permanent fibrin clot.

Platelet numbers can be determined readily, and only a single blood sample is needed. Platelets are usually evaluated as part of a routine complete blood count (CBC) that also evaluates the red blood cell and white blood cell components of blood. A marked decrease in total platelet numbers (termed *thrombocytopenia*) may result in episodes of bleeding. There are many causes of *thrombocytopenia,* including immune-mediated disease, bone marrow disorders, and infectious causes, among others.

"...*thrombocytopenia* may result in episodes of bleeding."

While changes in the red and white blood cells on a CBC do not provide specific information about coagulation, they may alert your veterinarian to investigate further. A reduction in red cell numbers *(anemia)* may occur as a consequence of coagulation factor or platelet deficiency, while changes in the white blood cell numbers or types may indicate an underlying inflammatory condition that may be responsible for the *thrombocytopenia*. Because clotting factors are made in the liver, and because many diseases can result in thrombocytopenia, a serum biochemistry panel that evaluates liver function may be helpful.

The buccal mucosal bleeding time (BMBT) is a test which can be performed in the clinic and which evaluates the ability of platelets to form a platelet plug. A spring-loaded cassette is used to produce a small, precise cut on the inside of the upper lip, and the length of time required for bleeding to stop is measured. This time may be lengthened by a decreased platelet count or by decreased platelet function. The BMBT is usually reserved for patients that have normal platelet numbers but have questionable platelet function.

The ACT (activated clotting time) test can be performed in the veterinary clinic. To perform this test a blood sample is added to a special ACT tube containing a substance (usually diatomaceous earth) that activates the coagulation factors in both the intrinsic and common pathways. A severe decrease (less than 5 per cent of normal activity) in these clotting factors or a severe decrease in platelet numbers will lead to an increase in the length of time it takes the blood to clot after it has been added to the ACT tube. The ACT is not very sensitive to milder decreases in clotting factors. What specific tests are used to measure the activity of coagulation factors?

> "More specific coagulation tests are sent to a veterinary or hematological (blood) reference laboratory..." These more specific coagulation tests are sent to a veterinary or hematological (blood) reference laboratory and require a single blood sample.

The PTT (activated partial thromboplastin time) measures the functional activity of the coagulation factors involved in the *intrinsic* and common coagulation pathways. The PTT measures the time that it takes for a fibrin clot to form after calcium and an activator are added to a blood sample. The results of the PTT will be increased (that is, the time required for a clot to form will increase) when there is at least a 70 per cent decrease in the activity of a single factor in either of the intrinsic or common coagulation pathways. Smaller decreases in multiple factors may also result in an increase in the PTT. Anti-coagulant therapy such as heparin will increase the PTT.

The PT (prothrombin time) measures the functional activity of the coagulation factors involved in the *extrinsic* and common pathways. The PT does this by measuring the amount of time it takes for a fibrin clot to form after calcium and a tissue-activating factor are added to a blood sample. The results of the PT will be increased (that is, the time required for a clot to form will increase) when there is at least a 70 per cent decrease in the activity of a single factor in either of the extrinsic or common pathways. Because of the specific factors involved in the extrinsic coagulation pathways, an increase in PTT is often noted with conditions such as vitamin K deficiency and rodenticide (rat poison) toxicity.

"...Increase in PTT is often noted with conditions such as vitamin K deficiency and rodenticide (rat poison) toxicity."

The TT (thrombin time) measures the functional activity of the *common* coagulation pathway, and more specifically of *fibrinogen*. The conversion of fibrinogen to a fibrin clot is the end point of both the intrinsic and extrinsic pathways in the body. Both pathways converge to the final common pathway that results in fibrin clot formation. The TT measures the amount of time it takes for a fibrin clot to form after calcium and thrombin (a coagulation factor) is added to a blood sample. Since the TT is dependent upon both the amount and the normal functional activity of fibrinogen, any condition that depletes the amount of fibrinogen or makes it unable to function properly will cause an increase in TT. Examples of such conditions include hereditary deficiencies in the amount or functional activity of fibrinogen and increased use/consumption of fibrinogen in the body because of excessive blood coagulation (clotting). Such excessive coagulation can occur because of shock, severe infections, and tumours, to name a few examples.

Von Willebrand's factor testing at a veterinary reference laboratory involves the evaluation of a blood sample for the presence of von Willebrand's factor, a protein that assists in the adherence or 'stickiness' of platelets to sites of blood vessel injury. Von Willebrand's factor also helps to stabilise one of the coagulation factors (Factor VIII) in circulation so that this factor is not lost prematurely. Von Willebrand's disease is one of the most common hereditary bleeding disorders of dogs, affecting over 50 breeds and resulting in variable deficiencies of this factor.

"Von Willebrand's disease is one of the most common hereditary bleeding disorders of dogs..."

> In addition to von Willebrand's factor testing, can the individual coagulation factors be evaluated?
>
> Yes. Specific coagulation factor analysis is not commonly done, but it is available in Specialised veterinary or hematological laboratories. Specific coagulation factor analysis is typically used to evaluate the most common inherited deficiencies, namely von Willebrand's factor, factor VIII deficiency (hemophilia A) and factor IX deficiency (hemophilia B).

"Coagulation testing is not usually done in isolation."

Coagulation testing is not usually done in isolation. Typically, a CBC and a biochemical profile are first evaluated. Then a coagulation panel consisting of a combination of PT, PTT and possibly von Willebrand's factor testing is performed. The *combination of results* from these coagulation tests will indicate what part of the coagulation pathway is affected. Once these results have been assessed, the necessity for additional testing can be determined.

Antithrombin III is one of the most commonly measured inhibitors of the coagulation system. While measurement of this protein requires only a single blood sample, antithrombin III determination is performed only at Specialised laboratories. Antithrombin III measurement is usually undertaken if a pet is at risk of increased coagulability (increased chance of clot formation). Increased coagulation of blood may be a complicating factor of many diseases including cancer, severe inflammation, Cushing's disease, and kidney disease.

7

Research Areas and Targets

The discussion in earlier chapter highlights the areas and suggest priorities for application and continuing research for improving animal production from the available feed resources for livestock in developing countries. The targets are:

Maximisation of P/E Ratio in Nutrients Absorbed from the Rumen

Some methods/techniques to do this are listed below:

- By combinations of minerals, non-protein nitrogen and protein supplementation to support high efficiencies of rumen fermentation
- Improve microbial growth efficiency by manipulating the microbial populations
  - To obtain more efficient microbes
  - To remove protozoa
  - To adjust the p/e ratio with feed additives
  - To alter the genetic capacity of the microbes to synthesise protein or to produce higher biological value proteins
- Improve dietary protein bypass. Where protein is fed, to decrease protein and/or peptide and/or amino acid degradation in the rumen and allow a greater flow of amino acids, peptides and protein to the intestines from dietary origin
- Development of sources of supplements of protein meals that have natural protection or are manipulated to escape rumen fermentation. *This includes the need to*:
  - Identify protein sources that are protected naturally or in processing
  - Identify soluble protein sources and find economic and viable mechanisms for protection of the proteins
  - Develop protein crops or by-products that can be grown and processed at the site of ruminant population densities in countries where protein meals are scarce
  - Develop rumen manipulation studies to enhance the bypass of soluble proteins.

Maximisation of Digestibility of Fibrous Feeds

This is achieved by:

- Providing supplements of essential nutrients required by microbes
- Manipulating microbial populations in the rumen to increase digestibility
- Promote populations of selected, highly fibrolytic fungi in the rumen
- Defaunation
- Treatment of crop residues prior to feeding to enhance their digestibility
- Altering the physiology of the digestive tract (*e.g.* Rumen mobility, turnover etc.) *e.g.* Through the use of immunisation of somatotropin release inhibiting factor (SRIF).

Optimising the Partitioning of Nutrients into Product

This includes:

- By breeding more efficient animals
- Chemical intervention—hormonal implants or injections
- Injections of compounds such as b-agonists, bovine growth hormone
- Development of transgenic animals with particular characteristics *e.g.* High circulating bst or enzymes complements previously not present in animals.

PRIORITY RATINGS

Assigning priorities within this list is a most important aspect of this report. Clearly the research requires a differing level of sophistication of technology and different priorities will need to be assigned to different resource bases.

Simply stated, the priority ratings for research emphasis are in order of priority:

- To ensure an adequate P/E ratio in nutrients absorbed
- To improve the extent of digestion of low digestibility feeds that require microbial fermentation for digestion
- To improve the partitioning of available nutrients for product synthesis (meat, milk, wool etc.) Or drought power generation.

It is clear that an inadequate nutrition will not allow the expression of any manipulations in priority. It is also obvious that a super bug cannot be successful in the rumen that is deficient in critical nutrients (for example, ammonia).

PRESENT RESEARCH PRIORITIES AND CHANGE

Biotechnology research from its broadest definition (any biological manipulation) to its narrowest definition (recombi-nant DNA technology) requires the same mechanisms to optimise progress in livestock production.

They involve:

- The training of scientists in the known principles and practice of animal science
- Development of research and research technology to expand the knowledge base
- Documentation of information.

Major nutritional constraints to livestock production in developing countries may be categorised according to feed availability and quality. In the cropping areas, animals are sustained largely on crop residues and by-products in which deficiencies of nutrients is the major problem. In the rangelands, the feeds available are deficient in nutrients and there is a seasonal shortage of pasture in the dry season when the available feed resources are even more deficient in nutrients than they were during the grazing season. These problems may be overcome to some extent by supplementary feeding strategies which emphasise the balance of nutrition of animals and include methods to increase feed digestibility.

Although a wide range of biotechnologies can be brought to bear on these two strategies, within the nutritional emphasis of this report it is feed technology that is likely to produce the greatest advances for the small farmer in the developing countries. Recombinant DNA research in the developing countries is at a preliminary stage of development and is fraught with difficulties and lack of knowledge of, in particular, control of genetic expression. It is largely exploratory, even in the developed countries. In the advanced research institutes, and at the university level, it is most useful in expanding knowledge. On the contrary the large input by business interests, at the potentially practical, and therefore commercially applicable-level is highly secretive and often advanced.

The markets of multi-national companies are likely to be in the more wealthy developed world and are unlikely to have an impact upon the developing countries with its different interests and objectives and the largely unpredictable success rate of an innovation to increase animal production.

Biotechnology research in all developing countries lacks the infrastructure of, and skills in, the integrated sciences. There is a shortage of trained personnel and those that are trained are tending to develop along the lines that they began as trainees, Ph.D or Masters students.

What is more, a significant number of these people are ‘skimmed off’ by institutions in the developed world if they show aptitudes as there is a shortage of trained personnel in these countries. The developing countries must consider the balance of research within a country. The need to partition the available funds and resources into areas that are likely to increase productivity in a reasonably short term and more importantly are likely to be accepted by small farmers. The politics of research funding in every country where the majority of scientists are concerned only with the development of their own science, will ensure the dedication of government funds to recombinant DNA technology and in general, this will have priority over, what appears to be the more 'mundane' animal nutrition research. This seems inevitable even though feeding trials using basal poor quality feeds given to ruminants have indicated that balancing nutrition has the potential to increase animal productivity by 5–10 fold depending on location. On the other hand recombinant DNA technology has a high potential to fail; it is costly and breakthroughs will be at least as difficult to apply as the present research on supplementary feeding.

Developed countries have improved milk production per cow by 60% from 1976–1986, and this has been achieved by altering the feed base and simultaneously breeding of cows to take advantage of the 'improved' feed base. At the same time, Asia and Africa have improved their yield per cow by 13% and 7% respectively. This indicates the enormous unused potential and the priorities for application. These are the manipulation of feed base with simultaneous genetic improvement.

Research and application in India has already demonstrated that a change of feed base with the introduction of cows with a high potential for milk production results in the large increases in productivity needed to lift production towards the demand for high quality protein by humans. The research application by NDDB and by others in a number of countries has indicated that high, realisable yields from Friesians or other breeds fed on local feeds. This re-emphasises the 'less sophisticated' biotechnology research concepts that are available to improve animal production from the available resources and which can be applied now. The need is to fit the technology to local conditions.

REAL WORLD PROBLEMS OF CAPITALISING ON MODERN BIOTECHNOLOGY IN DEVELOPING COUNTRIES

Many authors have suggested that the developing countries, in order to participate in the wealth that might be generated by modern biotechnology, (in this case largely dealing with recombinant DNA technology) must develop their research capacity in this area.

A country obtains the benefits of such developments from the new technology packages which when applied, result in improved animal productivity. However, the developing countries will at the present time have to purchase many developed packages which have not considered the particular constraint to production in their country.

This may result in no benefit (or even a negative effect) as the purchase price of the technology will often be higher than the value of the increased productivity (*e.g.* the lift in milk yield of 25% by daily injections of BSt into buffaloes does not pay for the cost of the injections in India). The other way the country will benefit is by its scientists being the inventor, preserving the world patent rights or by preserving at least the production and distribution rights from any invention for the country. The major problems here will be the same as for small-return businesses in the industrial world attempting to develop with limited finance. The potential of large companies being able to move in, take over, buy out or simply compete for promising inventions are obvious with a recent example in the takeover of Genotec.

Unless the developing country concerned are prepared to act in the same way as a multi national company, then any potentially highly-profitable invention is likely to be lost to the industrialised giants. This can happen even before the research scientists have identified the importance of their research.

The developing countries in general have only 'embryonic' staff, trained in the new biotechnology largely by the scientists from the industrialised countries. The research groups in developing countries are centered around a few 'high quality' scientists who recognise the need to develop new areas (rather than to compete with the scientists with whom they were trained); they lack funding and they will have major problems if they make a major discovery with the scaling up of a development and in defending their resultant patents.

It is imperative that along with the development of modern biotechnology there must be development of expertise in patent application/patent protection, deciding on commercial partnerships, scaling up operations and market research.

Given the business ethos it would be highly improbable that a breakthrough in biotechnology that would be applicable on a world basis would be fully capitalised by the inventor or his/her country.

The greatest problems come after the inventive stage when commercialisation is needed. For example, to produce commercial amounts of a new chemical, scaling up of the laboratory research costs about 10 times the expenditure for the experimental research, the costs of commercialisation can be even 100 times higher than this figure.

The lessons of recent years from the take over of new biotechnology discoveries in developed countries suggest that funding of biotechnology research should:

- Recognise the need for good managers and lawyers
- Have good market research. In this respect specific in-country problem solving may be better than competing in a world market.
- Recognise the need for international co-operation specifically in start up inventions
- Recognise early the need for considerable increases in funding with development and scaling up from the laboratory level.

Modern biotechnology research that is funded by Aid-Agencies is unlikely to be kept secret, with the present requirements and extent of the need to report back to the agency.

The need for secrecy stems from the potential of discoveries to be valuable to commercial enterprise. Without support for patent development, scaling up operations etc. then any invention is likely to end up through a variety of ways as the property of a large company.

Secrecy in Industrialised Countries

The communication of information between scientists has long been recognised as a great facilitator of research. However, the high likely value of inventions (*e.g.* BSt was calculated to have an annual global market of US$500 million) in modern biotechnology has destroyed considerably the ethos of communication and study in science. At the present time even PhD graduates may be sworn to secrecy and their thesis only published when the data is "old hat" or a patent or process fully protected. This represents a considerable disadvantage for the scientists in developing countries who have restricted access to the literature, no access to industrial personnel and limited funds to travel.

Most of the modern biotechnology is now financed by commercial enterprise who have 'picked off' and employed the scientific experts in many fields and have tight security on their developments. For any 'start up' researcher to get ahead and stay ahead of such commercial research it will only be possible where the research is only of local interest or is aimed at sections of the community that do not have the capacity to pay and therefore the inventions/strategies are to be made available at no cost.

The Need for Expertise in Developing Countries to Capitalise on Various Developments

The development of a capacity for biotechnology research and teaching and for scientists with a depth of knowledge in the field allows a country to access product development and also to pick-up technologies applicable to local or small markets and discarded for economic reasons by large companies. It also allows that country to capitalise on inventions following patent expiration. The question now is how to retain such expertise in countries with limited ability to develop a research resource in modern biotechnology. The only option appears to be specialised national institutes funded from within a country.

ADJUSTING P/E RATIO IN THE NUTRIENTS ABSORBED BY RUMINANTS WITH PROTEIN SUPPLEMENTS

The effects of improving the P/E ratio in nutrients available to ruminants on low quality forages have been discussed above. Research into supplementary feeding is well developed in a number of countries along the lines of optimising fermentative digestion (using molasses urea blocks) and optimising the efficiency of use of nutrients from the rumen. It is estimated that about 50 countries are now testing molasses urea blocks as a means of supplementing ruminants on forage based diets with critically deficient nutrients. Some results of studies from Indonesia are given for the effects of introducing molasses urea blocks into ruminant production systems using cut/carry grass. Many countries that do not have a source of molasses within the country are looking for other means of giving the same mixture of nutrients to their indigenous livestock.

It is again stressed that both supplementation of the rumen with deficient nutrients (*e.g.* phosphorus, sulphur and non-protein nitrogen) and the animal (with a bypass protein) will improve the protein to energy ratios in the nutrients that are available to the animal.

This in turn will optimise production from the available resources. Even where the rumen is not optimised a bypass protein can still adjust the P/E ratio significantly.

In some respects, where a bypass protein is relatively inexpensive, and/or molasses urea blocks difficult to use or get animals to take, then, a sole supplement of bypass protein may be sufficient to improve efficiency of feed utilisation significantly. In addition the soluble protein that is always present in the practical bypass protein supplements, together with the recycling of urea-N back to the rumen often diminishes the effectiveness of urea/molasses blocks and many applied practitioners have taken advantage of this particularly when dairy cows are fed high levels of bypass protein supplements, the molasses/urea block can become only marginally beneficial. The theoretical calculations of P/E ratios are shown in Table. Obviously the best option is the use of both supplements.

Bypass Protein Supplements

Providing bypass protein to cattle under small farmer management is often difficult and at times it is too expensive. There is often little information on the locally available protein sources, particularly the level of protection of the protein in the rumen. As a rule-of-thumb, solvent extracted oilseed cakes, fish meal that has been flame dried (but not sun-dried fish meal or fish silage) and protein sources that have been heat treated, have some considerable protection from rumen degradation. The degree of protection is enhanced by pelleting the protein meal in the presence of free xylose, glucose or fructose, when a mild browning reaction occurs (unpublished observations).

The major requirements before wide spread use of these technologies can be promulgated in a country are:

- Determination of the extent of protection of proteins from rumen degradation in the available protein resources
- Identification of the potential protein sources together with development of technologies to inactivate anti-quality compounds and to protect protein
- In some countries there are no recognised protein crops at the centres of ruminant population densities. In these areas there is a need to find new sources of protein. This could include growing trees and forages for leaf, seed or pod production followed by development of appropriate technologies to harvest and protect these proteins when these are not naturally protected
- The development in ruminants of response relationships to increasing

levels of bypass protein supplementation on the available feed resources to allow economic assessment

- Development of the marketing and extension technologies to get the products to the farmers.

Table. Summarised Data on Growth and Milk Production Responses to UMB Technology in Both Large Ruminants (UMB 400–500 g/h/d) and Small Ruminants (UMB 100–150 g/h/d) in West Central Java in 1988–89. The Data are from Hendratno, N and Numerous Co-operators and were Summarised in Entwhistle (1989)

Species	Location	Trait measured	Treatment		Response to UMB
			Control	UMB	
Dairy cattle	W.Java	Milk yield (l/d)	7.44	9.92	
(Friesan)	C.Java		5.70	8.00	
		Average	6.57	8.96	+36%
Beef cattle	W.Java	1 Weight gain (kg/d)	0.182	0.400	
(Ongole)	"	2	0.333	0.526	
	"	3	0.277	0.439	
	"	4	0.478	0.465	
	"	5	0.200	0.278	
	C.Java	6	0.446	0.689	
		Average	0.319	0.466	+46%
Sheep	W.Java	Weight gain (kg/d)	0.130	0.320	+146%
(Garut)					
Goats	C.Java	Milk yield (l/d)	0.795	1.091	+37%
(Ettawa)					

ADJUSTING P/E RATIO BY MANIPULATION OF THE RUMEN

Microbial growth efficiency can very from as low as 10 g of dry cells/MJ of VFA produced in the rumen to as high as 30 g of dry cells/MJ of VFA. The reasons for these variations include differences in population mix of microbes and the deficiency of nutrients specific to micro-organisms that grow in the rumen. Under most management conditions where ruminants are on good quality forage based diets the P/E ratio theoretically is of the order of 17 g cells/MJ VFA; on diets of low quality forage the ratio may be between 4 and 10 g cells/MJ VFA; therefore there is considerable scope for manipulation of this ratio.

Supplementation of the Rumen Microbial Ecosystem

In ruminants correcting a chronic rumen deficiency of nutrients for microbial growth generally increases digestibility, feed intake and the quantities of microbial cells produced relative to VFA.

The technologies discussed below all have a prerequisite that the rumen ecosystem has been brought up to a high level of efficiency by supplementation before attempts are made to further manipulate P/E ratio.

Chemical Manipulation of Rumen Fermentative Efficiency

There are a number of chemicals available which, when added to a diet, improve the efficiency of feed utilisation by 5–20%. Among these, the most prominent ones are monensin (or rumensin), lasalocid and avoparcin. However, the improvement that is brought about by balancing the amino acid supply in a forage based diet may increase the efficiency of feed conversion to liveweight of a milch heifer by many times this value.

Even though the costs are high and the returns small, monensin is utilised extensively throughout the world in the feedlot industry based on grain. These chemicals have been considered as propionate enhancers (in the rumen) but in all probability they improves P/E ratios by decreasing peptide and amino acid degradation in the rumen and in addition possibly by inhibiting protozoal growth which improve the P/E ratio in the nutrients absorbed.

Because these chemicals tend to have side effects in that they reduce intake at least initially, which often removes any overall benefits when added to a diet, they have not been accepted for forage fed ruminants.

Methods that decrease peptide and amino acid degradation in the rumen potentially would be a very effective means of stimulating P/E ratios on moderate protein diets but would be highly significant where soluble protein sources are available and would circumvent the necessity to chemically protect proteins. In summary, there is potential for screening chemicals for activity against the micro-organisms that degrade peptides and amino acids as they appear to be different to the ones that degrade proteins to peptides and amino acids.

Manipulation of the Microbial Mix Within the Rumen

The rumen microbial populations are composed of protozoa, bacteria and anaerobic fungi as well as viruses and phages. The population density of each group can be highly variable depending on diet but, in general, the end products of fermentative digestion are qualitatively the same.

Although there has been major attempts to manipulate protozoal populations little success resulted until good laboratory systems for defaunation were invented so that large numbers of ruminant animals could be studied. There is little doubt that defaunation results in increased microbial cell outflow to the intestines (defaunation improves the P/E ratio in the nutrients absorbed). Jouany and Ushida have also clearly shown that on diets containing considerable true protein, a greater amount of dietary protein reaches the intestines in addition to the extra microbial protein in animals that are unfaunated compared with those having normal populations of protozoa.

Provided that the amount of bypass protein in the diet is below requirements of the faunated animal, an improvement in efficiency of feed utilisation results when protozoa are removed from the rumen. Defaunation has increased ruminant production levels by up to 50% at times. On high quality concentrate feeds high in bypass protein, the improvement in efficiency that results from defaunation may not be expressed but the level of feed protein can potentially be reduced by 20–50% with the same efficiency and production rates.

The potential for application of defaunation is highlighted by the improved efficiency of utilisation of the basal feed resource in defaunated or unfaunated animals. Defaunation and maintenance of the unfaunated state has resulted in 30–60% increases in growth rate of sheep, cattle and buffalo and a preliminary study indicates a promise of up to 2 litres/day more milk in Friesians.

The problems are:

- To identify suitable defaunating or protozoa suppressing treatments which are simple and economic
- To find mechanisms for administration of anti-protozoal compounds to ruminants under prevailing management systems.

Defaunating Agents

Rumen protozoa are susceptible to a wide range of chemicals, particularly those that disrupt cell membranes (*i.e.* they are surface active). From a very small survey of natural products (less than 100 forages were surveyed), two sources of anti-protozoal agents which can be used in small doses to suppress or eliminate protozoa in the rumen were identified (Assafa, G., Klieve, A. and Leng R.A. unpublished).

The rich tropical floras of many of the developing countries may be sources of many other anti-protozoal compounds or forages. A priority area for research is to establish a simple anti-protozoal assay in a number of laboratories in differing climatic zones and to quickly identify potential sources of antiprotozoal drugs.

Initially, it would be simple to look at the effects of increasing quantities of a soluble extract of a forage on the viability of protozoa incubated with the materials for, say, up to 2 hours. This would obviously have to be followed by animal experimentation and, finally, growth studies to determine whether the other effects of these anti-protozoal compounds could be detrimental to the animal.

Mechanisms of Defaunation

The only practical means for manipulating the protozoal population of the rumen is likely to be through strategic supplements containing a defaunating agent, either given daily or on a periodic basis.

As discussed earlier defaunation has a marked stimulating effect on P/E ratios and efficiency of feed conversion. Research will be needed to examine the administration of any potential defaunating agent through the basal feed, in a protein supplement or through a multi-nutrient block to the animal.

The latter will be potentially the most practical routes, but it limits the dose rate of the drug to quite small quantities as intake of blocks tends to be a small fraction of total intake. A highly active antiprotozoal agent might be delivered by an intraruminal device capable of sustained release of a drug but again costs are likely to mitigate against this approach.

Other Manipulations of Rumen Ecosystems

By chance, recent research has demonstrated that small amounts of a clay mineral (bentonite—a montmorillonite clay), added to a diet of sheep, improved wool growth by up to 20% in faunated sheep but only by 5% in unfaunated sheep.

The mechanism of action of the bentonite is unknown but it either improves the P/E ratio or specifically the outflow of sulphur amino acids from the rumen as these are the main controlling nutrients for wool growth.

The problems are:

- To understand the mechanisms of action of bentonite as this will be crucial in identifying the sources of bentonite to use and the systems in which it will improve animal productivity
- Finding a mechanism for administration of the bentonite through supplements.

Alteration of Protein and Amino Acid Composition of Rumen Microbes—Recombinant DNA Technology

Rumen microbial protein appears to have a relatively constant amino acid composition, independent of the mix of microbes in the whole population. The primary limiting amino acids for wool growth in sheep are methionine and cysteine and for growth are possibly the same amino acids plus lysine and threonine.

Undoubtedly, if rumen microbes could be engineered to produce protoplasmic proteins high in the deficient amino acids then improvements in wool production would result.

Methionine is relatively slowly broken down in the rumen and peptides and proteins high in sulphur amino acids appear to be also relatively slowly degraded by the resident microbes. Therefore, establishment of rumen organisms in the rumen that produce these amino acids could increase the outflow of the sulphur amino acids and hence the efficiency of wool growth.

The problems will be to isolate, identify DNA en-coding for the necessary enzymes; develop vectors and transform rumen microbes. Following this, the transformed rumen microbes must be able to grow extensively in the rumen and be retained, particularly during periods of nutritional stress for the rumen microbes.

ADJUSTING P/E RATIOS FROM THE RUMEN BY MANIPULATING THE FEED BASE

Feed Technology and Development of Supplements

Supplementary feeding to ensure an efficient digestion in the rumen of cattle on poor quality forages, undoubtedly increases the efficiency of productivity from local feed resources. This has been well demonstrated by research of the National Dairy Development Board (NDDB) of India.

The NDDB has developed molasses/urea multi-nutrient blocks that are available at cost to village farmers. Similar developments are now occurring in some 50 developing countries in the tropics. However, few countries have realised the potential to develop and use bypass protein concentrates. A specific case history of the application of these feed technologies in India is discussed below.

Supplementation with "Naturally" Protected Protein: A Case Study in Strategic Supplements

In two milk sheds (Kedah and Baroda), through their feed mills, a high (30%) protein concentrate that contains a high proportion of bypass protein is manufactured and sold (roughly 100 tonnes/day in Kedah alone).

The protein meals selected are all from the oil seed industry and have received a degree of protection from the processing techniques which include solvent extraction and application of heat.

In addition, the final protein concentrate is pelleted with about 8% molasses which appears to give additional protection (presumedly due to heat in the press and some browning reaction of sugar with the lysine units that provide from the protein surface). In a commercial operation and using a mill with a capacity for 100 tonnes/day, mixtures of proteins from different sources are necessary and quality control essential. It is well recognised that protein sources vary in the extent to which they escape the rumen and pelleting seems to ensure that protection is improved.

Providing Bypass Protein in Areas Without Protein Resources

In many countries of the developing world, proteins for livestock are scarce. Sometimes highly soluble and easily degradable proteins are available (*e.g.* lupins and whole cotton seed) but these are only as effective in altering the P/E ratio as supplementation with urea. There is a great need for the development of inexpensive technologies for protection of protein meals.

Proteins can be protected from degradation in the rumen by insolubilisation processes which include:

- Heat (depending on the protein source); temperatures from 120 to 180°C will denature the protein and the subsequent insolubility affords considerable protection from microbial attack when it is in the rumen.

- *Chemical reactions which include*:
  - Reactions with aldehydes, such as formaldehyde and gluteraldehyde or
  - Mixing with tannins or selection of plants with tannins.

Table. Some Practical Results from Commercial Milk Producing Systems where Feed Resources are Based on "Low Quality" Forages Fed to Friesians (1–3) and Cross Bred Cows (4)

Basal Feed	Supplements	Milk Production
1. Tropical grass/maize silage or other crops plus 1-2 kg rice straw/day	Free choice molasses /urea blocks + protein pellet (30% CP) (350 g/kg milk)	5000-6500 kg/305 d
2. Rice straw/millet straw (8 kg/d)	Bypass protein pellet 300 g/kg milk	25 l/day (at 3 months)
3. *ad lib.* mixture of cottonseed hulls (46%; molasses (17%); cottonseed meal (18%); sesame seed meal (15%); crude lecithin (4%) and 10 kg freshly harvested kikuyu grass (2 kg DM/d)		6200 kg/300 days (2nd calf cows); 5700 kg/300 days (1st calf heifers)
4. Cane tops (50% more than daily intake) + cut/carry grass as available	Cottonseed meal 250 g/kg milk	2800 kg/lactation/yr(4)

Most Likely Technologies

It is most likely in the future that to process proteins to ensure that they bypass the rumen, feed technology will make use of the 'browning reaction' or the use of calcium soaps of long chain fatty acids (particularly for dairy cows where the long chain fatty acids can be used in milk synthesis and fat is low in the diet) to coat the protein meals.

The use of aldehydes to protect proteins has undoubtedly been successful but is often not economic, nor readily applied in most developing countries. It has been phased out in some countries because of the potential carcinogenic effect of a volatile compound produced when formaldehyde and acids react. In recent years the development of mild treatment of protein meals with xylose (a 5 carbon sugar pentose) at low temperatures has become a possibility. Results from Prof.T. Klopfenstein's laboratory at the University of Nebraska, have clearly shown that small quantities of xylose heated with soyabean meal substantially protects the protein from rumen degradation and improves efficiency of feed utilisation of cattle fed forage/concentrate based diets.

This technology has been singled out because it is simple, the process has enormous scope for development by imaginative scientists and the sources of xylose are readily available in most developing countries. Processing technologies for generating the xylose, however, must be developed prior to application. Xylose is a major constituent of hemicellulose and a useful source includes sugar cane bagasse and cottonseed hulls. It can be released in a mixture of sugars by simple acid hydrolysis or by application of steam and pressure. It is also present in significant quantities in the black liquor (*e.g.* sulphite liquor) from the acid bleaching in paper manufacture. Where bleaching depends on alkali then the sugars are probably destroyed and absent from the black liquor. Unfortunately the latter process is the one mostly used in developing countries.

Methodology for protection of proteins must be a priority research area in countries where the proteins in the available meals are highly soluble; for example, where unprocessed oil seed cakes, seeds such as lupins or pressure extracted oil seed cakes, forages or tree forages are available. The application of heat also removes anti-quality factors and, therefore, broadens the potential protein feed base. Extrusion systems appear to be a potential manufacturing systems for the future.

Use of Protein Banks to Provide a Source of Bypass Protein

The concept of the 'protein bank' which is used strategically for supplementing grazing cattle when the pastures are dry and have low protein content, is an important development in some countries where extensive rangelands are an important source of animal products. These protein banks provide a ready source of nitrogen and minerals for the rumen organisms and the animal. The strategy involves the development of an area of land, within a range land, with a protein crop which is a legume and to feed or graze this strategically with ruminants in the dry season.

Small inputs of legumes into a diet of low quality pasture are undoubtedly beneficial, providing minerals and nitrogen for the rumen organisms and also stimulating digestibility of the lower quality feed that is the bulk of the diet. However, it is unlikely that such supplements alter the P/E ratio other than through its direct effect on the rumen environment and therefore is only equal in value to a molasses/urea block. A much more effective use of such protein banks would be made by harvesting and protecting the protein and possibly developing alternative sources of NPN, such as molasses/urea blocks to feed along with this protein. A legume with tannins may on the other hand provide substantial bypass proteins and a molasses/urea block would then be extremely complementary.

Protein banks can be forage legumes, tree leaves, seeds or seed pods of crops, forages or trees (*e.g. Enterolobium, Prosopis* and *Leucaena*) or any other source of leaf protein. There is a need to develop appropriate technologies to capitalising on such protein sources in those countries where proteins are expensive or unavailable. It may be necessary to commence with plant and agronomic studies to find suitable plants and to develop the correct method of harvest, followed by techniques to protect the protein.

Potential of Trees as a Source of Bypass Protein

The potential of tree leaves, tree seeds and pods or seeds has been vastly underestimated. For example mature trees of *Prosopis juliflora* have been shown to produce 400–600 kg pods/tree/year in the rainfall areas of 400 mm annually (range 200–600 mm) (F. Riveros *pers. comm.*) with 16–20% crude protein. Many rangelands in the semi-arid areas produce less than 2,500 kg/annum of pasture biomass of which only 200–400 kg is harvested by cattle. A few trees per acre therefore will have little effects on the available pasture biomass but a huge effect on available biomass and will also supply a soluble N source and provide the option of producing bypass protein meal.

Trees cultivated for protein sources have a huge potential in the range lands. The case for growing *Prosopis* spp. is obvious and has been put.

The step missing is to marry the approach with the recent advances in protein nutrition of ruminants and to develop:

- Harvesting techniques for pods/seeds.
- Technologies for drying grinding and protecting the protein (if necessary)
- Techniques to concentrate the protein and protect it
- Methods to market the feeds
- Research to demonstrate the response of cattle to using such feeds.

There are a large number of trees that have potentially similar attributes, however, in the semi arid zone the use of *Prosopis* to provide protein is a major opportunity. Fractionation of the pod to produce a high protein component would be a useful first step prior to developing a protection technology. It should be noted that in many areas *Prosopis* is regarded as a potentially dangerous weed. In these areas it must not be grazed when pods are falling because of the spread of seeds through the faeces of cattle which may result in its establishment and spread to extensive areas. However, this is rather easily managed in plantation culture.

Possibilities of Using Plant Biotechnology

Plant biotechnology may be very important to the use of trees as forage components, as there is considerable variability in seed production among trees, cloning and plant tissue culture of seedlings from high yielding varieties could be a considerable advance. However, similar attempts with coconuts and palm oil have resulted in poor or no inflorescence in plants produced by tissue culture and therefore some caution is needed. *Prosopis* spp. are only given as an example here and there are many other under-developed potential sources of protein for the purpose discussed. The potential of developing legumes with tannins at appropriate levels is a worthwhile objective as Barry and his colleagues have demonstrated that *Lotus* sp with 3–6% tannins apparently have greater bypass protein in the leaf than similar species without tannins. This has potential application within the legume bank concept. Again the problem may be met in gene expression since too much or too little tannins are both disadvantageous. The level of tannin is often directly related to the soil type and rainfall.

MAXIMISING DIGESTIBILITY OF FIBROUS FEEDS

Supplementation

A deficiency of any nutrient in the rumen must first affect the rumen ecosystem by reducing microbial growth efficiency which, as the deficiency becomes more acute, will eventually reduce microbial pool size and inevitably digestibility and intake of roughage by ruminants, Decreased digestibility will only be seen with time as the deficiency of the nutrient becomes progressively greater. Supplementation of a critically deficient animal with nutrients for the rumen will increase microbial growth efficiency, microbial pool size and digestibility of forage which will almost always increase feed intake. The feed intake effect, however, often depends on the degree to which the limiting nutrient is deficient. The most likely deficient nutrients, are non-protein nitrogen, P, S, Mg, Na and also trace elements such as Co, Cu, and Zn. Supplementation with multi nutrients of the type listed above is generally successful in increasing intake and digestibility but the large increases in productivity can be anticipated from combining such supplements with a source of bypass protein.

Sources of Mineral Nutrients and Molasses Urea Blocks

One of the best sources of multiple trace minerals in developing countries is a concentrated plant juice, such as molasses or palm oil sludge. Multi-nutrient blocks are no better than the mixtures of materials from which they are made. Blocks are useful because they form a package readily handled, marketed and used by the farmer with little impact on the time he has for other activities. The major problem with these multi-nutrient blocks occurs in the grasslands where there is a need for appropriate means of encouraging stock to consume them in sufficient amounts. In these areas molasses is often unavailable or is too expensive. More research is needed to produce suitable packages (*e.g.* blocks without molasses) for such localities.

The importance of block supplementation relates more to the access it allows to livestock managed by small farmers. It may be possible in the future to apply innovations through inclusions in the blocks of chemicals and other materials that will manipulate the rumen (*e.g.* antiprotozoal chemicals) and manipulate the animal (*e.g.* protected chemicals that are absorbed from the intestines) or even control disease and parasitism (anthelminthics). In this respect the production and testing of blocks incorporating anthelminthic is appropriate and being undertaken already by the Commomwealth Scientific and Industrial Organization in co-operation with the Australian Centre for International Agricultural Research (ACIAR).

Improving the Enzymatic Ability of Rumen Microbes to Degrade Fibre

This is an area that has received emphasis and has aroused considerable expectations. The concept is simple, if rumen microbes can be developed with greater abilities to degrade fibre, or its components, the microbes will be able to extract a greater amount of the available nutrients from the feed consumed.

This often receives a high priority because of the concept that animals fed low quality pastures are primarily energy deficient. In fact, these animals more often are inefficiently using the available nutrients. It must be stressed that the application of balanced nutrition is the first priority and if other perturbations of the system are to succeed an animal must have an efficient rumen and also metabolism. However, in an animal fed a roughage diet, with an efficient rumen and balanced for protein, it is possible that for every 5 units increase in digestibility of the basal roughage resource, there will be 50% increases in liveweight gain on the same basal feed resource. Silva and Ørskov demonstrated that the extent of breakdown of a fibrous feed was dependent on the rumen medium. Untreated ground straw placed in nylon bags, in the rumen of sheep fed ammoniated straw, was fermented to a greater extent than the same untreated ground straw placed in the rumen of sheep fed untreated straw. This difference might be due to a higher concentration of enzymes in the rumen of sheep fed ammoniated compared to untreated straw.

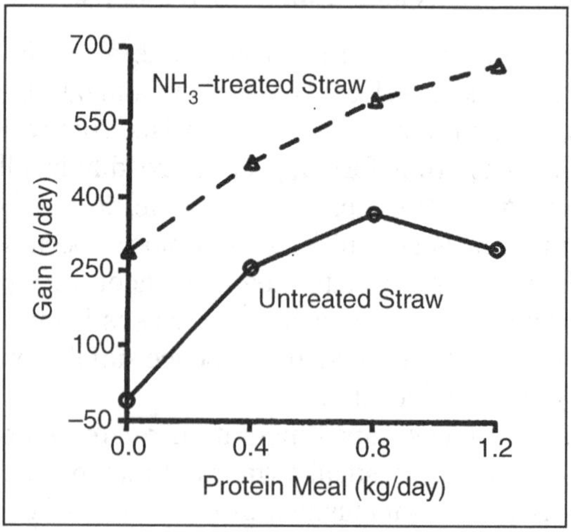

Fig. Growth Response to Different Levels of Protein Meal Supplementation of Cattle given Ammoniated (NH_3-Treated Straw) or Untreated Rice Straw (Untreated Straw)

The two observations discussed above when combined indicate the great potential for improvements in productivity from a successful establishment of a super bug in the rumen, *i.e.* a micro-organism engineered to produce more, or a greater variety, of enzymes for fibre digestion.

Potential Targets for Improving Fibre Digestion

There are potentially three ways to enhance the ability of rumen microbes to degrade fibrous feeds:

1. Selection of microbes, particularly with a high fibrolytic enzyme secretion or that secrete fibrolytic enzymes of high specific activity
2. Creation of microbes with greater spectrum of enzyme secretions by recombinant dna means, *e.g.* Create cellulolytic capacities in xylolytic organisms and vice versa
3. Create microbes with enhanced fibrolytic activity by recombinant DNA means.

In all cases, the prerequisite will be that the organisms are able to grow in and maintain their space in the rumen. These same prerequisites also apply to the production by genetic engineering techniques of high biological value proteins, other secretions of proteins, amino acids and peptides by rumen organisms (see earlier discussion).

State of the Art in Bioengineering of Rumen Organisms

There are number of well established ways of going about incorporating DNA encoding for specific enzymes into anaerobic bacteria by recombinant DNA technologies. Progress has been relatively swift, with at least 4 groups having now achieved transformation of rumen microbes with foreign DNA. Virtually all transformations have been achieved with plasmid constructs and through electroporation methods. None of the engineered organisms have been reintroduced into the rumen to test their stability and in only one case was the engineered organism a recent isolate from the rumen. The approach of using laboratory strains of rumen organisms which have definitely changed in culture clearly demonstrates that the research is at the basic level in which the transformation was the major object and not the improved digestibility that might result.

A major constraint has been the lack of suitable monitoring systems for identifying the engineered organism within the milieu of the rumen. DNA probes are not proving very appropriate because of the genetic diversity of bacterial strains within a species. The above discussion is intended to emphasise that their is a great need for considerable basic research before modified organisms that could survive in the rumen is developed. It should also emphasise the long time lag that is likely from the beginning, where virtually no information was available to application.

Selection of Anaerobic Fungi for Better Fibre Degradation in the Rumen

Filamentous structures of the rumen anaerobic fungi penetrate and substantially weaken the xylem cell walls of forages in the rumen, whereas the bacteria do not adhere to, nor degrade these highly resistant plant tissues to any significant extent. Rumen fungi, but not bacteria, penetrate the cuticle barrier that protects the leaf's surface. Research indicates that these fungi have unique enzymes, or enzymes with higher specific activities, that give them the ability to weaken and degrade the most limiting structural barriers to degradation.

On the basis of these observations it appears that research aimed at promoting the biomass of fungi in the rumen or the establishment of highly active rumen fungi (*e.g.* by selection) could be a major step forward in increasing the digestibility of poor quality forages by ruminants. The identification of strains of anaerobic fungi that most rapidly degrade the cell walls of forage plants is a necessary prerequisite to the successful inoculation of fungi into the rumen and which will nutritionally benefit the host.

Culture, selection of strains and the identification of new species of anaerobic fungi, testing of their ability to weaken plant fibre and improve the rate of digestion are worthwhile research areas for development. The developing countries may be well placed to initiate and develop this research as they have access to animals under extreme dietary conditions that have been adapted over long periods of time and therefore could have already selected fungi for high fibrolytic activity.

The research must include developments which allow selected strains to multiply in the rumen and to prevent the competition from wild strains. As rumen fungi are spread by resistant spores which are passed in faeces and then, when taken in by the animal in feed, multiply by sporulation in the rumen, the support of specific species to ensure the survival is a research area with a high priority. The selection criteria will include the measurement of the rate of solubilisation of fibrous carbohydrates by selected fungi and the weakening of the forage stems following a period of incubation with the forages.

Selection of Bacteria for Fibrolytic Activity

Selection of bacterial strains for improved cellulolytic activity appears to be less vital as it is the fungi that are relatively more important in the breakdown of the most resistant components of the forages, particularly the low quality forages.

Solubilisation of Lignin

Lignin is found within the cell walls of forage plants where it is closely associated with hemicellulose, forming a matrix surrounding the orderly cellulose microfibrils. Lignin is also found in high concentrations in the middle lamella between fibres where it functions as a binder for contiguous cells. Polymeric lignins are not degraded by any known anaerobic organisms. The aerobic white rot fungi *Basidiomycetes* degrade lignin more rapidly and extensively than any other studied microbial group. It is generally accepted that the delignification of a ligno-cellulose material will increase the rate of attack upon the cellulose/hemicellulose compounds when this enters the rumen.

Under aerobic conditions there are two mechanisms of biological delignification:

1. Mineralisation, with lignin being converted directly to carbon dioxide
2. Solubilisation when lignin is released (solubilised) from ligno-cellulose with a variable amount of hemicellulose material attached.

Solubilisation of lignins of grasses is particularly important for its degradation in soils. Something similar to solubilisation seems to occur in the rumen, as considerable lignin appears to be precipitated in the abomasum and therefore, is soluble in the rumen fluid (this is often referred to as acid-precipitatable polymeric lignin (APPL)). The enzymes for solubilisation of lignin, if present in rumen organisms, may be capable of being boosted by genetic means or by selection. In the event that they are not present in rumen organisms, the potential for inducing lignin-solubilising enzymes becomes a major possibility for improving digestibility of fibre in the anaerobic ecosystem of the rumen.

Detoxification of Anti-microbial, Toxic and Antiquality Factors in Plants

Plants in order to survive insect, fungal and bacterial attack, have developed secondary compounds which detract from these organisms colonising the leaf tissues. Some shrubs and trees respond to leaf damage as occurs by grazing and produce greater quantities of secondary compounds which often make them inedible. Recently it has been shown that the grazing of an Acacia tree caused it to release ethylene which within minutes, caused the adjacent acacias in the group to commence synthesising tannins which then caused the grazing deer to cease consumption of the leaves of these trees.

Many secondary plant compounds are toxic to the rumen microbes or directly or indirectly toxic to the animal following microbial metabolism in the rumen. This restricts the feed base of ruminants and, at times, prevents stocking of land. Goats and probably other grazing ruminants are able to detoxify many of these secondary plant compounds in the liver.

DEVELOPING DETOXIFICATION MECHANISMS IN RUMEN ORGANISMS

Research into the possibility of detoxification of secondary plant compounds was given impetus by the discovery that organisms in the rumen of goats in Hawaii that was able to degrade the breakdown product of mimosine (*i.e.* dihydroxypyridine) in *Leucaena leucocephala,* but ruminants in Australia were unable to do so as they had lost the specific rumen microbe with the necessary enzymes. The microbe isolated from the rumen of the Hawaiian goats degraded dihydroxy-pyridine, the toxic breakdown product of mimosine. Introduction of the microbe from goats in

Hawaii into ruminants in Australia prevented the symptoms of mimosine toxicity in previously susceptible ruminant livestock. This has raised the possibility of genetically engineering into rumen organisms the ability to degrade such toxic compounds. Research at the University of New England is in progress to attempt to introduce genes into bacteria for defluorination of fluoroacetate, a lethal compound present in *Acacia gidyea,* which often kills cattle in northern Australia when consumed in the dry season.

The successful transformation of rumen bacteria with a single gene for defluorination of fluoroacetate would indicate the possibility of the utilization of a range of other plants, which may be weeds (*e.g.* lantana), or potential high biomass producers (some legumes and legume trees) and also high protein crops (*e.g.* canavalia).

The problems are universally the same. The first is identification of bacterial DNA encoding for the suitable enzyme followed by development of methods to introduce this into an appropriate bacteria, stabilisation of the DNA in the cell and the last problem is whether the modified organisms will survive in the rumen and be capable of expressing the gene. The major research area would be in finding, isolating and packaging the DNA for the appropriate enzymes which must be capable of expression of being switched on easily and function in an organisms in the rumen ecosystem.

There is a danger in developing the ability of ruminants to degrade toxic compounds, in that often these are the last defence of plants being eaten and in the arid areas could lead to deforestation and soil erosion.

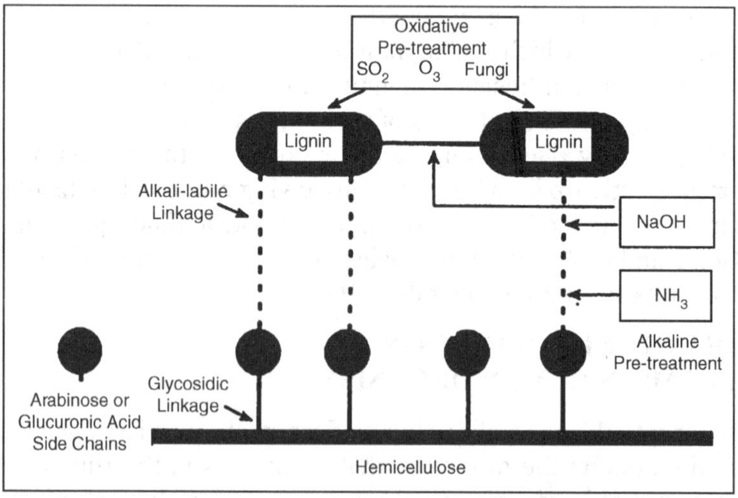

Fig. Sites of Action of Chemicals that, when Added to Straw, Improve its Digestibility

TREATMENT TO INCREASE DIGESTIBILITY

Improving the Digestibility of Crop Residues by Chemical Treatments

There are a number of acid and alkaline hydrolytic processes that will solubilise lignin, cause disruption of fibre by swelling or improve the potential digestibility of fibrous roughages in other ways. It seems that there is adequate information available on the technology of treatment and on the benefits of treatment of low quality forages.

There is therefore little stimulus in pursing research of the methods. A new and novel approach will at times, however, require research but at present it can be safely assumed that alkaline hydrolysis of wet straw by ammonia generated by urea (usually 4% of the dry matter) by microbes in the straw, is probably the most feasible treatment for application in developing countries. The use of anhydrous ammonia application is also potentially applicable.

The ammonia in the straw has two effects:

1. It improves the fermentability of the straw in the rumen by breaking some of the ligno-hemicellulose bonds and
2. It provides non-protein-nitrogen for growth of microbes in the rumen when the forage is consumed.

Although urea ensiling of straw can be economic and effective the technology has not been widely taken up by small farmers in developing countries in general, although there are a few reports of individual farmers regularly using the technology.

It is necessary for researchers to understand the reasons for non-acceptance of such technology which is almost always associated with a slow return on funds expended and sociologic constraints.

Microbial Treatment of Straw and Other Crop Residues to Improve Digestibility

In recent years considerable emphasis has been placed on the improvement of fibrous crops by the strategy of growing non-toxic fungi on the straw. In particular, the white rot fungi have been used because of their ability to delignify the plant material.

The major problem that has arisen is that the technology, although relatively simple, is more complex than that of urea treatment of roughages and although protein is produced and digestibility of the residue increased, a considerable proportion of the total biomass is lost, particularly when white rot fungi is allowed to proceed to the mushroom formation stage.

To some extent the loss of biomass can be prevented by a reduction in the incubation time of the straw and forages, such that biomass losses are reduced to less than 10%. Dr. B.N. Gupta and his colleagues at the National Dairy Research Institute (NDRI) in Karnal, India have developed a two stage process using an altophilic fungus (*Coprinus fimetorius*).

The technology is two-stage and relies on:

1. Alkali treatment (urea ensiling)
2. A second incubation period where a fungi is cultivated on the straw.

The technology is relatively simple, although the two stages make it more complex than the urea treatment alone for application by the small farmers. Both chemical and microbiological treatments may, however, be very effective where large amounts of feed must be stored and moved to areas where forages are scarce because of drought. However, again caution is needed in that to obtain maximum benefits from such feed, cattle will require supplements of bypass protein.

Potential for Increasing the Digestibility of Poor Quality Roughage by Manipulating the Digestive Physiology of the Animal

Goats compared with sheep, and buffalo compared to cattle, tend to retain fibrous materials in the rumen for longer periods and extract a few more units of digestibility at the same time. Within these comparisons, goats and buffaloes recycle a higher amount of urea-N back to the rumen. In the same way, *Bos indicus* cattle recycle more urea-N back to the rumen that *Bos taurus* cattle. Mechanisms that slow rumen turnover, increase rumen volume and allow greater recycling of urea-N may therefore improve the utilisation of poor quality forages. Immunisation against somatotropin release inhibiting factor (SRIF) has recently been demonstrated to increase flow rate through the gut, leading to increased digestibility and greater availability of protein to sheep on concentrate/forage diets. The effects of immunisation against SRIF on cattle on forage/bypass protein diets would be extremely interesting. However, the technology will not be easily applied to village farmers because of the numbers of injections required at the present time to effect immunity.

ALTERING THE PARTITIONING OF NUTRIENTS WITHIN THE ANIMAL

A whole range of injectable compounds will lead to more efficient utilisation of nutrients by livestock. In particular, repartitioning of nutrients into lean meat production or into milk production. These include anabolic steroids, growth hormone, and other hormonal growth factors, beta agonists and techniques such as the suppression of hormones by immunisation. These compounds in general, act through manipulation of hormone status and they lead to improved lean meat in the carcass and a greater efficiency of feed conversion into product. For a recent review of this area, the reader is referred to the publication by Buttery and Dawson.

Anabolic Steroids

Natural sex steroids are used to promote growth and reduce the fat/protein ratio in meat in many countries of the world but their use has been recently banned in Europe. The injected hormone alters the influences of endogenously secreted hormones (oestradiol injections into cattle usually lift growth hormone levels in blood) and growth hormone is more tightly bound to sites in the liver. As is usually the case there is a marked interaction with nutrition and on imbalanced diets in general the effect of exogenous hormones is less obvious than for instance when a diet of silage is balanced by a bypass protein (fish meal). Again this stresses the differences and therefore the need for a new approach to biotechnology in developing countries where ruminant diets are usually low in true protein.

Growth Hormone

Recent developments in fermentation technology together with recombinant DNA technologies have made it possible to produce large quantities of peptide proteins which appear to be the same as bovine or porcine growth hormone (BSt. or PSt.). These growth hormone injected into animals stimulates growth and dramatically decreases fat content of the animals carcass. They also stimulate milk production by some 20–25% in dairy animals.

In the initial studies with growth hormone injections milk production increases appeared to result from repartitioning nutrients and mobilisation of nutrients from tissue deposits in recent times a long term feed-intake effect has been reported.

In addition the stimulation of milk production was dependent on the level of management and was not apparent in herds with poor management. In Italy and India in well managed buffaloes, milk yield has been increased by exogenous growth hormone by up to 25% but the cost of the injections may limit this application.

β-Agonists

β-agonists given by mouth, increase lean meat deposition and reduce fat content of the carcass in pigs and ruminants but with only small increases in liveweight gain. Again it is more than likely that the responses are dependent on the nutrition of the animal.

Injected Growth Promotants Versus Supplementation to Balance Nutrition

There are strong similarities between the response observed to growth hormone/β-agonists etc. and the response to correcting the P/E ratio in nutrients absorbed. At least one paper reports an interaction of bypass protein and response to exogenous hormones. It is thus possible that the optimisation of P/E ratio in the nutrients absorbed elicits responses in hormonal release that mimic the injection of growth hormone etc. Conversely and if true, this means that effects of exogenous hormones may not be so obvious where the P/E ratio in nutrients absorbed is optimised. In addition the requirements for protein relative to energy in the transgenic animals expressing growth hormone will be much increased as will requirements for minerals and vitamins.

The important conclusion from the paper by Buttery and Dawson is that: "the current technology has given many exciting possibilities but there are, however, still major gaps in the knowledge of the major metabolic control processes associated with growth which will have to be filled before a universally accepted method of growth promotion is developed" This is a reservation which is repeatedly used by biotechnologists and indicates that there will be an ongoing requirement for basic research at the level of metabolic control.

CROSS BREEDING TO IMPROVE PARTITIONING OF NUTRIENTS INTO MILK

Many scientists believe that selection among individual breeds for milk production is too slow to produce the highly significant increases in milk production needed to meet increasing population growth and demand in developing countries. Cross breeding of native animals with temperate-country high yielding dairy cows is universally accepted as the way forward. The high yielding dairy cow is considered to have the ability to partition nutrients more efficiently into milk then the indigenous animals. The concept is accurate when management is optimum, nutrition balanced and the feed of high digestibility. To obtain effective milk production from cattle in the tropics it is highly essential to control disease and supplement the poor quality forage to balance nutrition otherwise, a low reproduction rate, coupled with a high death rate, often eliminates the advantages of cross-breeding.

Recent experiences in India, however, suggests that this is not necessarily the scenario of crossbreeding. Case Study (India). The milk yield of imported Friesians at The NDDB station in Anand, in India, is an outstanding example of the potential improvements in milk that can result when a package of technologies are applied. These cows are kept under institutional conditions, disease is under control and they are fed fresh forage (up to 40 kg daily), supplemented with maize silage and rice straw in the dry season and given 350 g of a bypass protein concentrate (30% CP) for each litre of milk produced. Average yields of first lactation heifers were above 5,000 litres/305 days with exceptional animals achieving 6,500. The animals are all in their second lactation now, with indications of an average milk yield in excess of 6,000 litres.

This level of production has been achieved by using molasses urea blocks and a bypass protein feed supplements. The only grain concentrate, representing 10% of the bypass protein mixture, is used for manufacturing purposes to provide a good pellet composition. This example is given here because it indicates that even in the most difficult climates in Asia, where temperatures often exceed 40°C, and reach 50°C at times, Friesians can produce to at least T! of their genetic capacity. It also indicates a very important concept that must be emphasised in this report; genetic improvement is not a panacea for livestock improvement in developing countries and improvement from breeding programmes will only be successful when nutritional and disease management is optimised.

TRANSGENESIS AND EMBRYO MANIPULATION

Although embryo transfer has little importance in nutritional manipulation, it is a required technology as a forerunner to the production of transgenic animals. The development of techniques to isolate, manipulate and transfer 'defined' pieces of DNA into early embryos removes the potential barrier for the movement of genetic information between totally different living organisms. For example, DNA encoding for enzymes normally produced by bacteria may be inserted into the genome of an animal and it may be expected to express the generation of the enzymes in the animal after birth.

The technology consists of the digestion and legation of appropriate sources of DNA with specific enzymes to accurately define and rearrange particular DNA fragments, the molecular cloning of these fragments into bacteria and phages or as plasmids, the nucleotide sequencing of cloned DNA and the technology to transfer the cloned DNA into cultured cells and early embryos.

Transgenesis research is largely aimed at developing new genomes (the total complement of genes in the animal) beyond the scope of the random assortment of genes during sexual reproduction, augmented by mutation, which is restricted by the available genetic variation and species boundaries. Furthermore, individuals selected for breeding often transmit some of its undesirable genes to its offspring. Transgenesis, which brings together the technologies of recombinant DNA, embryo manipulation and embryo transfer offers extra opportunities in the elaboration of new genomes.

The boundaries of potentially useful developments of new genomes in animals are only limited by the imagination of the researcher and the definition, isolation and packaging of the DNA with suitable methods for insertion into the early embryo. An example of the highly imaginative approach is the introduction of genes for the synthesis of S-amino acids into sheep, but again although transgenic animals have been produced they have not increased wool growth and expression of the genes is the most important problem facing such research.

Most emphasis, to date, has been on developing the technology and introduction of DNA for the expression of growth hormone. This has been successful in a wide variety of animals. In a recent review of these developments, however, Dr. C. Polge (1990, *pers. comm.*) concluded that the major problem for research into transgenesis is the inability to control the level of expression of a particular gene together with a very low success rate in achieving transgenesis and a low success in expression of the gene. The general conclusions are that a return to the study of the factors that allow or control expression of genes is needed before any potential development can be made.

This must be considered in any allocation of funds for this particular development. *Archibald (1989) recently concluded an article on transgenesis by the following statement*: "Transgenesis offers new opportunities to make new genomes. In the short term, transgenic animals are more likely to increase the understanding of the genetic control of performance than they are to make a contribution to agricultural production." This clearly indicates that at the present time research aimed at developing new genomes in bacteria, other organisms or animals should be clearly oriented to advancing fundamental knowledge. This is not to deny that these may have some practical application in the future but the future could be 50–100 years hence.

8

Nutrition and Metabolism of Animals

ANIMAL NUTRITION

The developing countries, in general, have severe constraints on food availability for humans and are often critically balanced in producing sufficient starch-based carbohydrates and high quality proteins to provide for their human population. Thus, the grains produced are generally required for the resident population, which is often increasing at a rate several times that of the populations of the industrialised countries. Short term food surpluses due to good seasonal growing conditions and/or application of plant/soil research results, will inevitably be converted to deficits by the growing population's demand for food.

The only exception to this will be if birth rate is reduced and death rate accelerated in these countries. The impact of the presently untreatable viral disease HIV (or AIDS) will be significant in this area but no predictions are yet available on its effects on future population densities in developing countries.

The likely small surpluses of grains over and above that needed by humans indicates that the production of monogastric animals which compete with humans for the basic feed resources (grain) must have good political and or trade advantages before it can be encouraged. However, production of monogastric animals on sugar based products and various by-products may be a future direction for considerable research effort. There is, of course, a middle class in all developing countries which demands meat from poultry and pigs and can afford to pay the relatively high costs of production. This group of people is expanding in the countries that are rapidly industrialising, and this together with the influx of tourists in such countries will increase demand for these products.

There is a high correlation between meat consumed and cash income or standard of living. The husbandry of monogastric animals is already at a very high level and, in general, research on grain-fed domestic animals is probably best left to the industrialised countries where surplus grains are generally available and their production is subsidised (*e.g.* approximately 40% of the value of grain production throughout the EEC and USA is met by subsidies). In most developing countries pig and poultry production is either based on a scavenger system, (which is restricted to village farmers), or a high cost technology system as used, and transferred from, temperate countries (which is used by the large farmer).

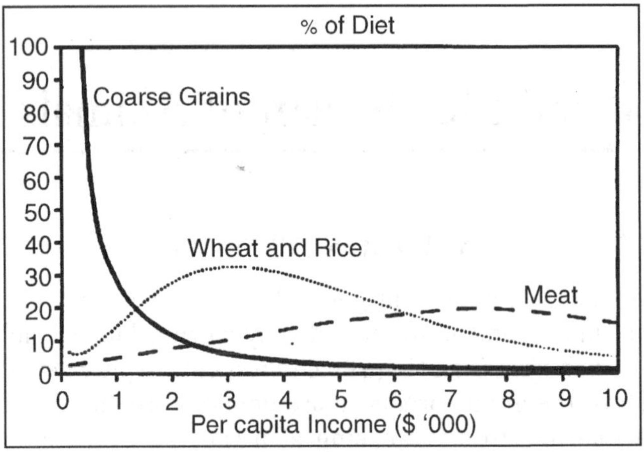

Fig. Food Consumption/percentage of Diet for Meat, Wheat and Rice, and Coarse grains as *Per capita* Income Increases.

Monogastric nutrition cannot be omitted from consideration, however, as the appropriate integration of monogastric animals with ruminants in cropping areas is potentially the most efficient systems that might be (or are being) developed to increase animal production overall. Within these systems the production of pig and chicken meats from non-conventional feed sources (*e.g.* sugar cane, molasses, household swill, tubers, roots and by-products) integrated with such systems as protein production from aquatic plants should be the major consideration in the future.

The ruminant animal, because it has pre-gastric fermentative digestion of feed, generally does not compete with humans for vital quality-feed resources and must therefore have the focus of the discussions. Ruminant animals (biomass) in developing countries far outnumber all other domestic animal not only as a source of high quality human food (meat and milk, with blood in some areas), but of fuel (from dung) and draught power.

The continuing use of ruminants as domestic animals resides in their ability to:

- Convert fibrous carbohydrates through fermentative digestion, into nutrients that can be used for growth, and milk synthesis
- Efficiently utilise low protein feeds and non-protein nitrogen in the rumen and synthesise proteins with a high biological value for human consumption
- Convert the carbohydrates of fibrous feeds into nutrients that can be used to carry out work-functions (*e.g.* Ploughing)

- More efficiently use dietary protein for tissue synthesis than monogastric animals provided it is in a form protected from microbial attack in the rumen but digestible by gastric and intestinal enzymes.

Any biotechnology developments will undoubtedly have to target the improvement of efficiency of these attributes under practical conditions pertaining particularly to the small farmer.

There are five major ways by which any technology may significantly improve livestock production:

- By altering the feed base to provide a better quantity and balance of nutrients to the animal
- By altering the digestibility of the feed base by treatment so that more nutrients are extracted.
- By manipulating the fermentative, gastric and post-gastric digestive processes to extract more and a better balance of nutrients for the animal from the basal feed.
- By manipulating the efficiency of partitioning of absorbed nutrients into productive processes including those that are involved in life-time productivity
- By removing or ameliorating constraints that are part of the environment (largely disease, but also the effects of temperature and humidity stress)

Strategies for the future use of animals for work and food production cannot ignore the growing environmental crisis and the need to reduce gaseous emissions from farming systems.

DEFINITION OF BIOTECHNOLOGY OR HIGH TECHNOLOGY

Biotechnology is a much used "in word" in research submissions since it conjures up images of research at the cutting edge of science. It also has an overtone of application, potentially patentable products or processes and therefore returns on investment. The promises have been much overrated in recent times and in general the promises for application from, for instance, recombinant DNA technology have failed to materialise in terms of animal production. In general, the results of recombinant DNA technology have been disappointing. For example transgenic animals have been produced but failure to control expression of the introduced genes has resulted in adverse effects often of a nature that horrifies animal welfare groups. This has been given 'bad press' but it has highlighted the need to study the basic aspects of control of gene expression and cell physiology.

This does not mean however, that the future for and importance of such work is debatable. In fact, the contrary is true, but it has indicated a major requirement for basic research to understand gene expression and that more time and funds will be needed before many new concepts can be applied. Biotechnology in the context of this report cannot be restricted to recombinant

DNA technology. Biotechnology is in reality, a science of great antiquity having its origins in processes such as brewing and wine making.

The Broad Definition Used here is the Application of Biological Organisms, Systems or Processes to Production of Animal Products

These include meat, milk, hides, wool or hair and draught power. In particular, biotechnology stresses the integration of microbiology, biochemistry and chemical and process engineering. It is always multi-disciplinary, and its strongest aspect is that it is directed to application. It usually requires disciplinary scientists working together and shepherded by person(s) with major integrative abilities. Young scientists (or disciplinarians) caught up in biotechnology and working in isolation often lose the direction for application or seek out compromise objectives to justify their approach which may or may not be rational.

On the tour of institutions prior to the writing of this report, it was an observation that a number of young, newly trained (overseas) scientists in the less well developed countries, were still working in the area of their overseas training without true recognition of the potential application of their work. They were, thus, in some ways competing with their previous supervisors and are therefore unlikely to produce novel innovations. For the purposes of this report biotechnology research is regarded as a multi-level activity.

In animal nutrition this includes research that aims to improve the efficiency of production through manipulation of:

- The feed base
- The animal's digestive system
- The animal's metabolism

It must also consider the potential for augmenting the feed base with critically deficient nutrients that may be produced locally, particularly from non-conventional sources (*e.g*. production of protein meals from aquatic plants (algae) grown on biodigestor effluent). It must also consider the possibility of decreasing protein fermentability of plants consumed by ruminants by genetic engineering of plants and other techniques applied to the plant, the microbial digestion system and the animal. The narrower definition will be referred to here as the new biotechnology. This is defined as the application of recombinant DNA technology to the improvement of animal production through improving nutrition.

THE PROMISE OF THE NEW BIOTECHNOLOGY

The beginning of recombinant DNA technology arose from the work of Crick and Watson and their colleagues at Cambridge. Research in this area is often seen as being superior to other forms of biological research. However, like all research it is often the acquisition of technology and instrumentation which triggers development or progress in this field. Example of developments which allowed many groups to begin or progress in their work include the development of techniques to split the ovum, to introduce foreign DNA into chromosomal DNA or to force a plasmid into a cell where it will replicate along with other DNA. This is not meant to be a criticism of modern biotechnology research but it is stated to point out that the new biotechnology is supported by a large group of 'normal scientists' led largely by a few highly capable and creative persons in the same way as every other field of research endeavour. The concept of the new biotechnology as a science for the gifted and the imaginative promises of biotechnology put forward in most reviews, have undermined many other fields of research which have then suffered from financial stringencies. These fields often regain prominence when, for example, innovative gene transfer methodology has failed to produce the expected applied technology (*e.g.* higher productivity in domestic animals expressing genes for growth hormone). In this case there has been little recognition of nutritional principles; an animal capable of growing say to twice the size and at twice the rate because of the acquisition of a gene for growth hormone may need a totally new nutritional approach. For example, in order to provide for growth and normal bone growth in such animals it will be perhaps necessary to provide more calcium and phosphorus in forms more easily absorbed and assimilated; protein to energy ratios in the nutrients absorbed may have to be increased substantially as may be the availability of vitamins and other minerals.

The need is for a suitable balance of research which must be maintained. The new biotechnology needs to advance along with the fundamental and applied research that is needed to ensure that the application of molecular genetic research reaches the end user, in this case the farmer. It is a major theme of this report that it is imperative that research on nutrition must not compete for limited funds with the new biotechnology. It is also a major conclusion that concepts of nutrition transferred from temperate countries have been misleading. Recently developed understanding of nutrition, which has massive effects on productivity, is the area with most promise and with potential immediate application. The great need is for research to find ways of applying these concepts in production systems under differing environmental conditions within countries. With a likely doubling of food requirements of developing countries by the year 2000 the need for research which will result in strategies that can be quickly applied is paramount.

THE TARGET ANIMALS

This dissertation must deal largely with the "economically" (in its broadest sense) important ruminants in developing countries. These are largely cattle, buffaloes, sheep and goats. Other animals that pre-ferment their feed, include camels, alpaca, llama, yak, thimin and certain monkeys as well as certain deer species, and post-gastric fermenters such as the horse, donkey, guinea pig and rabbit must be kept in mind as they are often of major importance in some areas. However, the latter group have not been targeted because of the predominance of ruminant herbivores. Research on the use of non-conventional feeds is given a brief mention but the major research requirements here are to develop the systems which depend on locally available resources and particular within an integrated farming systems concept.

CONDITIONS OF RUMINANTS IN THIRD WORLD COUNTRIES

The reasons for keeping ruminants in developing countries are not always easily understood by the outsider.

They are kept for a number of reasons, which change in priority depending on their location and owners including the following:

- For food (*e.g.* Meat, milk and blood or any of these combinations) and also as a reliable food store for years of drought
- As status symbols of wealth
- As a means of accumulation of wealth to be cashed for a number of purposes (*e.g.* Life threatening events; to meet marriage costs; to provide for pay-back etc.)
- As an edge against inflation
- For fuel (dung for sale or to provide for household cooking)
- For fertilizer production (*e.g.* Dung)
- Drought power
- For religious purposes and/or entertainment (*e.g.* The fighting rams of indonesia)
- Work purposes (ploughing, puddling of soil for rice etc.)
- Transport
- Hides for leather
- As investment by city business men to create a stake in agriculture which is often motivated by the possibility of tax relief
- To make use of poor lands which would not otherwise be used for agricultural purposes.

The desire of the farmer to increase productivity of his animals, is highly dependent on the purpose for keeping the livestock. It is sometimes an advantage to maintain a low level of productivity. For example, if animal numbers are more important than production per animal, it is advantageous to have stunted, thin animals which require low management inputs. In this presentation the target animals are the animals in the herds of small farmers where meat, milk, work, or any combination of these (meat/work, meat/milk, milk/work) are the major objectives as these are the major owners of livestock in developing countries and the target for many of the aid-sponsored projects.

PRODUCTIVITY OF LIVESTOCK IN DEVELOPING COUNTRIES

Few developing countries have surplus tracts of land that can be regarded as fertile and therefore produce high quality fodder.

In general, human population pressures and the primary need to supply human food ensures that livestock are restricted to:

- Poor quality (often overgrazed) pasture lands, either infertile or with terrain that makes them impossible to utilise for crops or where erosion has made them unusable.

Table. Average Meat Production (kg) Per Animal of Total Population of Cattle/ buffaloes in Europe (Representative of the Concentrate/forage Feeding Systems) and in Asia/Pacific (1986)

	Cattle	Buffalo
Europe	68	50
Asia/Pacific	5	7

- Standing crop residues or weeds following cropping when environmental conditions are poor for plant growth and a further crop in that year cannot be taken.
- Crop residues (cut and stored)
- Agro-industrial by-products
- Extensive pastures of poor quality and otherwise sparse (*e.g*. The Llanos of Colombia and Venezuela).

The net result is in general an extremely low rate of productivity with animals often at 5 years of age at maturity and productivity at 0.1–0.25 of that of ruminants in temperate countries grazing fertilised pastures or fed high quality feeds based on grain and immature pasture plants. A comparison of the levels of production of cattle between developed and developing countries is shown in Tables.

Table. Average Carcass Weight (kg) Per Animal Slaughtered (1986 Statistics)

	Cattle	Buffalo
Europe	185	206
Asia/Pacific	120	161

Table. The Change in the Average Milk Yield Per Cow in Industrialised and Third World Countries

Country/Region	Average Yield/Cow (Kg/Year)		Percentage Increase (%)
	1976	1986	(1976 to 1986)
North America	3,250	5,200	60
EEC Countries	2,900	4,100	35
Asia	620	700	13
Africa	322	354	7

THE IMPLICATION OF LOW PRODUCTIVITY

Biotechnology research in industrialised countries is not generally aimed at low yielding animals. In addition to poor nutrition, adverse climate and disease, other stresses are also generally high, particularly in those countries situated in the tropics. These additional constraints are likely to affect and often remove any advantage of biotechnology transferred from developed countries. The considerable differences in feed resources available in developing countries compared to developed countries (where most biotechnology research is presently centered) and the low cost of production systems employed in the developing world as compared with the industrialised world indicates that direct technology transfer is unlikely to be successful.

FEED RESOURCES AVAILABLE TO RUMINANTS

The feeds that are available to ruminants in developing countries are fibrous and relatively high in ligno-cellulose. They are usually of low digestibility and they are often deficient in critical nutrients, including protein, non-protein nitrogen and minerals.

As a generalisation, the forages consumed by ruminants in developing countries are almost always below 55% (usually 40–45%) digestibility and are often less than 8% crude protein and this protein level is more often around 3–5%, *e.g.* cereal straws. The only exception to this is in the early growth phase of pasture and when stocking rates are extremely low and the animals are able to select for leaf material.

The low levels of production per head and per acre of most grazing systems are indicated by the summary of data given by Walker (1987). Without supplements, these low levels of production lead to a highly inefficient use of the available feed, with a possibility that up to 30% of the feed consumed is dissipated as heat.

This heat has at times great effects on feed intake particularly in the tropics. It is necessary, therefore in discussing the nutrition of ruminants, to appreciate the digestion of forage based diets and the constraints to the utilisation of nutrients that arise largely from a fermentative digestion system, since this knowledge must considerably influence research priorities.

CHEMICAL COMPOSITION OF LOW QUALITY FORAGES

In the literature concerned with the nutritional value of forages, considerable emphasis is placed on the crude chemical composition of the forage. Although analyses that indicate cell solubles and cell wall materials are highly useful for studying the fermentative characteristics of a forage, they bear little relationship to its feeding value to the animal.Considerable efforts is often put into feed analysis which is often totally unwarranted particularly in the developing countries. In this report the overriding effects of a balanced nutrient approach to feeding are emphasised. It is suggested that in most production systems for ruminants based on a poor quality forage, it is the balance of those nutrients providing the major building blocks for tissue synthesis and milk production, that should be the primary concern. With most forages and contrary to the assertations in the past that energy deficiency is the primary constraint to ruminant production on low quality feeds, the efficiency of feed utilisation is the major determinant of the production levels achieved. Therefore in reviewing the need for biotechnology research, this is the area for most consideration.

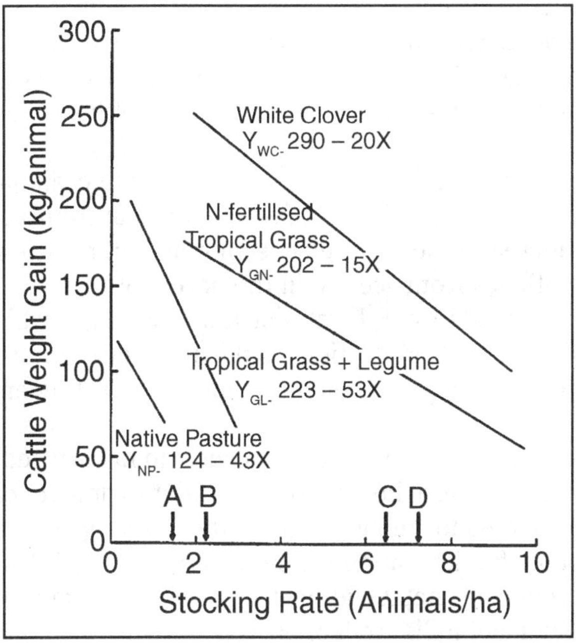

Fig. Cattle Growth on Pasture is a Function of Pasture Type, Fertilizer Applications and Legume Content. Productivity Per Unit Area is Maximised for the Different Pastures at Different Stocking Rates: 89 kg/ha for Native Pastures, 223 kg/ha for Tropical Grass with Legume, 682 kg/ha for Tropical Grass with Fertilizer and on Temperate Pasture (Clover) 105 kg/ha.

Recent evaluation of data from studies in tropical countries has indicated that medium to high levels of production at very high feed conversion efficiencies can be achieved by ruminants on poor quality forages adequately supplemented with critical nutrients.Of more importance is that the efficiency of utilisation of the metabolizable energy of a straw based diet appropriately supplemented can be higher than that of grain based diets. This suggests that the efficiency of utilisation of metabolisable energy of a forage can be markedly improved simply by supplementation (by up to 10 fold). It also discounts theories that the digestible nutrients from such feeds are less efficiently utilised than from grain based diets.

IMPLICATIONS OF AN INCREASED NUTRIENT REQUIREMENTS FOR WORK

Light work requires acetogenic substrate probably acetate for muscle contraction but heavy work is probably dependent on long chain fatty acids mobilised from adipose tissue. All working muscles use some glucose and there is always a concomitant increase in glucose utilisation when free fatty acid metabolism is increased by the work load. Imbalanced diets fed to draught animals which result in a low P/E ratio in the nutrients absorbed are not so disadvantageous as they are for a lactating or growing animal.

The excess acetogenic substrate is used for work removing the necessity to otherwise enzymatically dispose of the substrate. However, the increment in requirements for glucose oxidation in muscles although small could be a limitation.

In addition the need in heavy work to supply long chain fatty acids which can be oxidised to produce ATP at a faster rate than from acetate, indicates that there is an increased need for glucose not only in muscle metabolism but also to aid fat synthesis from acetate in the period of rest.

An imbalanced feed (low P/E ratio or low G/E ratio), which is associated with a high metabolic heat production, could also reduce the recovery of body temperature of draught animals when the animal is resting and, thus, reduce feed intake.

A decreased fat deposition because of such an imbalanced diet during the non working season may also be a major constraint to draught capacity because of lack of body reserves for mobilisation in the working season.The P/E ratio required to support fat deposition (in periods of low work load) or to reduce heat stress by reducing metabolic heat is likely to be much lower than for example for growth and milk production.

A draught animal fed poor quality forage probably requires little more nutrients than can be supplied from an efficiently functioning rumen. This is attained for example by supplying the animal with a molasses/urea multi-nutrient block.

Indian farmers soon found the benefits of molasses/urea block for draught animals when these became available (personal observation) and recently the beneficial effects of feeding molasses/urea blocks to draught buffalo have been demonstrated in Vietnam (T.R. Preston personal communication). The results of Preston's studies in Vietnam are given in Table.

Implications for Areas of Research

This discussion highlights the manipulable aspects of ruminant nutrition, where substantial improvements in productive efficiency of animals fed largely on fibrous feeds could result.

The differences between temperate and tropical conditions also indicate opportunities which are often not apparent in temperate countries and mitigates against direct transfer of results from the former to the latter. In tropical conditions, protein nutrition of ruminants is more crucial than in temperate areas.

Table. Liveweight Change and Work Capacity of Buffaloes given Rice Straw Supplemented with a Urea/molasses Block. There were 22 Animals in the Trial

Observation	Control (no Supplement)	Block
Live weight (kg)		
Dry season (no work)		
Beginning	354	381
After 1 month	346	395
Change	-814	+ 14
Wet season (ploughing)		
Beginning	346	372
After 1 month	334	370
Change	-11.5	-2
Work capacity		
Area ploughed (m^2/day)		
Beginning	1919	2243
After 1 month	1508	2141
Ploughing speed		
(2 buffaloes) (m/min)		
Beginning	36	44
After 1 month	32	41
Recovery time (min)		
Beginning	14	12
After 1 month	16	13

The general conclusions are that:

- The primary constraint to ruminant production from fibrous feeds (in the tropics) is the low efficiency of feed utilisation often coupled with an environmental/physiological effect which results in a reduction in potential feed intake.
- In practice the most effective mechanisms for improving productivity will be to improve the p/e ratio in the nutrients absorbed because of the large effect on efficiency of feed utilisation.
- Draught animals will also benefit from technologies that increase microbial growth efficiency in the rumen and at times improve digestibility, intake and p/e ratio in the nutrient absorbed.
- Contrary to many statements in authoritative reviews, only when p/e ratios have been optimised does the energy density of the feed become a primary constraint.
- As the primary constraint is an inefficiency due to a low p/e ratio in the nutrients absorbed it is unlikely that other inputs [*e.g.* agents to repartition nutrients or to stimulate growth (B-agonists, BSt)] could be successful without first applying strategic supplementation.

THE MINERALS

Mineral elements have a great diversity of uses within the animal body. The following mineral elements are recognized as essential for body functions in fish: calcium, phosphorus, sodium, molybdenum, chlorine, magnesium, iron, selenium, iodine, manganese, copper, cobalt and zinc. To these may be added fluorine and chromium which have also been shown to be essential for land animals.

The prominence of each mineral element in body tissues is closely related to its functional role. As constituents of bones and teeth, minerals provide strength and rigidity to skeletal structures. In their ionic states in body fluids they are indispensable for the maintenance of acid-base equilibrium and osmotic relationship with the aquatic environment, and for integration activities involving the nervous and endocrine systems. As components of blood pigments, enzymes and organic compounds in tissues and organs they are indispensable for essential metabolic processes involving gas exchange and energy transactions.

CALCIUM AND PHOSPHORUS

Distribution

Calcium and phosphorus are usually discussed together because they occur in the body combined with each other for the most part and because an inadequate supply of either limits the nutritive value of both.

Almost the entire store of calcium (99 per cent) and most of the phosphorus (80 per cent) in the fish's body are present in bones, teeth and scales. There appears to be little variation in the composition of bone ash even though bone ash will decrease as a result of dietary deficiency in either calcium or phosphorus. This composition consists of calcium and phosphorus in the ratio of approximately 2:1.

The one per cent extra-skeletal calcium is widely distributed throughout the organs and tissues. Calcium in body fluids exists in two distinguishable forms, diffusable and non-diffusible. Non-diffusible calcium is bound to protein whereas the diffusible fraction is present largely as phosphate and bicarbonate compounds. It is this diffusible fraction that is of significance in calcium and phosphorus nutrition. Ionized calcium in the extracellular fluids and in the circulatory system participate importantly in muscle activity and osmoregulation.

Large amounts of extra-skeletal phosphorus are present mostly in combinations with proteins, lipids, sugars, nucleic acids and other organic compounds. These phosphocompounds are vital exchange currencies in life processes and are distributed throughout the organs and tissues of the fish. The skin, like the skeleton, also appears to be an important repository for dietary phosphorus in some species.

ABSORPTION AND METABOLISM

Although their natural diets are rich in calcium, most fish are also capable of extracting dissolved calcium directly from their aquatic environment through the gills.

After a 24-hour acclimatization period, channel catfish have been shown to efficiently extract calcium from rearing water containing 5 ppm of the mineral element. On the other hand, gill extraction of phosphorus is negligible and fish rely mainly upon dietary sources for this mineral element. Phosphorus present in plant phytate is poorly absorbed by fish.

Absorption of dietary calcium and phosphorus begins in the upper gastro-intestinal tract. Absorbed calcium is rapidly deposited as calcium salts in the skeleton but absorbed phosphorus is distributed to all the major tissues: viscera, skeleton, skin and muscle.

Phosphorus absorption is enhanced by increasing water temperature and by the presence of glucose in the diet. Its recovery from tissues also increases with increasing dietary levels of the element. On the other hand, increasing dietary calcium is not accompanied by correspondingly higher retention of the mineral element in the tissues.

Studies with common carp, Cyprinus carpio, and rainbow trout, Salmo gairdneri, have also shown that the absorption of dietary phosphorus is not affected by calcium in the diet. The level of phosphorus in the diet, however, sets the rate at which calcium is retained in the body.

An increasing level of dietary phosphorus will be accompanied by increasing: retention of both mineral elements in body tissues, thus maintaining the ratio of calcium and phosphorus within narrow limits. In the common carp, whole body Ca/P ratio is about 1.4 except when phosphorus is severely lacking in the diet. Vertebral Ca/P ratio is about 2.0. Fish appear to have an ability to balance Ca/P ratios by controlling the absorption and excretion of calcium for optimal utilization of both mineral elements.

The dietary level of phosphorus for maximum growth in the common carp and the red sea bream, Chrysophrys major,has been shown to be 0.7 per cent. This corresponds well with the level for maximum conversion of the mineral element in the trout.

As stated earlier, most cultured species show efficient gill extraction of calcium from rearing waters although red sea bream fingerlings exhibit better growth with dietary supplementation of calcium.

In general, the nutrition of calcium and phosphorus of both salt and freshwater fish species are very similar. Vitamin D plays an essential role in intestinal calcium absorption in land animals.

A similar role for fish has not been established. The ability of fish to sequester calcium from water through the gill membrane possibly reduces the importance of such a role.

DEFICIENCY SYMPTOMS

Deficiency symptoms of calcium have not been described in fish although poor growth is observed with diets limited in phosphorus (which leads to reduced accretion of calcium by body tissues).

Prolonged feeding of phosphorus-deficient diets to common carps resulted in deformed backs (lordosis) and heads due to abnormal calcification of bone. Bone growth was reduced in the skull and operculum regions. Recent studies with this species and the red sea bream have also shown fatty infiltration of liver and muscle tissues related to dietary phosphorus deficiency.

CALCIUM AND PHOSPHORUS IN FEEDS

Feed ingredients vary widely in their calcium and phosphorus content. Fish meal, a principal ingredient in fish feeds, is rich in both calcium and phosphorus. On the other hand, feed ingredients of plant origin usually lack calcium and, despite a fairly high content of phosphorus the latter is predominantly in the form of phytin or phytic acid which is not readily available for absorption by fish.

Animal sources of calcium and phosphorus are generally better absorbed, although the stomachless carp cannot utilize bone phosphate present in fish meal as well as fish with functional stomachs.

Dicalcium phosphate has the highest availability (80 per cent). Phosphorus availability of common feedstuffs varies from 33 per cent for grains to 50 per cent for fish meal and animal by-products. Soybean meal has an intermediate phosphorus availability of 40 per cent.

MAGNESIUM

Magnesium is closely associated with calcium and phosphorus both in its distribution and its metabolism. The bulk of magnesium in fish (60 per cent in the carp) is stored in the skeleton. Magnesium constitutes a little over 0.6 per cent of the ash content of bones compared with 30 per cent calcium and 15 per cent phosphorus.

The remaining 40 per cent of the body's magnesium is distributed throughout the organs and muscle tissues (where it plays vital roles as enzyme co-factors, and as an important structural component of cell membranes) and in extracellular fluids.

ABSORPTION AND METABOLISM

Fish are capable of extracting magnesium from the environment, although studies with the common carp showed that, in this species, gill extraction of this element is very limited. Due to the comparatively low concentrations of the mineral element in fresh water, non-marine fish appear to depend upon dietary sources to meet their requirement of magnesium.In the common carp, as well as in the rainbow trout, dietary magnesium levels do not affect calcium and phosphorus composition in the whole body or skeleton despite sharp reductions of up to 50 per cent of tissue magnesium when this mineral element was lacking in the diet (80 ppm) and retarded growth and behavioural abnormalities observed.

DEFICIENCY SYMPTOMS

The symptoms of magnesium deficiency in the common carp and rainbow trout are very similar to those described for magnesium deficient land animals: loss of appetite, poor growth, sluggishness and convulsion followed by tetany. Mortality is often high. Histo-logical changes have also been observed in muscle, pyloric caeca and gill filaments of trout fed magnesium-deficient diets.

MAGNESIUM IN FEEDS

Although natural waters are a good source of dissolved magnesium, fish do not extract this mineral element in sufficient quantities to meet dietary needs. Natural foods, as well as most artificial feed ingredients of both animal and vegetable origin, are adequate sources and deficiency under ordinary rearing conditions has not been observed to date.

INORGANIC ELEMENTS

Dietary requirements of fish for most of the trace mineral elements have not been established. Iron deficiency in the red sea bream results in a form of microcytic, hypochromic anaemia similar to iron deficiency anaemia in land animals. Common carp fed a semi-purified diet without supplementary iron grew normally but exhibited sub-clinical symptoms of hypochromic microcytic anaemia.

Iodine deficiency produces a goitrous condition in trout. Rainbow trout fed a semi-purified diet deficient in zinc (1 ppm) had increased mortality rate, cataracts in the eyes and erosion of the fins and of the skin. Protein digestibility was also reduced. Manganese has also been shown to be essential for growth and survival ofTilapia mossambica and the rainbow trout.

The roles of trace elements in fish, although not clearly defined, are probably similar to those described for land animals. Fish in their natural habitats are probably adequately provided for to meet the requirements for all the mineral elements.

However, the intensive culture of certain fish species in man-made ponds and raceways, together with reliance on artificial feeding, make it necessary to incorporate adequate quantities of mineral nutrients in the feed. For the most part, where exact requirements are not known, levels are arbitrarily based on land animal requirements.

Table. Summary of Information on Mineral Requirements

Mineral element	Principal metabolic activities	Requirement symptoms	Requirement/ kg dry diet
Calcium	Bone and cartilage formation; blood clotting; muscle contraction	not defined	5g
Phosphorus	Bone formation; high energy phosphate esters; other organo-phosphorus compounds	Lordosis, poor growth	7g
Magnesium	Enzyme co-factor extensively involved in the metabolism of fats, carbohydrates and proteins	Loss of appetite, poor growth, tetany	500 mg
Sodium	Primary monovalent cation of inter cellular fluid; involved in acid-base balance and osmoreg-ulation	not defined	1-3g
Potassium	Primary monovalent cation of intra-cellular fluid; involved in nerve action and osmoregulation	not defined	1-3g
Sulphur	Integral part of sulphur amino acids and collagen; involved in detoxification of aromatic compo-unds	not defined	3-5g
Chlorine	Primary monovalent anion in cellular fluids; component of digestive juice (HCl); acid-base balance	not defined	1-5g
Iron	Essential constituent of haeme in haemoglobin, cytochromes, peroxidases, etc.	Microcytic, homochronic anaemia	50-00 mg
Copper	Component of haeme in haemo-cyanin (of cephalopods); co-factor in tyrosinase and ascorbic acid oxidase	not defined	1-4g
Manganese	Co-factor for arginase and certain other metabolic enzymes; involved in bone formation and erythrocyte regeneration	not defined	20-50 mg
Cobalt	Metal component of cyanocoba-lamin (B_{12}). Prevents anaemia; invo-lved in C_1 and C_3 metabolism	not defined	5-10 mg
Zinc	Essential for insulin structure and function; co-factor of carbonic anhydrase	not defined	30-100 mg
Iodine	Constituent of thyroxine; regulates oxygen use	Thyroid hyperplasia (goiter)	100-300 mg
Molybdenum	Co-factor of xanthine, oxidase, hydrogenases and reductases	not defined	(trace)
Chromium	Involved in collagen formation and regulation of the rate of glucose metabolism	not defined	(trace)
Fluorine	Component of bone appatite	not defined	(trace)z

THE RUMEN AND ITS MICRO-ORGANISMS

As the utilisation of forages by ruminants depends on microbial fermentative digestion, the principles of digestion in the rumen are discussed as a framework to view the requirements for biotechnology innovations in nutrition. The rumen is the dominant feature of the digestive tract of cattle. This maintains a medium that supports a dense and varied population of microorganisms. These organisms ferment feed materials to produce mainly shortchain organic acids or volatile fatty acids (VFAs), methane and carbon dioxide and the process provides substrate (the feed) and ATP (energy) for the growth of micro-organisms. The microbial mix in the rumen is complex and highly dependent on diet. The main agents that break down fibre, sugars, starches and proteins in the rumen are all anaerobic and include bacteria, protozoa and fungi. The bacteria are the principal organisms that ferment plant cell-wall carbohydrates but the anaerobic phycomycetous fungi may at times be extremely important.

Protozoa are now recognised as having an overall negative effect in the rumen, particularly where ruminants are fed forage diets low in true-protein. Protozoa ingest and digest bacteria and reduce the bacterial biomass in the rumen and consequently the protein supply to the animal. Thus, they decrease the protein to energy ratio in the nutrients absorbed (see later) and increase the requirement of animals for true protein. The net result of the presence of protozoa is an increased requirement for dietary bypass protein and on low protein diets a decreased efficiency of utilisation of feed for growth and milk production. The presence of protozoa in the rumen may also reduce the rate at which bacteria colonise and degrade the ingested feed particles. In studies with sheep fed straw based diets, it has been found that the apparent digestibility of dry matter was increased by 18% after protozoa had been removed from the rumen (*i.e.* defaunated). This research indicates that large increases in productivity may be achieved with ruminants fed fibrous diets, particularly those low in true protein by controlling or removing protozoa from the rumen. Other workers have not seen the differences in digestibility and in some instances removal of protozoa from the rumen has led to decreased digestibility of mixed, starch containing diets.

FERMENTATIVE EFFICIENCY IN THE RUMEN

A deficiency of a nutrient needed by rumen micro-organisms reduces microbial growth efficiency which reduces microbial biomass and eventually reduces digestibility and feed intake, particularly of fibrous feeds.

The first priority in feeding ruminants is to ensure no deficiencies in the diet of nutrients for microbial growth in the rumen. Of major importance is that the efficiency of microbial growth (that is, the amount of microbial biomass available for digestion in the intestines per unit of digestible carbohydrate entering the rumen) also determines the proportion of digested feed that is converted to methane and VFA. Methane production accompanies the formation of acetate or butyrate, whereas methane and VFA production are inversely related to microbial cell production.

MEETING THE REQUIREMENTS FOR EFFICIENT MICROBIAL GROWTH IN THE RUMEN

On most diets based on crop residues and low-digestibility forages, the primary limitation to the growth of rumen micro-organisms is probably the concentration of ammonia in rumen fluid The second consideration is deficiencies of minerals, particularly sulphur, phosphorus, magnesium and certain trace minerals. Ammonia in the rumen must be above a critical level for a considerable period of the day to ensure a high rate of microbial growth and digestion and therefore feed intake. The level of ammonia that supports the optimal population of micro-organisms in the rumen the highest protein to energy ration in the nutrients absorbed, and therefore maximum digestion, will vary among diets. In general on forage based diets the ammonia level should be above 200 mg nitrogen/litre. It must be stressed, however, that any nutrient, (including many minerals required in the growth of micro-organisms), that is deficient in a diet will result in low microbial cell yield relative to VFA and lead to a low protein (from microbes) to energy (from VFA) in the nutrients absorbed. The ratio of protein digested and absorbed from the intestines to the VFA produced in and absorbed from the rumen is termed the P/E ratio.

CONSEQUENCES OF THE RUMINANT MODE OF DIGESTION

One of the consequences of the ruminant mode of digestion is that fermentation results in up to 20% of the digestible energy intake being lost as heat and methane. A second major disadvantage is that proteins that are fermented in the rumen are not then sources of amino acids for the animal because they are hydrolysed and their constituent amino acids deaminated by microbes. In general, where ruminants are fed forage based diets typical of that available in tropical developing countries, small amounts of extra nutrients are needed to balance nutrient availability to requirements. Proteins which are directly available to the animals and are protected from degradation increase the efficiency of anabolism of the absorbed nutrients in growth, pregnancy, lactation or work.

QUANTITATIVE ASPECTS OF FERMENTATIVE DIGESTION IN THE RUMEN

The end products of rumen fermentative digestion are governed by the feed, the rate of consumption of feed, the balance of nutrients in the feed for microbial growth and the balance of micro-organisms that develop in the rumen (bacteria, protozoa and fungi). In general, a proportion of the digestible feed dry matter is converted to VFA, methane and carbon dioxide and the balance is assimilated into microbial cells. The pathways of these reactions are well known and a schematic outline is shown in Figure. Microbial cells, that are synthesised from the feed resource use the ATP that is generated in the formation of VFA from the feed to provide the energy for synthesis. The microbes are lost from the rumen pool either by passage out of the rumen to be partially digested in the intestine or by death and breakdown within the rumen (with formation of VFA, CO_2 and methane). Lysis and degradation in the rumen is inefficient as it makes the protein of microbes unavailable as such to the animal. Because microbial cells are more reduced than the substrate fermented, the quantity of microbial cells leaving the rumen per unit of carbohydrate consumed is related to methane production. The efficiency of microbial growth is then a primary determinate of the quantity of methane produced.

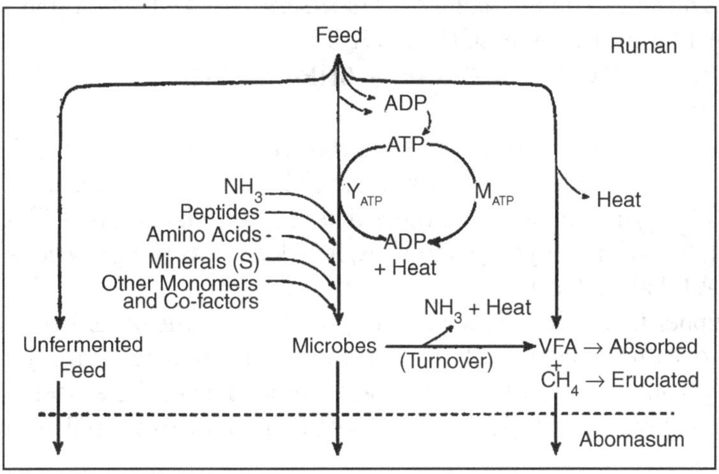

Fig. Energetics of Rumen Fermentation

A Model of Fermentation in the Rumen

For the purposes of the present discussion and to demonstrate the underlying principles of the concepts developed, a model for a 200 kg steer will be used to illustrate the quantitative availability of nutrients from rumen fermentation. The steer consumes 4 kg which represents 25 Mole anhydroglucose or organic matter which is completely fermented in the rumen.

It is assumed:

- That the fermentation of 1 mole of carbohydrate gives rise to either 2 mole acetate, 2 mole of propionate or 1 mole of butyrate, according to the following stoichiometry:

Hexose	→	Pyruvate + 2ATP + H_2
2Pyruvate + $2H_2O$	→	2HAc + $2CO_2$ + 2H2 + 2ATP
2Pyruvate + $8H_2O$	→	2HPro + $2H_2O$ + 2ATP
2Pyruvate + $4H_2O$	→	H Bu + $2H_2$ + $2CO_2$ + 2ATP
CO_2 + H_2	→	CH_4 + $2H_2O$ + 2ATP

- In the stoichiometry, H_2 indicates reduced co-enzymes, HAc is acetic acid, HPro is propionic acid and HBu is butyric acid
- That the animal's rumen is functioning at "normal" level of

fermentative efficiency in which one-third of the organic matter fermented is converted to microbial cells and the rest to VFA, CO_2 and CH_4.

- That the moles ATP generated per mole of end-product are for acetate 2, butyrate 3, propionate 3, and methane 1.

On chemical principles, the equation of substrate use and end products from fermentation of 4 kg of carbohydrate is:

- *Carbohydrate to* VFA: 16.7 CHO → 21 HAc + 6HPro + 3HBu + $7.5CH_4$ + 78ATP
- *Carbohydrate to microbial cell precursors*: 8.3CHO → 1.4 polysaccharide + 13.8 pyruvate + $2CH_4$ + 17ATP
- *Overall*: 25CHO → 21HAc + 6HPro + 3HBu + $9.5CH_4$ + 1300 g dry cells.

In the example, one-third of the carbohydrate provides the substrate for microbial cell synthesis 1300 g dry microbial cells are produced at a Y_{ATP} of about 14.5 (Y_{ATP} is a measure of the efficiency of utilisation of ATP generated in fermentation of carbohydrates to VFA; it is defined as the g dry cells produced per mole ATP available.)

The upper level of efficiency has a Y_{ATP} of 26. On the other hand the lowest efficiency of a microbial growth in the rumen that is deficient in, say, ammonia, is possibly below a Y_{ATP} of 4. The relative efficiency of the system (indicated as Y_{ATP}) is governed largely by the availability of essential nutrients for microorganisms.

The ranges of Y_{ATP} are shown for:

A. A relatively inefficient rumen (*i.e.* Ammonia deficient)
B. A 'normal' rumen with no deficient nutrient for microbial growth
C. A rumen free of protozoa with no deficient nutrient for microbial growth
D. The theoretical optimum microbial growth efficiency.

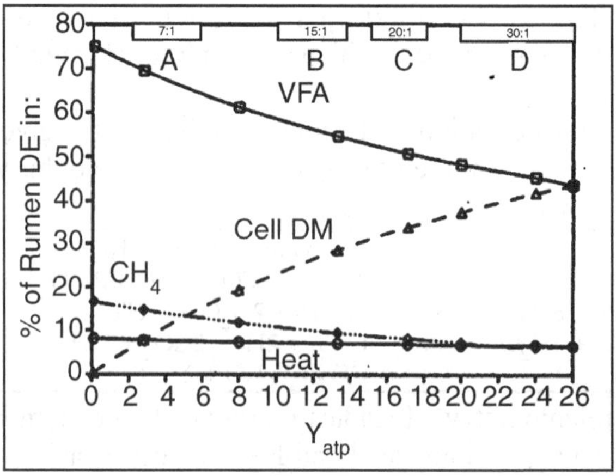

Table. The Effect of Different Efficiencies of Microbial Growth on the Ratio of Protein to VFA Energy (P/E Ratio) Available from the Rumen of a Steer Consuming 4 kg of Organic Matter which is Totally Fermentable.

	Y_{ATP}			
	8	14	19	25
Microbial protein* synthesised (g/d)	500	800	1010	1212
VFA produced (MJ/d)	41	34	30	26
Methane produced (MJ/d)	9.4	8.5	8.0	7.6
Heat (MJ/d)	6.4	5.1	4.3	3.1
P/E ratio (g protein/MJ)	12	25	34	47

* Microbial protein may be only 75–85% digestible and this will change the P/E ratio markedly in the animal.

Based on this model, but assuming a varying efficiency, the microbial cells produced relative to VFA and methane production change are shown in Table. The main point to emphasise is that, depending on the efficiency of utilization of ATP, the amount of carbohydrate converted to microbial cells can be highly variable. It is the efficiency of microbial growth that largely controls the amount of methane produced by an animal.

PROTEIN UTILISATION BY RUMINANTS

Protein that is fermented in the rumen is largely wasted as a source of amino acids to the animal because:

- Dietary protein is degraded and essential amino acids are deaminated to form ammonia and VFA
- Fermentation of 1 g of protein generates only half the ATP that would be produced from 1 g of carbohydrate and therefore anaerobic microbial growth on protein is approximately half that on carbohydrate.

In combination these effects result in only 30 to 60 g of microbial protein becoming available to the animal for digestion for every kilogram of dietary protein that is fermented in the rumen.

The fermentation of protein is, however, associated with relatively small amounts of methane production. On the other hand methane is not generated when protein bypasses the rumen.

Protein that is insoluble, or has a high component of disulphide bonds or is associated with tannins tends to bypass rumen fermentation but is digested in the intestines and in this way it augments the microbial protein and alters the ratio of protein to energy (P/E) in the nutrients absorbed.

The better the balance of nutrients for microbial growth the higher the ratio of P/E in the nutrients produced in fermentation. The higher the content of bypass protein in the diet the higher the P/E ratio in the absorbed nutrients.

Ensuring a Balanced Nutrition For Ruminants on Forage Based Diets

From the above discussion the first priority for improving the utilisation of a low digestibility forage by ruminants is to optimise the availability of nutrients from fermentative digestion by:

- Ensuring that there are no deficiencies of microbial nutrients in the rumen and therefore the microbes in the rumen grow efficiently and, through fermentative activity, extract the maximum possible amounts of nutrients from the forage (*i.e.* The ratio of microbial cells to vfa produced is high as are production rates of these end products)
- Ensuring that the microbial cells (which provide most of the protein to the animal) synthesised in the rumen are not lysed and fermented in the rumen but are available for digestion and absorption as amino acids from the intestines.

The second objective of a feeding strategy should be to optimise the efficiency of partitioning of absorbed nutrients into product by:

- Supplementation with critical nutrients that escape or bypass rumen fermentation to augment and balance the nutrients absorbed to those required for maintenance of homeostasis, maintenance of body temperature, exercise (or work), and the particular physiological or productive function.

As the nutrients needed for different functions differ in priority, supplementation strategies will need to vary according to climate, environment, management and production targets in any one location.

OPTIMISING MICROBIAL GROWTH IN THE RUMEN

Mineral Requirements of Rumen Microbes

The rumen microbes have specific requirements for both macro and micro minerals to meet the needs of structural components of cells and for components of enzymes and co-factors. Little is known about the requirements of the microbial milieu for trace elements and as a 'rule of thumb' it is accepted that if the animal is not deficient then it is unlikely that the rumen microbes will be deficient.

As Suttle has so aptly put the situation, "it will rarely be possible to approach a suspected mineral deficiency situation with a table of minor nutrient requirements or biochemical criteria in the hand, and define a scale of the animal health (microbial health) problems".

In practice, either no mineral supplements are used or a "shot gun" mixture is given as a salt licks or as molasses (which is concentrated plant juice rich in minerals) suitably fortified with minerals. As with any deficiency of a nutrient the likely scenario of a mineral deficiency for rumen organisms is first a reduced growth efficiency of microbes (lowered ratio of cells to VFA produced) with or without a decrease in digestibility. As the deficiencies become more extreme the digestibility of forage must decrease along with the decrease in microbial pool size and it is only then that feed intake will decrease. Feed intake however, will be decreased as P/E ratio decreases if the animal is heat stressed (see later). Correction of deficiency will obviously reverse these effects.

Requirements for Ammonia

Ensuring adequate ammonia N in the rumen to supply the majority of nitrogen for microbial growth is the first priority in optimising fermentative digestion of forage. Satter and Slyter suggested that 50–80 mg NH_3-N/1 of rumen fluid was the optimum for maximising microbial growth yield and this has been widely accepted.

However, recent studies from two laboratories in Australia have clearly indicated that the minimum level of ruminal fluid ammonia for optimum voluntary intake of low N, low digestibility forage by cattle is about 200 mg N/1, even though the digestibility of the forage (in nylon bags) was optimised below 100 mg NH_3-N/1. All these studies were carried out in hot environments and the effects on feed intake are possibly explained by an improving P/E ratio in the nutrients absorbed, which reduces the metabolic heat load.

The effects of increasing ruminal fluid ammonia by infusion of urea into the rumen of steers on the intake of rice straw and its digestibility in nylon bags in the rumen are shown in Figure.

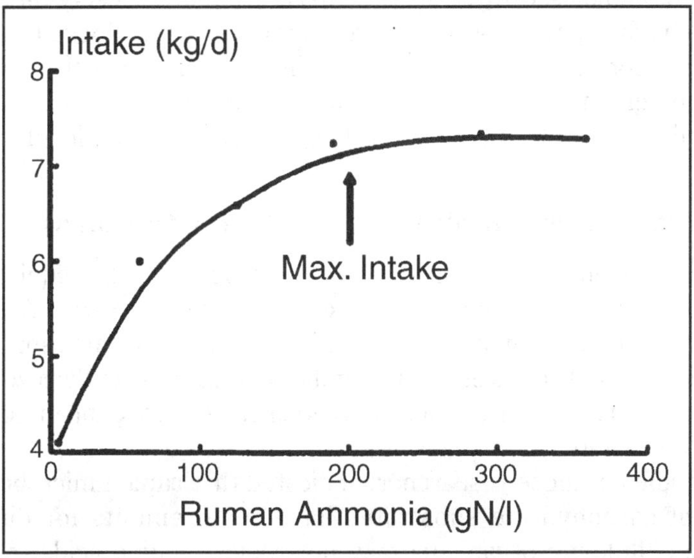

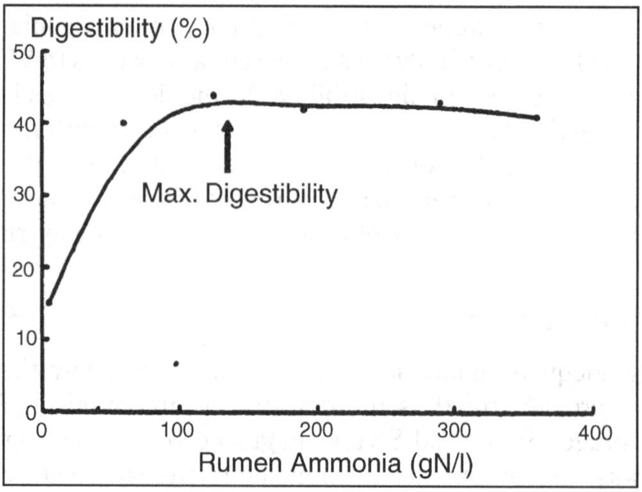

Fig. The Effects of the Level of Ammonia in the Rumen on the Intake and *in Sacco* Digestibility of Straw by Cattle. The Ammonia Levels were Adjusted by Infusing Urea in the Rumen.

Timing of Urea Supplements and the Ratio of Sugars and Starches to Fibre in a Diet

Supplements must provide adequate levels of ammonia in the rumen for continuous growth of both fibrolytic and saccharolytic organisms. The only satisfactory approach to meeting these changing requirements for ammonia is to provide ammonia continuously. One way of doing this is to provide salt/urea or molasses/urea licks and allow the animal to take these as needed. There are indications that cattle and buffaloes given continuous access to multi-nutrient blocks based on molasses/urea are able to control fairly closely their intake of urea. Once buffaloes were accustomed to molasses/urea blocks they adjusted their intake according to the N content of the basal diet (NDDB—unpublished data). Lambs given wheat straw and molasses/urea blocks also had similar abilities and consistently maintained their rumen ammonia levels above 200 mg N/1.

Requirements for Amino Acids/Peptides by Rumen Organisms

There has been considerable controversy concerning the requirements for peptides/amino acids by rumen microbes for efficient growth. A number of studies, however, have reported results of *in vivo* studies which appear to have indicated no apparent requirement for amino acids for efficient growth of rumen organisms. The results of studies by Maeng *et al.* may explain some of the contradictory results.

The studies of these researchers indicated that rumen microbes growing on different carbohydrate substrates have requirements for different N-substrates; celluloytic organisms may not require amino acids to the same extent as organisms growing on starches or sugar as the major substrate. For microbes utilising sugars growing on starches there was an apparently high requirement for preformed amino acids/peptides but this was not so for cellulolytic organisms. Maeng *et al.* also showed an increase in efficiency of microbial growth on fibrous carbohydrates with decreasing dilution rate of rumen contents. If true this may be advantageous to ruminants given low quality forages that must be retained in the rumen for a considerable period to allow digestibility to be optimised. At the same time the improved ratio of cells: VFA yielded (*i.e.* P/E ratio) along with the increased availability of the total nutrients are both advantageous.

Such a mechanism would advantage an animal with:

- A comparatively slow turnover rate of rumen contents (*i.e.* Buffalo vs. Cow or goat vs. Sheep
- Fauna-free vs. faunated animal or animals at high environmental conditions versus cold stressed animals.

Amino Acid Requirements of Microbes Digesting Fibre

The organisms in the rumen that are largely responsible for the fermentation of cellulose (*Ruminococcus albus, Ruminococcus flavefaciens* and *Fibrobacter succinogenes* (previously called *Bacteroides succinogenes*) appear to have minimal requirements for amino acids and grow on ammonia. Conversely, organisms important in starch hydrolysis (*Butyrivibrio fibrisolvens, Bacteroides ruminicola, Selenomonas ruminantium, Streptococcus bovis* and *Ruminobacter (Bacteroides) amylophilus* readily incorporate amino acid N and in many cases peptides.

Supplementation of sheep fed a poor quality forage with branched chain VFA has been reported to increase the apparent flow of microbial-N to the duodenum. The apparent stimulation of microbial growth with branched chain VFA has also been shown to increase feed intake on occasions. This together with the suggested requirements for peptides/amino acids by rumen organisms (which on the basis of the results of Maeng *et al.*

must now be questioned) has tempted many scientists to explain the increased feed intake of ruminants, on poor quality forages that are supplemented with bypass protein, to the slow release of amino acids, peptides and branched chain fatty acids to the rumen milieu from the protected protein, even though in most studies there was no evidence of increased digestibility with such supplements in predominately fibre based diets.

The above discussion indicates that the cellulolytic organisms in the rumen even of cattle on straw based diets, are rarely if ever deficient in amino acids, peptides or branched chain VFA in the rumen.

This is not to deny that these organisms may still need these nutrients in "catalytic" amounts but that they are rarely if ever at such low concentrations in rumen fluid to bring about a deficiency.

The Roles of Small Amounts of Fresh Forage in Straw Based Diets

Farmers in developing countries have generally recognised the benefits to cattle of adding a small amount of fresh green herbage to straw based diets. These practices, which have evolved through trial and error, may have a number of beneficial effects which include the supply of vitamin A, essential minerals, ammonia, peptides/amino acids in an otherwise unsupplemented diet.

Recently it has been shown that where the supplemental forage in a straw based diet given to sheep is of high digestibility a boost to digestibility of the basal diet occurs even at relatively small levels of supplementation. The rate of digestibility of straw depends on the rate and extent of colonisation of fibre and the biomass of adherent organisms and the high digestibility forage supplement may act to seed microbes onto the less digestible straw. On the other hand, other influences cannot be ruled out. For example, in the studies of Silva and Ørskov in the absence of an effect of supplemental forage on digestibility, the rumen ammonia levels were often not significantly below 200 mg NH_3-N/1. Where increases in digestibility of the basal forage occurred to supplemental forage the ammonia levels in the rumen were significantly below 200 mg N/1 and the supplement apparently improved the concentration to above the critical level.

Elimination of Rumen Protozoa and Preservation of the Fauna-Free State

The physiological research which has shown that there is an increased availability of microbial protein for digestion in fauna-free as compared to faunated ruminant has supported the feeding trials with large numbers of animals which has demonstrated significantly high feed conversion efficiencies and wool growth rate in sheep without rumen protozoa as compared to control animals.

Fauna free cattle on the same intake of a low protein, molasses/urea based diet grew at a 43% greater rate than faunated cattle on the same feed intake. The improved production was therefore an effect of a higher efficiency of feed utilisation.

The discussion to follow, on the implications of environmental temperature/humidity for the nutrition of ruminants, will indicate why a major change in P/E ratio in the nutrients absorbed (*i.e.* the major difference between faunated and fauna-free ruminants) will be more effective in improving ruminant production in the tropics as compared to temperate/cold countries. In the tropical areas the available forages used to feed to ruminants are generally lower in digestibility, lower in true protein and animals are rarely cold, but heat stress at times may be severe. It should also be noted that animals brought into animals houses from fairly could environments may at times suffer severe heat stress through a combination of a well insulated fleece or coat and an imbalanced diet.

METABOLISM

In order for an animal to perform any functions it must have energy. Animals acquire energy through food, which can be acquired in several ways. After acquiring food, it must be broken down and absorbed. Animals use energy to support all life processes, including breathing, circulation, movement, nerve function, and temperature regulation. Animals use several physiological and behavioural mechanisms to maintain their body temperature and minimize the loss of energy.

Metabolism is the total of all physical and chemical changes that take place within an organism, and according to the Laws of Thermodynamics, all of these changes will ultimately release heat. Therefore, metabolic rate is a measure of the heat production of an animal. Very few organisms can survive in extreme thermal conditions (notable exceptions are bacteria).

Less extreme but variable conditions are made tolerable through thermal regulation of body heat that is achieved through varying degrees of metabolic activity. For most animals it is essential that the body temperature be maintained within certain parametres, regardless of external thermal conditions.

ENERGY METABOLISM AT THE CELLULAR LEVEL

Most of the information on energy metabolism at the cellular level has been obtained from cellularly homogeneous, purified preparations enriched in astrocytes, neurons, or vascular endothelial cells. Currently, most studies are conducted in primary cultures prepared from neonatal or embryonic rodent brain tissue. A cautionary note is always necessary when attempting to extrapolate results obtained in vitro to in vivo situations. It is, however, generally accepted that important insights may be gained from these cellularly homogeneous preparations.

Brain energy metabolism is often considered to reflect predominantly, if not exclusively, neuronal energy metabolism. However, it is now clear that other cell types, namely neuroglia and vascular endothelial cells not only consume energy but also can play an active role in the flux of energy substrates to neurons. First, there is a quantitative consideration; although it is arduous to provide a definitive ratio between neurons and nonneuronal cells given the variability in figures obtained in various species, brain areas, and developmental ages using methods that are not easily comparable, it is clear that neurons contribute at most 50% of cerebral cortical volume. In addition there is clear evidence indicating that the astrocyte-to-neuron ratio increases with increasing brain size; this is an important consideration when approaching the study of the cellular bases of brain energy metabolism in humans. It is therefore clear that glucose reaching the brain parenchyma through the circulation should provide energy substrates to a variety of cell types, only a portion of which are neurons.

DIFFERENT METHODS OF FEEDING

In order to sustain life all organisms must have some way of attaining food. This process can occur by means of filtering, piercing, seizing or grazing. The amount of energy put into attaining food can determine the efficiency of the method used for acquiring the food. If a lot of energy is put into acquiring food then the amount of energy coming from the food must also be great. Whereas, if very little energy is put into getting food then the amount of energy from the food does not have to be very great. The processes by which organisms acquire food are important because it is through these means that the organisms are able to survive. One way organisms acquire food is by the process of filter feeding. Organisms such as sponges, brachiopods, lamellibranchs and tunicates are found in aquatic environments and use filter feeding to acquire food. This method requires very low energy expenditure if any at all.

In some cases, water flowing across an opening in the organism can result in a decrease in pressure (the Bernoulli effect), causing water to flow out of this opening and drawing water into another opening, therefore bringing food to the mouth. Mucus is also another important feature for filter feeders. This sticky mucus covers the ciliated epithelium of the organism and traps the microorganisms, phytoplankton or zooplankton. The trapped organism is then transported to the oral parts by the beating motion of the cilia. The extra water that is taken in is squeezed back out. The largest of these feeders are the baleen whales. This animal opens its mouth and sucks the water in. Its hair-like teeth, made of keratin, strain the food. When the mouth is closed the water is then squeezed back out through the hair-like teeth. The food that was obtained through this process is swallowed and digested for energy.

Another way organisms obtain food is through a process of fluid feeding. *There are two main areas to fluid feeding*:

- Piercing and sucking,
- Cutting and licking.

The organisms associated with piercing and sucking are platyhelminths, nematodes, annelids and arthropods. These organisms have distinct mouth parts which bore into their prey. The organisms then suck out the prey's body fluids with their pharynx. Enzymes secreted from the pharynx help facilitate the digestion of the fluids. One of the most common piercing mouthparts, found in insects, is the proboscis which has two canals formed by the maxillae. The first canal carries in the victims blood and the other carries saliva and anticoagulants.

The process of fluid feeding by means of cutting and licking are associated with some invertebrates (such as black flies) and a few vertebrates (such as vampire bats). The fluid feeder will feed by cutting the prey's body with sharp mouthparts or teeth and then lick the fluids as they flow from the body. Anticoagulants injected into the wound helps prevent blood from clotting. A third method of obtaining food is by seizing of prey. The organisms associated with this form of feeding have jaws, teeth or beaks, and some also use toxins. Many invertebrates that don't have true teeth use a beak-like structure for feeding. The beak-like structure is driven into the prey, and some of these organisms also inject venom to paralyse their prey. Other non-mammalian vertebrates, such as sharks, tear their prey apart with successive rows of pointed teeth. The prey are then swallowed. Many poisonous snakes have modified teeth, called fangs, which can fold back when not in use. The fangs pierce the prey and inject venom. The snakes mouth, made of bones linked with elastic ligaments, spreads open and allows it to swallow its prey whole.

Mammals have various shapes of teeth, which serve different purposes. Some of the teeth types include incisors for gnawing, tusks for fighting and piercing, canines for tearing and piercing, and molars for grinding. Some gastropod mollusks have a radula, for tearing or grazing. Birds on the other hand, have horny beaks, which vary in shape and size according to the type of food they eat. The beak will capture the food which is then swallowed and passed into a crop for storage, and then on to the gizzard, which often contains small stones, for grinding.

Some animals also rely on toxins to immobilize prey for feeding. There are two different forms of toxins, which are made of proteins, associated with feeding. The first are nematocysts which are stinging cells which contain a toxin that immobilize prey and are found on tentacles of coelenterates. Another type of toxin is neurotoxin, which is associated with organisms such as scorpions and spiders. Neurotoxins interfere with nerve impulses at the motor endplate in muscles, which leaves the prey paralysed. Alpha-bungarotoxin is one of the neurotoxins associated with this group of toxins. All of these toxins require great amounts of energy to make, and thus the amount of toxin used on a prey is given in measured doses. Special enzymes in the host protect it from its own toxin.

ALIMENTARY SYSTEM

The alimentary system plays a key role in the process of digestion, absorption, excretion and provision of energy/nourishment. The two forms of digestion are extracellular and intracellular. Extracellular deals with digestion which occurs outside of the cell in the true alimentary system.

Whereas, intracellular digestion breaks down nutrients within the cells and is mainly associated with unicellular organisms. Extracellular digestion can be categorized as either being a batch reactor (coelenterates), continuous-flow reactor (all phyla higher than flatworms),or a plug-flow reactor (most mammals). The batch reactor system brings food in batches. The food is then digested and excreted before another batch of food is taken in.

The continuous-flow reactor continually carries in and mixes food and excretes food products. The last form of extracellular digestion is the plug-flow reactor. In this type, food is taken in and digested while it winds through long tubes in the digestive system. The alimentary system is broken up into different structural divisions and within each division there is a specialization in the process of digestion.

For each organism, the structure of each division varies with length, width, or winding. The first structural division of the digestive system is the headgut. It is the most anterior portion of the digestive system which includes the external opening and specializes in receiving ingested food. In this area digestion begins and salivary glands that secrete a lubrication, mucus, to help the organism swallow food.

Tongues, a specialization found in the headgut of chordates, help in chemoreception, grasping food and manipulation during chewing. The foregut is the division which follows the headgut and specializes in conducting, storing, and digesting food. The esophagus brings the food to the area of digestion. This process of transportation occurs by peristaltic movement and in certain animals, like birds, the food is passed into a crop where it is stored before digestion. The food material is then passed into the stomach which is a storage site and the area where most chemical digestion begins in animals. In the stomach, enzymes and muscular movements mix and break down food particles. The stomach is specialized for the type of food that the organism eats, and it is either monogastric, which is associated with carnivores and omnivores, or digastric, which is associated with mammalian ruminants.

The midgut follows the foregut in the alimentary system. In vertebrates this is the primary site for chemical digestion of proteins, fats, and carbohydrates. Food leaves the stomach through the pyloric sphincter and moves into the small intestine. The vertebrate midgut is divided into the duodenum, jejunum, and the ileum.

The liver and the pancreas secrete fluids, through a duct, into the duodenum that digest food particles. The liver secretes bile salts which emulsify fats and neutralize acidity in the duodenum. The pancreas produces a juice containing protease, lipase, and carbohydrates. The midgut varies from species to species in function and structure. Carnivores have a shorter small intestine than herbivores because the plants takes longer to digest than meat.

The midgut is structured to allow for full absorption. The hindgut functions mainly as a storage unit for undigested food particles. While food is in the hindgut, inorganic ions and excess water are re-absorbed into the blood. Organisms require water for many physiological functions, therefor they try to conserve as much water as they can.

The feces of some insects are almost dry when they are expelled. This enables them to retain most of the water that they ingest. Also in the hindgut, bacterial digestion occurs in birds, herbivorous reptiles, and most herbivorous mammals. In all animals feces pass into the cloaca or the rectum and are expelled through the anus.

TYPES OF EXOCRINE SECRETIONS

There are various exocrine glands that secrete chemicals. These chemicals further digest and break down food particles so that they can be absorbed. Exocrine glands include the salivary glands, secretory cells of the stomach, intestine, liver, and pancreas. These glands are divided into three categories according to what they secrete: water and electrolytes, bile, and digestive enzymes. Most exocrine secretions are largely water based enzymes and chemicals. An aqueous mucus solution is produced in the goblet cells of the stomach and intestine. The mucus lubricates to prevent mechanical and enzymatic injury. Bile is secreted by the liver and is essential for the digestion of fats. Bile is a mixture of water and a weak basic solution of cholesterol, lecithin, inorganic salts, bile salts, and bile pigments. The bile is transported to the gallbladder via the hepatic duct where it is concentrated and stored.

Bile buffers the acidity in the intestines introduced by gastric juices fro the stomach. Secondly, it facilitates enzymatic fat digestion. Finally, bile contains substances removed from the blood which is then digested or excreted. Digestive enzymes aid in the hydrolysis of large food particles into smaller compounds enabling them to cross cell membranes of the intestinal barrier. Digestive enzymes are substrate specific, sensitive to temperature, pH, and ions. There are three types: protease, carbohydrases, and lipase.

Proteases break peptide bonds of proteins and polypeptides. Whereas, carbohydrases break long chain carbohydrates and disaccharides into smaller carbohydrates. Lipase emulsifies fats, thereby decreasing the surface area. In addition, and with the aid of bile salts they produce fatty acids, monoglycerides, and diglycerides from fats. Most glands of the alimentary canal are stimulated by another chemical secreted by another gland in the alimentary system. The secretion of saliva, in the mouth, is stimulated when food is present in the headgut. The secretion of gastrin is in turn stimulated in the lower stomach by the presence of saliva. Gastrin, then, stimulates the secretion of hydrochloric acid. Hydrochloric acid is a major secretion of the stomach. The secretion of HCl is stimulated by vagal motor discharges, gastrin, and paracrine actions synthesized in the mast cells of the gastric mucosa. HCl breaks down peptide bonds, activates gastric enzymes, and kills microorganisms in the stomach.

UNICELLULAR EXOCRINE GLANDS

These consist of single cells, specialized for secretion, which are interspersed amongst other, non-secretory epithelial cells. Although, being unicellular, they lack ducts, they are nevertheless considered to be exocrine because they secrete their products directly on the free surface of open body cavities. The most common unicellular exocrine glands are the goblet cells (mucus secreting cells) found in the epithelium of the trachea and the digestive tube.

MULTICELLULAR EXOCRINE GLANDS

These are formed by invagination, or in-pouching, of an epithelial sheet. The epithelium grows down from the surface into the underlying tissues to form either a simple or compound tube. The blind end of the tube constitutes the secretory parts of the gland and may stay tubular or expand to form round bags called acini or alveoli. The various structural types of endocrine glands are shown in the illustration.

There are three different ways in which exocrine glands secrete their products. These modes of secretion are called merocrine, apocrine, and holocrine. Merocrines glands (e.g., salivary glands) secrete their product from intact cells.

Apocrine glands (e.g., mammary glands) accumulate their secretory product at the apical surface of each cell, which then separates from the remainder to from a secretion in the lumen of the gland. The cells then repair themselves. Holocrine glands (e.g., sebaceous or oil glands) are those in which entire cells and their secretions accumulate as the gland's secretory product. Discharged cells are replaced by new ones.

ABSORPTION IN ELECTROLYTE BALANCE

Once food particles are broken down the products (amino acids) must be transported from the gut to cells and tissues of the organism. In multicellular organism amino acids must be transported across absorptive epithelium into the blood and then into tissues. The structure of the intestinal epithelium aids in the success of absorption. The small intestines of vertebrates are specialized to increase surface area. The first level are the folds of Kerckring that project into the lumen of the small intestine.

They increase surface area and slow the progress of food, allowing time for digestion. Villi sit on circular depressions on the folds of Kerckring. These circular depressions are called the crypt of Lieberkuhn. Within each villus is a network of blood vessels and lymph vessels through which nutrients are absorbed. At the apical surface of the absorptive cells is the brush border. The brush border contains digestive enzymes for the final digestion. The type of transfer depends on the type of molecule.

Passive diffusion is used to transport fatty acids, monoglycerides, cholesterol, and other fat-soluble substances across the brush border. Water, some sugars, alcohols, and small water-soluble molecules passively diffuse through water filled pores. Carrier-mediated diffusion is responsible for transporting large molecules like monosaccharides and hydrophilic amino acids. Protein channels transport sugars by coupling sodium gradients and electrical gradients. A sodium/potassium pumps out $Na+$, creating a gradient that powers the transport of large or hydrophilic molecules. The molecules move down concentration gradients.

Active transport can be one of four non-competing systems depending on the category of amino acids:

1. Lysine, arginine, and histidine,
2. Glutamate and asparatate,
3. Glycine, proline, hyrooxyproline,
4. The remaining amino acids.

Each group uses a different method to transfer various types of amino acids across the brush border.

Lipids are an exception to the rule of absorption. Products of broken down lipids (fats, monoglycerides, fatty acids, and glycerol) diffuse through the brush border and are reconstructed on the other side. They are collected with phospholipids and cholesterol into chylomicrons. They're coated with proteins and contained in vesicles formed by the golgi apparatus which are then expelled by exocytosis. Digested particles enter the blood or the lymph system from the alimentary system.

Lipids, for example, enter the lymph as chylomicrons. The lymph is returned to the blood via the thoracic lymph duct located near the heart. Sugars and amino acids generally enter directly into the blood.

METABOLISM

Metabolism is the sum total of all the chemical reactions occurring in an organism at any given time. Anabolism requires energy and is associated with building complex molecules whereas catabolism is involved in the breakdown of complex molecules into simpler ones. Metabolic rate is a measurement of the conversion of chemical energy into heat, or heat energy released per unit time.

Measuring metabolic rate is not only useful to physiologists, but also to ecologists, animal behaviourists, evolutionary biologists, and many other fields of study because the metabolic rate can yield information on the energy requirements of animals. In order to learn more about the heat conserving and heat releasing mechanism of animals, metabolic rates can be measured at different temperatures. Metabolic rate can tell us how much energy an animal needs to expend to fly, swim, run, or walk. It can also tell us something about the processes of tissue growth and repair, chemical, osmotic, electrical, and mechanical internal work, and external work that is necessary for such things as locomotion and communication.

The basal metabolic rate is the stable rate of energy metabolism measured in mammals and birds under conditions of minimum environmental and physiological stress, or essentially at rest with no temperature change. Standard metabolic rate refers to an animal's resting and fasting metabolism at a given body temperature, whereas field metabolic rate is the average rate of energy utilization as the animal goes about its normal activities, which may range from complete inactivity while the animal is at rest to exerting maximum energy.

To measure the metabolic rate of an organism directly, one must determine how much heat is flowing from the organism, for this is the true measure of metabolic rate. These measurements can be made using a calorimetre and the process is called direct calorimetry, but this method is often hard to employ, especially when measuring the metabolic rates of large animals. Thus, there must be other ways in which metabolic rate can be measured. These methods are called indirect calorimetry, which involves measuring the amount of food an animal ingested compared to the amount it excreted, respirometry, which involves measuring an animal's respiratory exchange, and the isotopic technique, which measures the water flux in animals using deuterium or tritium labeled water.

Because animals do not ingest food steadily, there is not a moment to moment balance between the intake of food and the expenditure of energy. Food is obtained in bursts, and when an animal feeds, its immediate energy requirements are fulfilled with much being left over. The left over is not thrown out as waste but rather stored for later use, especially in the form of fats and carbohydrates. In 1885, Max Rubner concluded that an increase in metabolic rate was evident soon after the ingestion of food, independent of other activities. He gave this phenomenon the name specific dynamic action, or SDA. SDA has since been observed in all five vertebrate groups, along with invertebrates.

EFFECT OF SIZE

Body size is one of the most important factors that affects metabolism and the study of how body size affects physiological processes is called scaling. It has become clear that small animals must respire at higher rates per unit body mass than larger animals. Also, there is an inverse relationship between O2 consumption per gram of body mass and the total mass of the animal. When the log of the metabolic rate is plotted against the log of the mass for a variety of animals, the slope of the line always seems to correspond to, known as Kleiber's law. Changes in body size affect metabolic rates immensely, namely because increases in body size are not always simple and proportional.

The surface hypothesis, proposed by Max Rubner in 1883, states that the metabolic rate of birds and mammals that maintain a more or less constant body temperature should ultimately be proportional to their surface area. Since body size affects metabolic rate, and surface area is related to metabolic rate as well, there must be a correlation first between surface area and body mass. When animals of different size are compared to one another, their surface area varies to a. Power of their body mass. This is due to the fact that different size animals within the same species follow the rule of isometry, or proportionality of shape regardless of the animal's size. This concept does not hold for animals of different species and varying size. When this relationship is looked at, it can be found that the animal's surface area varies to a power of body mass. This is because when animals of different size and different species are compared to one another, they tend to follow the principle of allometry, which states that systematic changes in body proportions increases with a species size. When the basal metabolic rates of different size animals within the same species is plotted against body mass, the metabolic rate is proportional to the body mass raised to the power, which is the same degree to which surface area and body mass are correlated among animals within the same species.

But when basal metabolic rate in animals of different species are plotted against their body mass, the exponent relating the metabolic rate to the body mass is found to be. This is referred to as Kleiber's law. The surface hypothesis holds true when metabolic rates are plotted against body size in animals belonging to the same species, but it does not hold true when metabolic rates are plotted versus body mass of animals within different species. When one is comparing different species, the metabolic rate cannot be determined simply on differences in body surface area.

ANIMALS BODY TEMPERATURE EFFECT

The temperature of an animal depends on the amount of heat that is contained within the animals' body. Body heat is generally defined as the amount of heat produced by the body through metabolism added to any thermal exchange between the animal and the environment. There are several ways that an animal can absorb or lose heat from or to the environment: conduction, convection, radiation, and evapouration. Conduction is the transfer of heat between objects and substances that are in contact with each other.

The transfer of heat from the skin surface to molecules of gas in the air is an example of conduction. Convection is the transfer of heat contained in a mass of a gas or liquid, by the movement of that mass. A simple example of this is when you sit in front of a fan on a hot day and the movement of air takes the heat away. Radiation is the transfer of heat through electromagnetic radiation without objects coming into contact.

An example of radiation is the warming that can occur to animals in sunlight. Evapouration is a change in state from liquid to gas, which requires energy. Heat is dissipated from the body during evapouration because large water molecules with high energy content accumulate at the skin surface and enter the gaseous phase. When the larger molecules vapourize, they take thermal energy with them and any water left behind becomes cooler. Animals have the ability to gain and store heat from the environment which can result in an increase in body temperature. The amount of heat that will transfer into or out of an animal depends on surface area, temperature difference, and the specific heat conductance of an animals body surface. A large animal (elephant) has a small surface-to-mass ratio and will heat up more slowly in response to environmental heat, whereas an animal with a larger surface-to-mass ratio will heat up faster. If the temperature difference between the environment and an animal's body is small, very little heat will flow into or out of its body. Insulators like fur, feathers, and blubber have a very low thermal conductivity and help to reduce the rate of heat flow. In addition to these thermal regulating characteristics, animals can also regulate the exchange of heat between themselves and the environment using behavioural control and/or autonomic control. Behavioural control is used by animals when they move to a part of the environment where heat exchange favours the attainment of optimal body temperature. An example of this is when snakes or other reptiles choose to bask in the sun during daylight hours, but may avoid basking during midday, when the suns rays are most intense.

Autonomic control is being used when the temperature of the skin and extremities is controlled by the amount of blood flow to these areas of the body. Constriction of arterioles leading to the skin keeps warm blood from reaching the colder extremities and conserves heat at the body core. Autonomic control can also be used to absorb heat by increasing the amount of blood that flows to the surface tissues. Near the skin surface, blood will approach temperature equilibrium with the environment. The insulating properties of the blubber layer in whales is a good example of how autonomic control affects body temperature regulation.

Whales at the surface of the ocean will increase the flow of blood to their blubber layer to absorb radiant heat from the sun. When diving into colder depths, whales constrict their blood vessels and decrease the blood flow to the blubber layer so that heat is conserved at the core and not lost at body surfaces. Acclimatization is also a method of regulating heat exchange, but it involves changes in insulation quality or heat dissipation effectiveness due to long term exposure to either high or low temperatures.

TEMPERATURE CHANGES AFFECT

Temperature variation can cause changes at the molecular level. Homeoviscous membrane adaptations occur as a result of temperature changes. The cell membrane and many functions associated with the cell membrane are sensitive to temperature change. Low temperatures cause the membrane to enter a gel-like phase with very high membrane viscosity. High temperatures, on the other hand, cause the membrane to enter a hyperfluid phase with very low viscosity. Initially, acute temperature changes cause changes in membrane polarity and fluidity. On the other hand, after acclimation to both high and low temperatures, the resulting homeoviscous adaptations cause similar lipid polarization and membrane viscosity at both temperatures.

Temperature variation causes certain changes in enzymes. The rate of enzymatically controlled reactions changes due to temperature. This process is called enzyme acclimation. Enzyme acclimation can occur due to changes that occur in the molecular structure of one or more enzymes, changes in the quantity of the enzyme, or other factors that affect enzyme kinetics (for example nerve conduction). Ectotherms are animals that produce metabolic heat at low rates and rely primarily on thermal conditions of their surroundings. They maintain body temperature that is often equal or dependent on the temperature of the surrounding environment, and tend to have lower metabolic rates at low temperatures and higher metabolic rates at higher temperatures. Ectotherms that normally live in cool temperatures have a low body temperature, maintain adequate metabolism at very low levels of enzyme activity, and have enzymes that can function at low temperatures.

Ectotherms that normally live in warm temperatures function at very low levels of metabolism and rely heavily on behavioural regulation to control their body temperature. Certain reptiles also use autonomic control to regulate body temperature. For example the Galapagos marine iguana regulates its heart rate and blood flow during dives into cold water to reduce the amount of heat lost at its surface tissue (skin). It is often more difficult for ectotherms to survive in extreme conditions of cold or hot environments. Extremely hot conditions are not frequented by ectotherms.

Most ectotherms never experience such extremes due to the existence of the critical thermal maximum, a temperature above which long-term survival is not possible. Freezing and cold temperatures are dangerous to all living organisms because if ice crystals begin to form within a cell, the crystals will continue to grow in size as freezing progresses until eventually causing the cell to rupture. No animal is known to survive complete freezing of its tissues, but some ectotherms have come close. Freeze tolerance mechanisms are used by some ectotherms that actually freeze and remain alive. Some species of beetles can withstand freezing temperatures because they have extracellular fluid that contains a substance that accelerates crystal formation. As a result of more rapid crystal formation outside of the cells, the solute concentration inside the cell increases, lowering the intercellular freezing point. Red blood cells, yeast, and sperm can withstand freezing temperatures using this mechanism, provided that intercellular ion concentrations do not get high enough to cause damage to the cell organelles.

Freeze avoidance strategies are used by other ectotherms to prevent freezing. Freeze avoidance is usually characterized by supercooling or the presence of antifreeze substances. Supercooling is observed in fish that live in water temperatures below the freezing point of their bodily fluids. They remain unfrozen because ice crystals are unable to form due to lack of nuclei which are needed to initiate crystallization. Antifreeze substances are characterized by their capacity to lower the freezing point of body fluids. Glycerol, which is present in various species of arthropods and insects, is an example of an antifreeze that has been shown to lower the freezing point to as low as -47°C.

Heterotherms are animals capable of varying degrees of endothermic heat production, but they generally do not regulate body temperature within as narrow a range as endotherms. Heterotherms are broadly broken into two categories, temporal and regional heterotherms. Temporal heterotherms are a broad category of animals whose temperatures vary widely over time and may exhibit daily temperature fluctuations. Camels behave like temporal heterotherms because they allow their body temperatures to fluctuate throughout the day - absorbing heat during the day, and releasing it at night. Regional heterotherms are characterized by the fact that they can achieve high core temperatures, while peripheral tissues and extremities approach ambient temperatures.

The most common form of regional heterothermy is found among animals that are able to conserve heat generated by muscle activity. Certain species of flying insects require their flight muscles to be pre-warmed to a specific temperature before they are able to fly successfully. During flight, these insects can achieve relatively high body temperature, while at rest their body temperatures will reach equilibrium with ambient temperatures. Certain fish, like tuna and some sharks are referred to as warm-bodied heterotherms because of their ability to maintain relatively constant, high core temperatures. The ability of these fish to attain such temperatures is dependent on the organization of the vascular system. Blood vessels in ectothermic fish are located centrally, while heterothermic fish have blood vessels located under the skin. The location of the blood vessels in heterothermic fish allows for countercurrent heat exchange to be utilized, minimizing the loss of heat. The location of swimming muscles in heterothermic fish also influences the retention of body heat. These muscles are located near the central part of the fish and since most of these fish do not stop swimming, the muscles do not cool down. Other types of fish have specialized thermogenic structures that maintain a specific heat in a certain region of the body. An example of this is the swordfish which is able to maintain the temperature of its brain and eyes about 10 degrees higher than its surroundings.

AINMAL ENDOTHERMS

One trait that distinguishes the major groups of vertebrates from one another is the way in which they control their body temperature. Most fish, amphibians, and reptiles have body temperatures that are close to the temperature of their environment.

Fish, amphibians, and reptiles are ectotherms. An ectotherm is an animal whose body does not produce much internal heat. Its body temperature changes depending on the temperature of the environment. For example, when a turtle is lying in the sun on a riverbank, it has a higher body temperature than when it is swimming in a cool river. Ectotherms are sometimes called "cold-blooded," but that is misleading. The blood of ectotherms is often quite warm.

In contrast to the turtle, a beaver would have the same body temperature whether it was in cool water or on warm land. The beaver is an endotherm. An endotherm is an animal whose body controls and regulates its temperature by controlling the internal heat it produces. An endotherm's body temperature usually does not change much, even when the temperature of its environment changes. Mammals and birds are endotherms. They have a stable body temperature that is typically much warmer than their environment. Endotherms are often called "warm-blooded" animals.

ENDOTHERMS

Endotherms are animals that generate their own body heat and are able to maintain internal temperatures that are often stable within a few degrees (between 37°C – 38°C in mammals and about 40°C for birds). This is achieved through elevated basal metabolism in conjunction with heat-conserving and heat dissipating mechanisms. At stable, moderate temperatures regulation is maintained by enough metabolic activity to exactly balance the heat that is lost to the environment. The range of temperatures in which an endotherm can maintain the basal rate of heat production is called the thermal neutral zone. As the temperature drops below the endotherms' lower critical temperature (LCT), the basal metabolic rate is no longer sufficient to balance heat loss to the environment.

The endotherm must increase heat production by means of thermogenesis, which is the production of heat through either shivering or non-shivering methods. Heat production will increase linearly as temperatures continue to decrease so that colder temperatures yield greater rates of metabolic regulation to produce more heat. Eventually if the temperature drops too much, metabolic systems fail to compensate and the animal will die.

Endotherms are able to survive in cold environments through different mechanisms of adaptation. Fur or feathers are useful in reducing convection and the loss of body heat at the body surface of different animals that have fur or feathers. Thick layers of insulation can also reduce loss of heat. For example, blubber (fatty tissue found under the skin of whales) is a good insulator because it has a lower thermal conductivity than water, is metabolically inactive, and requires little profusion of blood.

Endotherms are generally larger animals than ectotherms and this quality is useful in extremely cold environments because large animals generally have a lower specific heat conductance and relatively smaller surface areas which will reduce surface heat loss. Countercurrent heat exchange is also utilized by endotherms to drastically reduce heat loss from appendages. As environmental temperatures rise above the endotherms' internal temperature, metabolic rate decreases with increasing temperatures.

When external temperatures exceed the thermal neutral zone the endotherm must be able to release, or dissipate excess body heat through passive or active heat-dissipating mechanisms, such as evapourative cooling by sweating or panting. All living animals are continuously producing heat at a basal level. If the body temperature can not be controlled and the heat dissipated, it is possible for the animal to overheat and die.

9

Care and use of Animals

REGULATIONS

The regulations that apply to animals in Labouratories vary across species. In the U.S., under the provisions of the Animal Welfare Act and the *Guide for the Care and Use of Labouratory Animals* (the *Guide*), published by the National Academy of Sciences, any procedure can be performed on an animal if it can be successfully argued that it is scientifically justified.

In general, researchers are required to consult with the institution's veterinarian and its Institutional Animal Care and Use Committee (IACUC), which every research facility is obliged to maintain. The IACUC must ensure that alternatives, including non-animal alternatives, have been considered, that the experiments are not unnecessarily duplicative, and that pain relief is given unless it would interfere with the study.

Larry Carbone, a Labouratory animal veterinarian, writes that, in his experience, IACUCs take their work very seriously regardless of the species involved, though the use of non-human primates always raises what he calls a "red flag of special concern." However, a study published in Science magazine on July 27, 2001 confirmed the low reliability of IACUC reviews of animal experiments.

Funded by the National Science Foundation, the three-year study found that animal use committees that do not know the specifics of the university and personnel do not make the same approval decisions as those made by animal use committees that do know the university and personnel.

Specifically, blinded committees more often ask for more information rather than approving studies.The IACUCs regulate all vertebrates in testing at institutions receiving federal funds in the USA. Although the provisions of the Animal Welfare Act do not include purpose-bred rodents and birds, these species are equally regulated under Public Health Service policies that govern the IACUCs. Animal Welfare Act regulations are enforced by the USDA, whereas Public Health Service regulations are enforced by OLAW and in many cases by AAALAC.

Numbers

Accurate global figures for animal testing are difficult to obtain. The British Union for the Abolition of Vivisection (BUAV) estimates that 100 million vertebrates are experimented on around the world every year, 10–11 million of them in the European Union. The Nuffield Council on Bioethics reports that global annual estimates range from 50 to 100 million animals. None of the figures, including those given in this article, include invertebrates, such as shrimp and fruit flies. Animals bred for research then killed as surplus, animals used for breeding purposes, and animals not yet weaned (which most Labouratories do not count) are also not included in the figures.

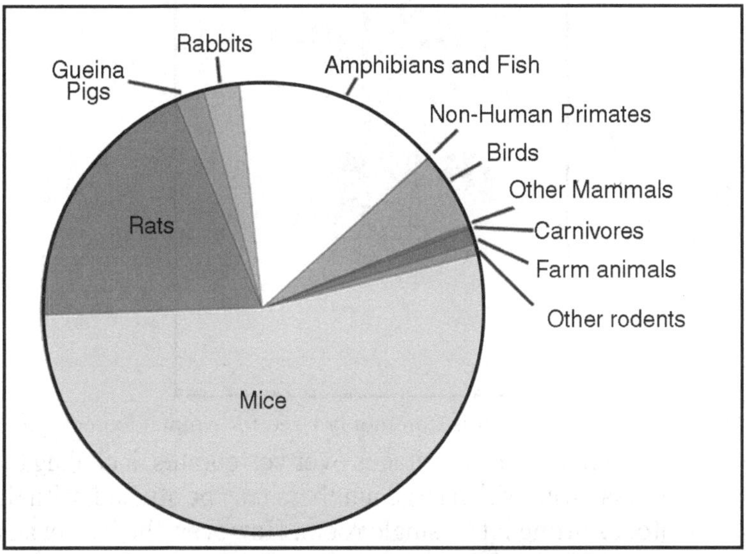

According to the U.S. Department of Agriculture (USDA), the total number of animals used in that country in 2005 was almost 1.2 million, but this does not include rats and mice, which make up about 90 per cent of research animals. In 1995, researchers at Tufts University Centre for Animals and Public Policy estimated that 14-21 million animals were used in American Labouratories in 1992, a reduction from a high of 50 million used in 1970.

In 1986, the U.S. Congress Office of Technology Assessment reported that estimates of the animals used in the U.S. range from 10 million to upwards of 100 million each year, and that their own best estimate was at least 17 million to 22 million.

In the UK, Home Office figures show that nearly three million procedures were carried out in 2004 on just under the same number of animals. It is the third consecutive annual rise and the highest figure since 1992. Most animals are used in only one procedure: animals either die because of the experiment or are euthanized afterwards. A "procedure" refers to an experiment that might last minutes, several months, or years.

SPECIES

Invertebrates

Although many more invertebrates than vertebrates are used, these experiments are largely unregulated by law. The most used invertebrate species are *Drosophila melanogaster*, a fruit fly, and *Caenorhabditis elegans*, a nematode worm. In the case of *C. elegans*, the worm's body is completely transparent and the precise lineage of all the organism's cells is known, while studies in the fly *D. melanogaster* can use an amazing array of genetic tools.

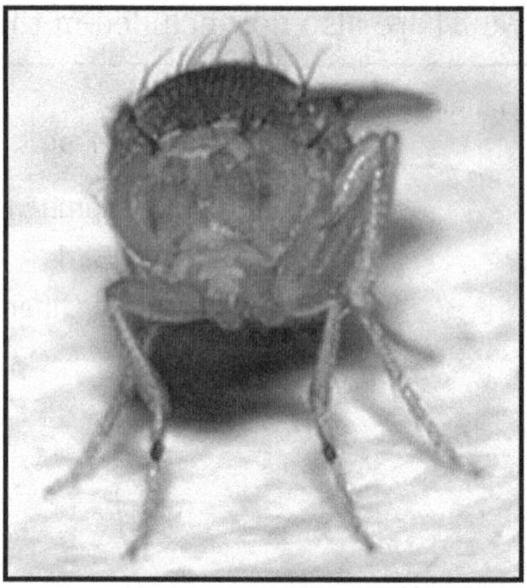

Fig. Drosophila Melanogaster is Commonly Used for Animal Experimentation.

These animals offer great advantages over vertebrates, including their short life cycle and the ease with which large numbers may be studied, with thousands of flies or nematodes fitting into a single room. However, the lack of an adaptive immune system and their simple organs prevent worms from being used in medical research such as vaccine development. Similarly, flies are not widely used in applied medical research, as their immune system differs greatly from that of humans, and diseases in insects can be very different from diseases in vertebrates.

Non-Primate Vertebrates

In the U.S., the numbers of rats and mice used is estimated at 20 million a year. Other rodents commonly used are guinea pigs, hamsters, and gerbils. Mice are the most commonly used vertebrate species because of their size, low cost, ease of handling, and fast reproductionThe water is within 1 cm of the small flower pot bottom platform where the rat sits. At the onset of REM sleep, the rat would either fall into the water only to clamber back to its pot to avoid drowning, or its nose would become submerged into the water shocking it back to an awakened state. Mice are widely considered to be the best model of inherited human disease and share 99 per cent of their genes with humans.

With the advent of genetic engineering technology, genetically modified mice can be generated to order and can provide models for a range of human diseases.

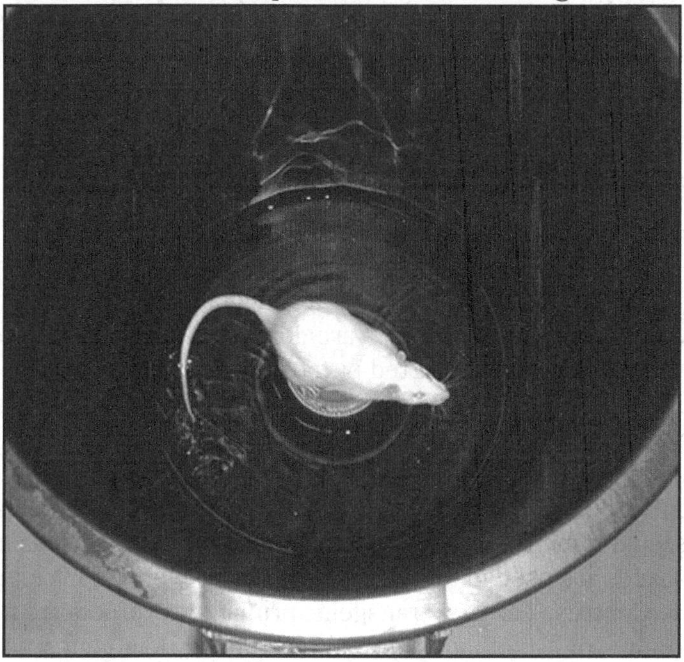

Fig. This Rat is Being Deprived of Restful REM Sleep by a Researcher Using a Single Platform ("flower pot") Technique.

Rats are also widely used for physiology, toxicology and cancer research, but genetic manipulation is much harder in rats than in mice, which limits the use of these rodents in basic science.Nearly 200,000 fish and 20,000 amphibians were used in the UK in 2004. The main species used is the zebrafish, *Danio rerio*, which are translucent during their embryonic stage, and the African clawed frog, *Xenopus laevis*. Over 20,000 rabbits were used for animal testing in the UK in 2004. Albino rabbits are used in eye irritancy tests because rabbits have less tear flow than other animals, and the lack of eye pigment in albinos make the effects easier to visualize. Rabbits are also frequently used for the production of polyclonal antibodies.

Cats and Dogs

Cats are most commonly used in neurological research. Over 25,500 cats were used in the U.S. in 2000, around half of whom were used in experiments which, according to the American Antivivisection Society, had the potential to cause "pain and/or distress". Dogs are widely used in biomedical research, testing, and education — particularly beagles, because they are gentle and easy to handle. They are commonly used as models for human diseases in cardiology, endocrinology, and bone and joint studies, research that tends to be highly invasive, according to the Humane Society of the United States. The U.S. Department of Agriculture's Animal Welfare Report for 2005 shows that 66,000 dogs were used in USDA-registered facilities in that year. In the U.S., some of the dogs are purpose-bred, while most are supplied by so-called Class B dealers licensed by the USDA to buy animals from auctions, shelters, newspaper ads, and who are sometimes accused of stealing pets.

Non-Human Primates

Non-human primates (NHPs) are used in toxicology tests, studies of AIDS and hepatitis, studies of neurology, Behaviour and cognition, reproduction, genetics, and xenotransplantation. They are caught in the wild or purpose-bred. In the U.S. and China, most primates are domestically purpose-bred, whereas in Europe the majority are imported purpose-bred.

Rhesus monkeys, cynomolgus monkeys, squirrel monkeys, and owl monkeys are imported; around 12,000 to 15,000 monkeys are imported into the U.S. annually. In total, around 70,000 NHPs are used each year in the United States and European Union. Most of the NHPs used are macaques; but marmosets, spider monkeys, and squirrel monkeys are also used, and baboons and chimpanzees are used in the U.S; in 2006 there were 1133 chimpanzees in U.S. primate Centres. The first transgenic primate was produced in 2001, with the development of a method that could introduce new genes into a rhesus macaque. This transgenic technology is now being applied in the search for a treatment for the genetic disorder Huntington's disease. Notable studies on non-human primates have been part of the polio vaccine development, and development of Deep Brain Stimulation, and their current heaviest non-toxicological use occurs in the monkey AIDS model, SIV. In 2008 a proposal to ban all primates experiments in the EU has sparked a vigorous debate.

SOURCES

Animals used by Labouratories are largely supplied by specialist dealers. Sources differ for vertebrate and invertebrate animals. Most Labouratories breed and raise flies and worms themselves, using strains and mutants supplied from a few main stock Centres. For vertebrates, sources include breeders who supply purpose-bred animals; businesses that trade in wild animals; and dealers who supply animals sourced from pounds, auctions, and newspaper ads. Animal shelters also supply the Labouratories directly. Large Centres also exist to distribute strains of genetically-modified animals; the National Institutes of Health *Knockout Mouse Project*, for example, aims to provide knockout mice for every gene in the mouse genome.

In the U.S., Class A breeders are licensed by the U.S. Department of Agriculture (USDA) to sell animals for research purposes, while Class B dealers are licensed to buy animals from "random sources" such as auctions, pound seizure, and newspaper ads. Some Class B dealers have been accused of kidnapping pets and illegally trapping strays, a practice known as *bunching*. It was in part out of public concern over the sale of pets to research facilities that the 1966 Labouratory Animal Welfare Act was ushered in — the Senate Committee on Commerce reported in 1966 that stolen pets had been retrieved from Veterans Administration facilities, the Mayo Institute, the University of Pennsylvania, Stanford University, and Harvard and Yale Medical Schools.

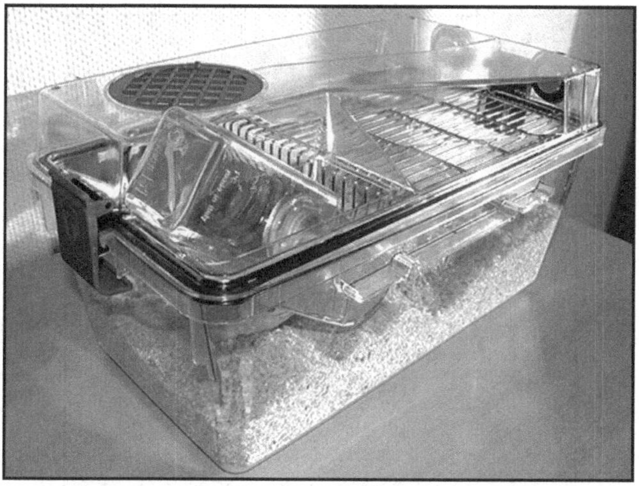

Fig. A Labouratory Mouse Cage. Mice are Either Bred Commercially, or Raised in the Labouratory.

The USDA recovered at least a dozen stolen pets during a raid on a Class B dealer in Arkansas in 2003.Four states in the U.S. — Minnesota, Utah, Oklahoma, and Iowa — require their shelters to provide animals to research facilities. Fourteen states explicitly prohibit the practice, while the remainder either allow it or have no relevant legislation. In the European Union, animal sources are governed by *Council Directive 86/609/EEC*, which requires lab animals to be specially bred, unless the animal has been lawfully imported and is not a wild animal or a stray. The latter requirement may also be exempted by special arrangement. In the UK, most animals used in experiments are bred for the purpose under the 1988 Animal Protection Act, but wild-caught primates may be used if exceptional and specific justification can be established. The United States also allows the use of wild-caught primates; between 1995 and 1999, 1,580 wild baboons were imported into the U.S. Over half the primates imported between 1995 and 2000 were handled by Charles River Labouratories, Inc., or by Covance, which is the single largest importer of primates into the U.S

Pain and Suffering

The extent to which animal testing causes pain and suffering, and the capacity of animals to experience and comprehend them, is the subject of much debate.

According to the U.S. Department of Agriculture, in 2006 about 670,000 animals (57 per cent) (not including rats, mice, birds, or invertebrates) were used in procedures that did not include more than momentary pain or distress. About 420,000 (36 per cent) were used in procedures in which pain or distress was relieved by anesthesia, while 84,000 (7 per cent) were used in studies that would cause pain or distress that would not be relieved.

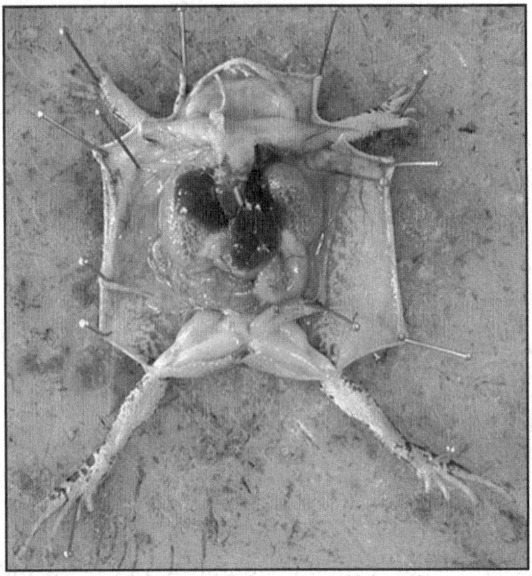

Fig. Prior to Vivisection for Educational Purposes, Chloroform was Administered to this Common Sand Frog to Induce Terminal Anesthesia.

In the UK, research projects are classified as mild, moderate, and substantial in terms of the suffering the researchers conducting the study say they may cause; a fourth category of "unclassified" means the animal was anesthetized and killed without recovering consciousness, according to the researchers. In December 2001, 39 per cent (1,296) of project licenses in force were classified as mild, 55 per cent (1,811) as moderate, two per cent (63) as substantial, and 4 per cent (139) as unclassified. There have, however, been suggestions of systemic underestimation of procedure severity.

The idea that animals might not feel pain as human beings feel it traces back to the 17th-century French philosopher, René Descartes, who argued that animals do not experience pain and suffering because they lack consciousness. Bernard Rollin of Colourado State University, the principal author of two U.S. federal laws regulating pain relief for animals, writes that researchers remained unsure into the 1980s as to whether animals experience pain, and that veterinarians trained in the U.S. before 1989 were simply taught to ignore animal pain. In his interactions with scientists and other veterinarians, he was regularly asked to "prove" that animals are conscious, and to provide "scientifically acceptable" grounds for claiming that they feel pain.

Carbone writes that the view that animals feel pain differently is now a minority view. Academic reviews of the topic are more equivocal, noting that although the argument that animals have at least simple conscious thoughts and feelings has strong support, some critics continue to question how reliably animal mental states can be determined. The ability of invertebrate species of animals, such as insects, to feel pain and suffering is also unclear.

The defining text on animal welfare regulation, "Guide for the Care and Use of Labouratory Animals" defines the parameters that govern animal testing in the USA. It states "The ability to experience and respond to pain is widespread in the animal kingdom.Pain is a stressor and, if not relieved, can lead to unacceptable levels of stress and distress in animals." The Guide states that the ability to recognize the symptoms of pain in different species is vital in efficiently applying pain relief and that it is essential for the people caring for and using animals to be entirely familiar with these symptoms.

On the subject of analgesics used to relieve pain, the Guide states "The selection of the most appropriate analgesic or anesthetic should reflect professional judgment as to which best meets clinical and humane requirements without compromising the scientific aspects of the research protocol". Accordingly, all issues of animal pain and distress, and their potential treatment with analgesia and anesthesia, are required regulatory issues in receiving animal protocol approval.

EUTHANASIA

There is general agreement that animal life should not be taken wantonly, and regulations require that scientists use as few animals as possible. However, while policy makers consider suffering to be the central issue and see animal euthanasia as a way to reduce suffering, others, such as the RSPCA, argue that the lives of Labouratory animals have intrinsic value. Regulations focus on whether particular methods cause pain and suffering, not whether their death is undesirable in itself. The animals are euthanized at the end of studies for sample collection or post-mortem examination; during studies if their pain or suffering falls into certain categories regarded as unacceptable, such as depression, infection that is unresponsive to treatment, or the failure of large animals to eat for five days; or when they are unsuitable for breeding or unwanted for some other reason.

Methods of euthanizing Labouratory animals are chosen to induce rapid unconsciousness and death without pain or distress. The methods that are preferred are those published by councils of veterinarians. The animal can be made to inhale a gas, such as carbon monoxide and carbon dioxide, by being placed in a chamber, or by use of a face mask, with or without prior sedation or anesthesia. Sedatives or anesthetics such as barbiturates can be given intravenously, or inhalant anesthetics may be used. Amphibians and fish may be immersed in water containing an anesthetic such as tricaine. Physical methods are also used, with or without sedation or anesthesia depending on the method. Recommended methods include decapitation (beheading) for small rodents or rabbits. Cervical dislocation (breaking the neck or spine) may be used for birds, mice, and immature rats and rabbits. Maceration (grinding into small pieces) is used on 1 day old chicks. High-intensity microwave irradiation of the brain can preserve brain tissue and induce death in less than 1 second, but this is currently only used on rodents. Captive bolts may be used, typically on dogs, ruminants, horses, pigs and rabbits. It causes death by a concussion to the brain.

Gunshot may be used, but only in cases where a penetrating captive bolt may not be used. Some physical methods are only acceptable after the animal is unconscious. Electrocution may be used for cattle, sheep, swine, foxes, and mink after the animals are unconscious, often by a prior electrical stun. Pithing (inserting a tool into the base of the brain) is usable on animals already unconscious. Slow or rapid freezing, or inducing air embolism are acceptable only with prior anesthesia to induce unconsciousness.

GENERAL USE

NHPs are used in research into HIV, neurology, Behaviour, cognition, reproduction, Parkinson's disease, stroke, malaria, respiratory viruses, infectious disease, genetics, xenotransplantation, drug abuse, and also in vaccine and drug testing. According to The Humane Society of the United States, chimpanzees are most often used in hepatitis research, and monkeys in SIV research. Animals used in hepatitis and SIV studies are often caged alone. Eighty-two per cent of primate procedures in the UK in 2006 were in applied studies, which the Home Office defines as research conducted for the purpose of developing or testing commercial products. Toxicology testing is the largest use, which includes legislatively required testing of drugs. The second largest category of research using primates is "protection of man, animals, or environment", accounting for 8.9 per cent of all procedures in 2006. The third largest category is "fundamental biological research,", accounting for 4.9 per cent of all UK primate procedures in 2006. This includes neuroscientific study of the visual system, cognition, and diseases such as Parkinson's, involving techniques such as inserting electrodes to record from or stimulate the brain, and temporary or permanent inactivation of areas of tissue.

Primates are the species most likely to be re-used in experiments. The Research Defence Society writes that re-use is allowed if the animals have been used in mild procedures with no lasting side-effects. This is contradicted by Dr. Gill Langley of the British Union for the Abolition of Vivisection, who gives as an example of re-use the licence granted to Cambridge University to conduct brain experiments on marmosets. The protocol sheet stated that the animals would receive "multiple interventions as part of the whole lesion/graft repair procedure."

Under the protocol, a marmoset could be given acute brain lesions under general anaesthetic, followed by tissue implantation under a second general anaesthetic, followed again central cannula implantation under a third. The re-use is allowable when required to meet scientific goals, such as this case in which some procedures are required as preparatory for others.

METHODS OF RESTRAINT

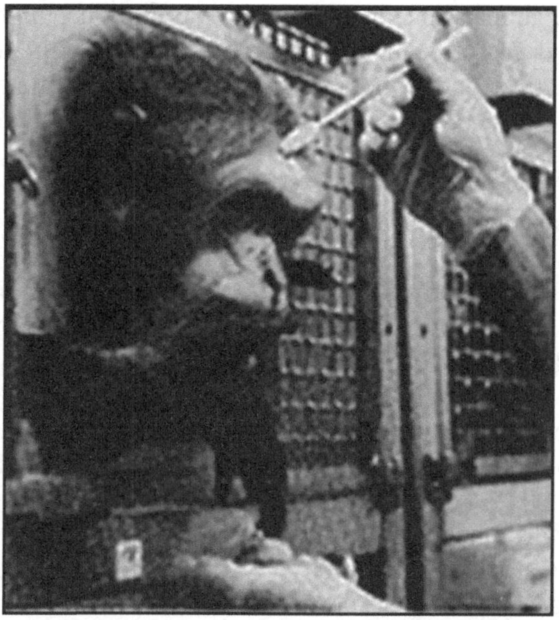

Fig. The Holes are Placed in Such a Way as to Allow the Primate to Reach for Food While Presenting his Head for the Experiment.

One of the disadvantages of using NHPs is that they can be difficult to handle, and various methods of physical restraint have to be used. Viktor Reinhardt of the Wisconsin Regional Primate Research Centre writes that scientists may be unaware of the way in which their research animals are handled, and therefore fail to take into account the effect the handling may have had on the animals' health, and thereby on any data collected. Reinhardt writes that primatologists have long recognized that restraint methods may introduce an "uncontrolled methodological variable", by producing resistance and fear in the animal. "Numerous reports have been published demonstrating that non-human primates can readily be trained to cooperate rather than resist during common handling procedures such as capture, venipuncture, injection and veterinary examination. Cooperative animals fail to show behavioural and physiological signs of distress."

Reinhardt lists common restraint methods as: squeeze-back cages, manual restraint, restraint boards, restraint chairs, restraint chutes, tethering, and nets. Alternatives include:

- Chemical restraint; for example, ketamine, a sedative, may be given to the animal before a restraint procedure, reducing stress-hormone production;
- Psychological support, in which an animal under restraint has visual and auditory contact with the animal's cage-mate. Blood pressure and heart rate responses to restraint have been measurably reduced using psychological support.
- Training animals to cooperate with restraint. Such methods have been used and resulted in unmeasurable stress hormone responses to venipuncture, and no notable distress to being captured in a transport box.

Chimpanzees in the U.S.

There are around 1133 chimpanzees in research Labouratories in the United State as of October 2006, and this number has been monotonically decreasing since the breeding ban of 1996. Many have been used in hepatitis research, often caged alone because of the design of the research protocol. Chimps routinely live 30 years in captivity, and can reach 60 years of age.

Most of the labs either conduct or make the chimps available for invasive research, defined as "inoculation with an infectious agent, surgery or biopsy conducted for the sake of research and not for the sake of the chimpanzee, and/ or drug testing.

" Two federally funded Labouratories use chimps: Yerkes National Primate Research Centre at Emory University in Atlanta, Georgia, and the Southwest National Primate Centre in San Antonio, Texas. Five hundred chimps have been retired from Labouratory use in the U.S. and live in sanctuaries in the U.S. or Canada.

Their importation from the wild was banned in 1973. From then until 1996, chimpanzees in U.S. facilities were bred domestically. Some others were transferred from the entertainment industry to animal testing facilities as recently as 1983, although it is not known if any animals that were transferred from the entertainment industry are still in testing Centres. Animal sanctuaries were not an option until the first North American sanctuary that would accept chimps opened in 1976.

In 1986, to prepare for research on AIDS, the U.S. bred them aggressively, with 315 breeding chimpanzees used to produce 400 offspring. By 1996, it was clear that SIV/HIV-2/SHIV in macaque monkeys was a preferred scientific AIDS model to the chimps, which meant there was a surplus.

A five-year moratorium on breeding was therefore imposed by the U.S. National Institutes of Health (NIH) that year, and it has been extended annually since 2001. As of October 2006, the chimp population in US Labouratories had declined to 1133 from a peak of 1500 in 1996. Chimpanzees tend to be used repeatedly over decades, rather than used and killed as with most Labouratory animals. Some individual chimps currently in U.S. Labouratories have been used in experiments for over 40 years. The oldest known chimp in a U.S. lab is Wenka, who was born in a Labouratory in Florida on May 21, 1954. She was removed from her mother on the day of birth to be used in a vision experiment that lasted 17 months, then sold as a pet to a family in North Carolina. She was returned to the Yerkes National Primate Research Centre in 1957 when she became too big to handle. Since then, she has given birth six times, and has been used in research into alcohol use, oral contraceptives, aging, and cognitive studies.

With the publication of the chimpanzee genome, there are reportedly plans to increase the use of chimps in labs, with scientists arguing that the federal moratorium on breeding chimps for research should be lifted. Other researchers argue that chimps are unique animals and should either not be used in research, or should be treated differently.

Pascal Gagneux, an evolutionary biologist and primate expert at the University of California, San Diego, argues that, given chimpanzees' sense of self, tool use, and genetic similarity to human beings, studies using chimps should follow the ethical guidelines that are used for human subjects unable to give consent.

Stuart Zola, director of the Yerkes National Primate Research Labouratory, disagrees. He told *National Geographic*: "I don't think we should make a distinction between our obligation to treat humanely any species, whether it's a rat or a monkey or a chimpanzee. No matter how much we may wish it, chimps are not human."

A list of facilities holding chimpanzees and the numbers:

- Alamogordo Primate Facility (affiliated with the National Institutes of Health and Charles River Labouratories) at Holloman Airforce base (245)
- M.D. Anderson Cancer Centre, affiliated with the University of Texas (133)
- New Iberia Research Centre, affiliated with the University of Louisiana (342)
- Primate Foundation of Arizona (a holding facility), affiliated with M.D. Anderson/University of Texas (73)
- Southwest National Primate Research Centre, affiliated with the Southwest Foundation for Biomedical Research (236)
- Yerkes National Primate Research Centre, affiliated with Emory University and Georgia State University (109 held); BIOQUAL, Inc. (15)
- Language Research Centre, Georgia State University (4)
- Centres for Disease Control and Prevention (18)
- Food & Drug Administration (11 held) National Institutes of Health (11).

NOTABLE STUDIES

Polio

In the 1940s, Jonas Salk used Rhesus monkey cross-contamination studies to isolate the three forms of the polio virus that crippled hundreds of thousands of people yearly across the world at the time. Salk's team created a vaccine against the strains of polio in cell cultures of Green monkey kidney cells. The vaccine was made publicly available in 1955, and reduced the incidence of polio 15-fold in the USA over the following five years. Albert Sabin made a superior "live" vaccine by passing the polio virus through animal hosts, including monkeys. The vaccine was produced for mass consumption in 1963 and is still in use today. It had virtually eradicated polio in the USA by 1965. It has been estimated that 100,000 monkeys were killed in the course of developing the polio vaccines, and 65 doses of vaccine were produced for each monkey.

Split-Brain Experiments

In the 1950s, Roger Sperry developed split-brain preparations in non-human primates that emphasized the importance of information transfer that occurred in these neocortical connections. For example, learning on simple tasks, if restricted in sensory input and motor output to one hemisphere of a split-brain animal, would not transfer to the other hemisphere. The right brain has no idea what the left brain is up to, if these specific connections are cut.

Those experiments were followed by tests on human beings with epilepsy who had undergone split-brain surgery, which established that the neocortical connections between hemispheres are the principal route for cognition to transfer from one side of the brain to another. These experiments also formed the modern basis for lateralization of function in the human brain.

Vision Experiments

In the 1960s, David Hubel and Torsten Wiesel demonstrated the macrocolumnar organization of visual areas in cats and monkeys, and provided physiological evidence for the critical period for the development of disparity sensitivity in vision (ie: the main cue for depth perception). They were awarded a Nobel Prize for their work.

Deep-Brain Stimulation

In 1983, designer drug users took MPTP, which created a Parkinsonian syndrome. Later that same year, researchers reproduced the effect in non-human primates. Over the next seven years, the brain areas that were over- and under-active in Parkinson's were mapped out in normal and MPTP-treated macaque monkeys using metabolic labelling and microelectrode studies. In 1990, deep brain lesions were shown to treat Parkinsonian symptoms in macaque monkeys treated with MPTP, and these were followed by pallidotomy operations in humans with similar efficacy. By 1993, it was shown that deep brain stimulation could effect the same treatment without causing a permanent lesion of the same magnitude. Deep brain stimulation has largely replaced pallidotomy for treatment of Parkinson's patients that require neurosurgical intervention. Current estimates are that 20,000 Parkinson's patients have received this treatment.

AIDS

The non-human primate models of AIDS, using HIV-2, SHIV, and SIV in macaques, have been used as a complement to ongoing research efforts against the virus. The drug tenofovir has had its efficacy and toxicology evaluated in macaques, and found longterm-highdose treatments had adverse effects not found using shortterm-highdose treatment followed by longterm-lowdose treatment. This finding in macaques was translated into human dosing regimens. Prophylactic treatment with anti-virals has been evaluated in macaques, because introduction of the virus can only be controlled in an animal model. The finding that prophylaxis can be effective at blocking infection has altered the treatment for occupational exposures, such as needle exposures. Such exposures are now followed rapidly with anti-HIV drugs, and this practice has resulted in measurable transient virus infection similar to the NHP model.

ALLEGATIONS

Many of the best-known allegations of abuse made by animal protection or animal rights groups against animal-testing facilities involve NHPs.

University of Wisconsin–Madison

The so-called "pit of despair" was used in experiments conducted on rhesus macaque monkeys during the 1970s by American comparative psychologist Harry Harlow at the University of Wisconsin–Madison. The aim of the research was to produce clinical depression. The vertical chamber was a stainless-steel bin with slippery sides that sloped to a rounded bottom. A 3/8 in. wire mesh floor 1 in. above the bottom of the chamber allowed waste material to drop out of holes. The chamber had a food box and a water-bottle holder, and was covered with a pyramid top so that the monkeys were unable to escape. Harlow placed baby monkeys in the chamber alone for up to six weeks. Within a few days, they stopped moving about and remained huddled in a corner. The monkeys generally exhibited marked social impairment and peer hostility when removed from the chamber; most did not recover.

University of California

On April 21, 1985, activists of the Animal Liberation Front (ALF) broke into the UC Riverside Labouratories and removed hundreds of animals.

According to Vicky Miller of PETA, who reported the raid to newswire services, UC-Riverside "has been using animals in experiments on sight deprivation and isolation for the last two years and has recently received a grant, paid for with our tax dollars, to continue torturing and killing animals." According to UCR officials, the ALF claims of animal mistreatment were "absolutely false," and the raid would result in long-term damage to some of the research projects, including those aimed at developing devices and treatment for blindness. UCR officials also reported the raid also included smashing equipment and resulted in several hundred thousand dollars of damage.

In Germany in 2004, journalist Friedrich Mülln took undercover footage of staff in Covance in Münster, Europe's largest primate-testing Centre. Staff were filmed handling monkeys roughly, screaming at them, and making them dance to blaring music. The monkeys were shown isolated in small wire cages with little or no natural light, no environmental enrichment, and subjected to high noise levels from staff shouting and playing the radio. Primatologist Jane Goodall described their living conditions as "horrendous."

A veterinary toxicologist employed as a study director at Covance in Vienna, Virginia from 2002 to 2004, told city officials in Chandler, Arizona, that Covance was dissecting monkeys while the animals were still alive and able to feel pain. The employee approached the city with her concerns when she learned that Covance planned to build a new Labouratory in Chandler.

She alleged that three monkeys in the Vienna Labouratory had pushed themselves up on their elbows and had gasped for breath after their eyes had been removed, and while their intestines were being removed during necropsies (autopsy). When she expressed concern at the next study directors' meeting, she says she was told that it was just a reflex. She told city officials that she believed such movements were not reflexes but suggested "botched euthanasia performed by inadequately trained personnel." She alleged that she was ridiculed and subjected to thinly veiled threats when she contacted her supervisors about the issue.

In the UK, after an undercover investigation in 1998, the British Union for the Abolition of Vivisection (BUAV), a lobby group, reported that researchers in Cambridge University's primate-testing labs were sawing the tops off marmosets' heads, inducing strokes, then leaving them overnight without veterinarian care, because staff worked only nine to five. The experiments used marmosets that were first trained to perform certain Behavioural and cognitive tasks, then re-tested after brain damage to determine how the damage had affected their skills. The monkeys were deprived of food and water to encourage them to perform the tasks, with water being withheld for 22 out of every 24 hours. The Research Defence Society defended Cambridge's research. The RDS wrote that the monkeys were fully anaesthetised, and appropriate pain killers were given after the surgery. "On recovery from the anaesthesia, the monkeys were kept in an incubator, offered food and water and monitored at regular intervals until the early evening. They were then allowed to sleep in the incubators until the next morning. No monkeys died unattended during the night after stroke surgery." A court rejected BUAV's application for a judicial review. BUAV has appealed and a decision is expected in 2006. In 2003, CNN reported that a post-doctoral veterinarian at Columbia University complained to the university's Institutional Animal Care and Use Committee about experiments being conducted on baboons by E. Sander Connolly, an assistant professor of neurosurgery.

Connolly was mimicking strokes by removing the baboons' left eyeballs and using the empty sockets to reach and clamp a particular blood vessel in their brains. He would then test a neuroprotective drug on the baboon. The baboons were kept alive after the surgery for observation for three to ten days in a state of "profound disability" which would have been "terrifying," according to neurologist Robert Hoffman. Connolly's published animal model states that animals were kept alive for three days, and that animals that were successfully self-caring were kept alive for 10 days. People for the Ethical Treatment of Animals published the description of one experiment:

On September 19, 2001, baboon B777's left eye was removed, and a stroke was induced. The next morning, it was noted that the animal could not sit up, that he was leaning over, and that he could not eat. That evening, the baboon was still slouched over and was offered food but couldn't chew. On September 21, 2001, the record shows that the baboon was 'awake, but no movement, can't eat (chew), vomited in the a.m.' With no further notation about consulting with a veterinarian, the record reads, 'At 1:30 p.m. the animal died in the cage.'"

An investigation by the U.S. Department of Agriculture found "no indication that the experiments.violated federal guidelines." The Dean of Research at Columbia's School of Medicine said that Connolly had stopped the experiments because of threats from animal rights activists, but still believed his work was humane and potentially valuable.

Attacks on Researchers

In 2006, activists forced a primate researcher at UCLA to shut down the experiments in his lab. His name, phone number, and address were posted on the website of the UCLA Primate Freedom Project, along with a description of his research, which stated that he had "received a grant to kill 30 macaque monkeys for vision experiments. Each monkey is first paralyzed, then used for a single session that lasts up to 120 hours, and finally killed." [13] Demonstrations were held outside his home. A Molotov cocktail was placed on the porch of what was believed to be the home of another UCLA primate researcher. Instead, it was accidentally left on the porch of an elderly woman unrelated to the university. The Animal Liberation Front claimed responsibility for the attack. As a result of the campaign, the researcher sent an email to the Primate Freedom Project stating "you win," and "please don't bother my family anymore." In another incident at UCLA in June 2007, the Animal Liberation Brigade placed a bomb under the car of a UCLA children's ophthalmologist, who performs experiments on cats and rhesus monkeys; the bomb had a faulty fuse and did not detonate. UCLA is now refusing Freedom of Information Act requests for animal medical records.

The house of UCLA researcher Edythe London was intentionally flooded on October 20, 2007 in an attack claimed by the Animal Liberation Front. London conducts research on addiction using non-human primates, although no claims were made by the ALF of any violation of any rules or regulations regarding the use of animals in research.

SURGERY

MULTIPLE MAJOR SURGICAL PROCEDURES

The ILAR Guide differentiates major from minor surgery as follows: "Major survival surgery penetrates and exposes a body cavity or produces substantial impairment of physical or physiologic functions. Minor survival surgery does not expose a body cavity and causes little or no physical impairment." Minimally invasive surgery such as laparoscopy may benefit the animal relative to traditional surgical techniques.

Performance of more than one major survival surgical procedure on a single animal is discouraged but may be necessary to ensure or maintain the health of the animal. Long-lived animals may undergo multiple major surgeries, such as a cow that requires surgery for correction of displaced abomasum and cesarean section for therapeutic purposes. Multiple major survival surgeries performed for nontherapeutic reasons should be performed only when justified and must be reviewed and approved by the IACUC. Multiple major surgeries that produce minor physiologic or physical impairment and reduce overall animal use, such as multiple endoscopic laparotomies in sheep for reproductive purposes, might be appropriate. Likewise, multiple surgical procedures might be justified when they are related components of the same project.

ANESTHESIA AND ANALGESIA

Certain animal husbandry-related procedures may be conducted without anesthesia after consideration and approval by the IACUC. These procedures should be performed early in the life of the animal in accordance with accepted veterinary practices. When surgery is performed on older animals, appropriate anesthesia and sterile instruments should be used, trauma minimized, and hemorrhage controlled. It is important that husbandry practices be established to minimize stress, prevent infection, and ensure the comfort of the animals during the recovery period. Specific recommendations for each species are provided in subsequent chapters. The attending veterinarian should advise investigators about the choice and use of analgesics and/or anesthetics or any other pain-or distress-relieving measure, including recommended times for withholding of food and water.

After being trained and subsequently supervised by a qualified scientist or veterinarian, technical personnel may administer anesthetics and analgesics as part of a research or teaching protocol. If a painful or distressful experimental procedure must be conducted without the use of an anesthetic or analgesic because such use would prevent collection of useful data, this must be scientifically documented in the animal care and use protocol and approved by the IACUC. Paralytic drugs are not anesthetics. They must not be used unless animals are in a surgical plane of anesthesia and thus unconscious.

Use of paralytic agents must be justified in the animal use protocol and appropriate monitoring for depth of anesthesia described. Tranquilizers are psychotropic substances that alter mental processes or behaviour but do not produce anesthesia. These medications can reduce the dose of anesthetic required. When used alone, tranquilizers should only be used to allay fear and anxiety. Their use may render restraint less stressful and enable animals to adapt more easily to novel situations.

SURGERY PERSONNEL

Inappropriately performed surgical techniques or inadequate postoperative care will result in unnecessary pain and distress. Experimental surgery on agricultural animals should be performed or supervised by an experienced veterinarian or his/her designee in accordance with established protocols approved by an IACUC. Institutions must provide basic surgical training and opportunities to upgrade surgical skills for persons who will conduct or assist with experimental surgery. The training programme must be reviewed by the IACUC and under the direction of the attending veterinarian or his/her designee. Training provided must be documented and the competency of personnel assured.

SURGICAL FACILITIES AND ASEPTIC TECHNIQUE

Major survival surgeries should be performed in facilities designed and prepared to accommodate surgery whenever possible, and appropriate aseptic surgical procedures should be employed. Good surgical practice includes the use of surgical caps, masks, gowns, and gloves, as well as aseptic surgical site preparation and draping. Sterile instruments must be used.

Manufacturers' recommendations must be followed for chemical sterilants. For nonsurvival surgeries, during which the animal is euthanized before recovery from anesthesia, it may not be necessary to follow all aseptic techniques, but the instruments and surrounding area should be clean. Minor surgical procedures that do not penetrate a body cavity or produce substantial impairment may be performed under less stringent conditions if performed in accord with standard veterinary practices. Therapeutic and emergency surgeries may sometimes need to be performed in agricultural settings that are not conducive to rigid asepsis. However, every effort should be made to conduct such surgeries in a sanitary or aseptic manner and to use anesthetics and analgesics commensurate with the risks to the animal's well-being. Research protocols that carry a high likelihood of the need for emergency surgery should contain provisions for handling anticipated cases. Surgical packs and equipment for such events should be prepared and be readily available for emergency use.

POSTSURGICAL CARE

Appropriate facilities should be available for animals that are recovering from general anesthesia and major surgery.

The following are required:

- Segregation from other animals until recovery from anesthesia;
- Clean and sanitary recovery area;
- Adequate space, with consideration for physical comfort and well-being of the animal, in a place suitable for recovery from anesthesia without injury;
- Environmental controls sufficient to ensure maintenance of environmental temperature within the thermoneutral zone and animal temperature within the normal range during postsurgical recovery; and
- Trained personnel for postsurgical observation to help to ensure a safe recovery.
- Postsurgical observation should be provided until the animal is fully recovered from anesthesia, ambulatory, and able to safely return to its original housing location.

SIGNS OF PAIN AND DISTRESS

Pain is a sensation of discomfort that may lead to distress and feelings of urgency. Although pain and distress in animals can often be detected by an experienced observer, these conditions can sometimes be unapparent, especially in stoic animals. When unanticipated pain and distress are detected, animal-care attendants or research staff should take immediate ameliorative action as necessary and contact the attending veterinarian.

Pain can be one of the earliest signs of disease or injury. Animals in pain may become less active, restless, may continually get up and down, and refuse to stay in one place, reduce feed consumption, grind their teeth, or vocalize. Some animals become less active, whereas others appear frightened or agitated. Animals in pain may resist handling or favour the painful area by adopting an abnormal stance or abnormal behaviour. In some cases, pain may not be noticed until a physiological act is induced such as swallowing, coughing, chewing, or defecating.

The observer should try to determine whether pain appears to be constant or associated with a provoking act. Sudden, severe pain is often associated with fractures, rupture or torsion of visceral organs, or acute inflammatory processes and should be considered an emergency. Relief of pain and/or distress in agricultural animals involves removing or correcting the inciting cause when possible, administering appropriate analgesics, and taking steps to reduce stimulation of pain receptors.

Relief of pain should be one of the first tasks of the attending veterinarian, adhering to the following principles:

- Relief of pain is a humane act;
- Relief of pain must be initiated promptly once it is deemed necessary;
- It may be necessary to protect animals in pain from self-injury.

The attending veterinarian must be familiar with analgesics labeled for use in agricultural animals and must be able to prescribe and establish withdrawal times for extra-label use of analgesics when indicated. Animals with severe or chronic pain that cannot be alleviated must be euthanized.

ZOONOSES

For the purposes of this guide, zoonotic diseases are defined as infectious diseases in agricultural animals used in research and teaching that can be transmitted to humans and a natural reservoir for the infectious agent is an agricultural animal. Zoonotic pathogens, mode of transmission, disease signs in ruminants, and disease signs and symptoms in humans. A current list and incidence of notifiable diseases such as Q-fever may be obtained from the US Centers for Disease Control and Prevention.

The attending veterinarian, working with the animal scientists, should establish appropriate preventive medicine programmes and husbandry practices to decrease the likelihood of transmission of zoonotic agents. Each institution must have an appropriate occupational health and safety programme for evaluating the human health risks associated with animal contact and must take steps to ensure that health risks for each individual are assessed and managed to an acceptable level.

RESIDUE AVOIDANCE

Residues of 3 groups of chemicals must be prevented from occurring in research animals if those animals, or their products, are going into the human food chain.

These are:

1. Approved drugs used according to directions on the label,
2. Drugs used in an extra-label fashion, and
3. Other chemicals such as herbicides, pesticides, and wood preservatives.

The Food Animal Residue Avoidance Database is a project sponsored by the USDA Cooperative State Research, Education and Extension Service. The FARAD *Compendium of FDA Approved Drugs* provides information about drugs that are available for treating animal diseases, the withholding times for milk and eggs, and preslaughter withdrawal times for meat. Information about the drugs approved for use in food animals in the United States is included in this online database. The FARAD compendium allows selection of over-the-counter products that satisfy particular needs as well as alerts to the need for veterinary assistance with prescription drugs; FARAD also supplies estimated meat and milk withdrawal times for extra-label use of drugs. Drug administration to animals destined to enter the food chain requires special consideration.Before animals may be slaughtered for human or animal food purposes, time must be allowed for medications, drugs approved by the Food and Drug Administration (FDA), or substances allowed by the FDA for experimental testing under the Investigational New Animal Drug (INAD) exemption to be depleted from the tissues. Such use is only permitted when it adheres to the regulations in the Animal Medicinal Drug Use Clarification Act of 1994, Public Law 103-396. A record of the product used, dose, route of administration, duration of treatment, and period of withdrawal must be maintained. Adherence to proper withdrawal times must be ensured before animals are transported to the auction, market, or abattoir.

DRUG STORAGE AND CONTROL

Pharmaceuticals intended for use in food-producing animals must be managed responsibly. Storage should be in an area that is clean and dry and that offers protection from changes in temperature, sunlight, dust, moisture, and vermin. The manufacturer's labeling should be consulted for specific information regarding appropriate storage conditions and product shelf-life. In addition, the integrity of product containers should be periodically evaluated to assess for potential leakage or contamination of the stored product.Products in damaged containers or with missing or illegible labels should be disposed of properly. To minimize the potential for treatment errors, products should be physically segregated according to indicated use, with special attention to separate drugs that are intended only for animals of a certain age or production state. For large inventories, separate storage cabinets for each group of products will further reduce the opportunity for errors in selection and use. When necessary, lockable storage units should be used to prevent access by unauthorized persons.

RECORD KEEPING

Records of all potentially harmful products used in the facility, their storage, their use, and their disposal should be maintained. Such record keeping should be similar to the quality assurance programmes used by responsible farmers in the food animal industry. If used in accord with the label and with allowance for the correct withdrawal time, approved drugs should not result in violative residues. Record-keeping and management should be audited and should confirm that drugs are not outdated and that the directions on the label have been followed. Records should be maintained for at least 3 months or in timelines consistent with state and federal requirements as they apply.

QUALITY ASSURANCE PROGRAMMES

The food animal industries have developed several quality assurance programmes such as:

- The Milk and Dairy Beef Quality Assurance Programme,
- The Beef Quality Assurance Programme,
- The United Egg Producers Five Star Quality Assurance Programme,
- The Pork Quality Assurance Programme, and
- The Veal Producer Quality Assurance Programme.

Agricultural research or teaching programmes using animals that may be slaughtered for human consumption must institute quality assurance programmes that are equivalent or superior to those used in the food animal industries. Many food animal industries, private corporations, and humane organizations have also developed animal welfare assurance programmes that should be referenced.

REGULATORY OVERSIGHT

In the event that animals are given a new animal drug for investigational purposes, no meat, eggs, or milk from those animals may be processed for human food, unless authorization has been granted by the FDA or the USDA, and an appropriate INAD exemption from the FDA has been obtained for use of the investigational drug. In such cases, the investigator must follow specifications outlined in the INAD.

The authorization to process meat, eggs, or milk from such animals for human food will depend on the development of data to show that the consumption of food from animals so treated is consistent with public health considerations and that the food does not contain the residues of harmful drugs or their metabolites. In the event that animals are given a new animal drug, no meat, eggs, or milk from those animals may be processed for human food consumption under any circumstances. Proper methods of disposal of such meat, eggs, and milk may include incineration, burial, or other procedures ensuring safety, sanitation, and avoidance of the human food supply.

EXTRA-LABEL USE

The use of different dosages, formulations, or routes of administration, or the treatment of animals for conditions not specifically mentioned on the product label, constitutes extra-label use. Such use may be considered by licensed veterinarians when the health of the animal is immediately threatened and when suffering or death would result from failure to treat the affected animal. Such use is only permitted when it adheres to the regulations promulgated by the FDA under the Animal Medicinal Drug Use Clarification Act (AMDUCA) of 1994, Public Law 103-396.

The major principles guiding such use are that:

- There must be a valid relationship between veterinarian, client, and patient, and
- There must be an adequate safety margin in the withdrawal time that is based on the most complete pharmacokinetic data available.

The FDA should be contacted whenever guidance is needed.

ORGANIC FARMING

Some institutions have organic farming components. The US National Organic Standards state that "producers must not withhold medical treatment from a sick animal to maintain its organic status. All appropriate medications and treatments must be used to restore an animal to health when methods acceptable to organic production standards fail." It is important that research animals managed under organic standards be provided prompt and adequate health care as necessary even if the animal will, as a result, be removed from organic production.

HAZARDOUS CHEMICALS

There are many chemicals used on farms and in agricultural research establishments that could potentially result in residues in the meat, milk, or eggs of animals exposed to these chemicals. Examples are pesticides for insect control, herbicides, poisons for rodent control, wood preservatives, and disinfectants. Harmful products should be properly labeled and stored, a record of their purchase and expiration dates should be kept, and personnel must be informed of potential hazards and wear appropriate protective equipment. Chemicals must be stored, used, and disposed of in a manner that prevents contamination of animals and residues in milk, meat, or eggs.

RESTRAINT

Brief physical restraint of agricultural animals for examination, collection of samples, and a variety of other experimental and clinical manipulations can be accomplished manually or with devices such as stocks, head gates, stanchions, or squeeze chutes. It is important that such devices be suitable in size and design for the animal being held and be operated properly to minimize stress and avoid pain and injury. Personnel should be trained on the use of hydraulically operated restraint devices to prevent potential injury. Extended physical restraint should be reviewed and approved by the IACUC.

TRANSGENIC AND GENETICALLY ENGINEERED AND CLONED ANIMALS

Recent years have seen a growing interest in the development and use of transgenic and genetically modified agricultural animals for agricultural and human therapeutic purposes. A transgenic animal is one that carries a foreign gene that has been deliberately inserted into its genome. Genetically engineered animal models require deliberate modification of the animal genome by moving a desired trait into the genome.

These modifications are accomplished by microinjection, retroviral transfection, and a variety of other techniques. It is important not to confuse genetically engineered animals with cloned animals. Genetically engineered animals may be produced by cloning as well. The progeny of cloned animals are not properly termed "cloned animals." It is also important to distinguish between research and commercial application of cloning techniques.

Cloning technology has been reviewed by the FDA and is one of several commercially available assisted reproductive technologies including in vitro fertilization and embryo transfer. As advancements in research continue and new technologies are developed, specific considerations may need to be made for the care and use of agricultural animals.

Both transgenic and genetically engineered animal models may have physiologic or phenotypic problems including abortions, large offspring, enlarged umbilicus, retained placenta, hydrops, multiple births, and placenta deformities. The scientist is responsible for identifying physiologic and phenotypic changes and must have a plan to address changes that affect animal health to facilitate and ensure animal welfare. The US FDA is responsible for approving the use of genetically modified foods in the United States under the Food, Drug, and Cosmetic Act of 1992.

EUTHANASIA

Protocols for euthanasia should follow current guidelines established by the American Veterinary Medical Association and copies of the protocols should be made available to all personnel who euthanize animals. The agents and methods of euthanasia appropriate for agricultural animals are available in the AVMA Guidelines for Euthanasia or subsequent revisions of that document. Euthanasia is the procedure of killing an animal rapidly, painlessly, and without distress.

Euthanasia must be carried out by trained personnel using acceptable techniques in accordance with applicable regulations and policies. The method used should not interfere with postmortem evaluations. Proper euthanasia involves skilled personnel to help ensure that the technique is performed humanely and effectively and to minimize risk of injury to people. Personnel who perform euthanasia must have training and experience with the techniques to be used. This training and experience must include familiarity with the normal behaviour of agricultural animals and how handling and restraint affect their behaviour.

The equipment and materials required to perform euthanasia should be readily available, and the attending veterinarian or a qualified animal scientist should ensure that all personnel performing euthanasia have demonstrated proficiency in the use of the techniques selected. Acceptable methods of euthanasia are those that initially depress the central nervous system to ensure insensitivity to pain.

Euthanasia techniques should result in rapid unconsciousness followed by cardiac or respiratory arrest and the ultimate loss of brain function. In addition, the technique used should minimize any stress and anxiety experienced by the animal before unconsciousness. For this reason, anesthetic agents are generally acceptable, and animals of most species can be quickly and humanely euthanized with the appropriate injection of an overdose of a barbiturate.

Certain other methods may be used for euthanasia of anesthetized animals because the major criterion has been fulfilled. Physical methods of euthanasia may be used. Every attempt should be made to minimize stress to the animal before euthanasia. Personnel must be trained on the proper use of the captive bolt per species, and the captive bolt device must be appropriately maintained. Electrocution is an acceptable means of euthanasia if the electrodes are placed so that the current travels through the brain and through the heart.

Methods in which the current is directed through the heart only are not acceptable. It is imperative to ensure that the animal is indeed dead. Techniques that apply electric current from head to tail, head to foot, or head to moistened metal plates on which the animal is standing are unacceptable. Agents that result in tissue residues cannot be used for euthanasia of animals intended for human or animal food unless those agents are approved by the FDA.

Carbon dioxide is the only chemical currently used for euthanasia of food animals that does not lead to tissue residues. The carcasses of animals euthanized by barbiturates may contain potentially harmful residues and should be disposed of in a manner that prevents them from being consumed by human beings or animals. No matter what method of euthanasia is performed, personnel must ensure that death has occurred. Assurance of death may include ascertaining the absence of heartbeat and respiration, lack of corneal or other reflexes, and lack of physical movement. Personnel should be trained on how to assure death in animals.

HUMANE SLAUGHTER

Slaughter of animals entering the human food chain must be accomplished in compliance with regulations promulgated under the federal Humane Methods of Slaughter Act. These regulations outline the requirements for the humane treatment of livestock before and during slaughter. The Food Safety and Inspection Service is the agency within the USDA responsible for ensuring compliance with this Act.

When stunning is used during slaughter, stunning must be done appropriately and effectively. All equipment for stunning must be properly maintained, and personnel performing stunning must be properly trained, including instruction in assessing insensibility. The use of carbon dioxide alone or in combination with other gaseous inhalants remains controversial.

KINDS OF ANIMAL HANDLING

DAIRY CATTLE HANDLING

Mature milking dairy cows can be handled in head stanchions or a management rail. A complete squeeze chute is not required. Diagrams and pictures in Sheldon *et al.* illustrate methods for restraining tame dairy cows when they are held in a head stanchion. Young dairy heifers that are not accustomed to close contact with people are often handled most efficiently and safely in beeftype facilities with a squeeze chute. Disturbances by veterinarians and other visitors can reduce milk yield.

If the cows are accustomed to many people walking through the milking parlor, there may be no effect because the frequent visitors have become part of their normal routine. Dairy animals are able to discriminate between people who have handled them in a negative manner and people who handled them in a positive manner. They were most likely to avoid the negative handler when he was seen in the same location where the aversive events occurred.

Dairy bulls are usually more dangerous than beef bulls. Bull attacks are a major cause of fatalities when people are working with livestock. One of the reasons beef bulls are safer is that they are reared in a social group on a cow. Price and Wallach found that beef bulls attacked more often when they were raised in individual pens. A dairy bull calf raised to maturity alone in a pen is more likely to be dangerous than a bull that was always kept with other animals.

If a bull is going to become dangerous, he is most likely to show aggression towards people at 18 to 24 mo. Handlers must learn to recognize signs of aggression that precede an attack such as the broadside threat. The bull will turn sideways to show how big he is before he attacks. Good descriptions are in Albright and Arave and Albright and Fulwider. Bulls that show aggressive tendencies towards people should be culled or transferred to a secure facility.

HORSE HANDLING

Teaching and research horses are usually handled using halters and lead ropes, and extra control may be achieved by using the chain of a lead shank placed over the horse's nose. Only trained horses should be tied and only to solid objects that will not give way if the horse pulls back. Lead ropes attached to the halter should be tied with quick release knot. Horses should never be tied with a chain looped across the top of the nose. Cross-ties attached to each side of the halter should be equipped with panic-snaps or safety releases. A twitch may be applied to the horse's upper lip as a short-term restraint procedure. The movement of a horse may be restrained in stocks and chutes. An equine stock or chute may be as simple as a rectangular structure with a nonslip floor.

Other methods of restraint that may be applied by experienced individuals include front foot hobbles, sideline or breeding hobbles, or leg straps, but should be carefully considered depending on the training of the individual horse and the degree of restraint necessary. Chemical restraint can be effective and should be administered by a qualified person. With some drugs, an apparently sedated horse may react suddenly and forcefully to painful stimuli. General or local anesthesia should be administered by a qualified person, preferably a veterinarian, for painful procedures such as castration.

BEEF CATTLE HANDLING

Animals that are extensively raised and have large flight zones may become agitated if people stand close to the chutes and pens in the handling facility. If this occurs, solid fences may need to be installed so the animals do not see the people that are deep in their flight zone. Further information on facility design is in Grandin and Grandin and Deesing. There are many different designs of restraining chutes. Squeeze chutes should permit all animals to stand in a balanced position and the squeeze sides are applied evenly on both sides.

Squeeze chutes may be hydraulic or manual models. Settings of pressure relief valves for hydraulic restraint chutes should be adjusted to prevent excessive pressure from being applied. The chute should automatically stop squeezing at a reasonable pressure even if the operator continues to pull on the squeeze lever. A separate pressure control is required on chutes that have a hydraulic device for restraining the head. To avoid animal injury, this device must be set at a lighter pressure than other parts of the chute.

Pressure should be applied slowly to avoid exciting the animal. Excessive pressure can cause injury and incite cattle to fight the restraint. If cattle bellow the moment pressure is applied by a hydraulic device, this is an indicator of excessive pressure. Bellowing during restraint is associated with higher cortisol levels. Cattle should be able to breathe normally during restraint. The head gate can be self-catching or manually operated.

Self-catching head gates are generally not recommended for use with horned cattle unless they are operated manually. Unless they are very young or tame, calves restrained for routine procedures should be handled by means of a calf chute equipped with a calf cradle. Roping of cattle is necessary under certain conditions. However, roping should be performed by trained and experienced personnel and in a manner that minimizes stress to both the individual and the total herd. For head restraint of cattle in a squeeze chute, a properly fitted rope halter is recommended.

Nose tongs may be used on fractious animals in conjunction with other means of cattle restraint but nose tongs can slip and tear out of the nose, causing injury to both animal and personnel, and therefore are not recommended as a sole means of restraint. Nose tongs are aversive and cattle may resist the attachment of the tongs in the future. For repeated procedures that require head restraint, a rope halter is strongly recommended.

Electroimmobilization must not be used as a method of animal restraint; cattle and sheep find this procedure very aversive. Plastic streamers or a grocery bag tied to the end of a stick is an effective device for moving cattle and changing their direction. Cattle temperaments vary among individuals and among breeds. Handling should be adjusted for genetic and phenotypic differences.

SHEEP AND GOAT HANDLING

Sheep and goats show strong flocking behaviour in pens as well as on pasture. Breed, stocking rate, topography, vegetation, shelter, and distance to water may influence flocking behaviours. Isolation of individual sheep or goats usually brings about signs of anxiety. Separations from the flock, herd, or social companions are important factors that cause sheep and goats to try to escape. Sheep and goats tend to follow one another even in activities such as grazing, bedding down, reacting to obstacles, and feeding. When handling sheep and goats, these characteristic behaviours should be considered and used advantageously and, more importantly, for the best interest of the animal's health and welfare. Transportation of sheep and goats should take into consideration the climatic conditions and productive stage of the animals. Care should be exercised in the transport of animals, and special consideration should be given during conditions of temperature extremes and high humidity.

Measures such as increasing the supply of nutrients immediately before long-distance transport that may reduce the risk of pregnancy toxemia and transport tetany in sheep and goats should be considered. Except for short distances when hauling is less physically taxing than trailing, transportation of ewes and does during late gestation should be avoided. When possible, animals should be gated off into smaller groups during transport to prevent pileups and death losses. Additionally, temperature extremes or exposures should be considered and adequate and appropriate crating provided. Preventative or prophylactic medicinal agents may also be administered in an effort to minimize diseases that are associated with shipping. Sheep can be easily trained to enter a squeeze tilt table. The Panepinto sling can also be used for sheep.

Some restraint devices are more aversive than others. Welldesigned restrainers support the animal's body and do not have sharp pressure points.

Both sheep and goats can be easily trained to enter head stanchions. Sheldon and Battaglia have illustrated guides on manual methods for holding sheep and goats. Designs for sheep races and corrals can be found in Barber and Freeman and American Sheep Industry Association.

POULTRY HANDLING

Poultry are handled in many experimental and teaching situations. Examples include wing-or leg-banding, immunization by intramuscular and subcutaneous injections, intranasal or intraocular application of drops and wing-web puncture, and removing or placing birds in different groups, cages, or holding and transportation crates. Injured, diseased or birds for transport should be euthanized on the farm. They should not be placed in transportation crates. People handling birds should be adequately trained so that stress to birds is minimal.

Poultry that are not familiarized to humans tend to struggle vigourously when caught. They can easily be injured if grasped improperly or subjected to excessive force. All poultry tend to flap their wings when caught, inverted, or caused to struggle for balance or footing. This tendency leads to risk of joint dislocation, bone fracture, or bruises when wings strike objects or other birds. The risk is particularly great for modern varieties of market-weight meat-type birds, which have powerful breast muscles but relatively weak joints due to their youth, or for caged light hybrid laying hens, which have fragile wing bones. Poultry should be handled in ways that minimize wing-flapping or its harmful consequences. Care should be taken to prevent birds from striking their wings on door edges when placing them into or pulling them from cages or compartments. Particular care should be exercised in handling caged laying hens, which are prone to osteoporosis. To minimize the risk of bone fracture, hens should be held by both legs when removing them from the cage.

The manner in which a bird is carried can affect its fearfulness and stress. Broilers carried even briefly in the inverted position by the legs show a greater corticosterone response than do birds carried in an upright position, and the response lasts for about 3h. Therefore, birds should be carried upright whenever possible. Birds struggle less if they have been socialized, the body is fully supported in an upright position with wings restrained, the environment is relatively quiet, and the lighting is subdued. Poultry should not be picked up or moved by one wing unless the wing is grasped near the base of the wing close to the body. They should quickly be released from such a hold, as when transferring birds from a coop to a floor pen. They should be shifted to a hold that firmly grasps both wings at their bases or that supports the body to minimize struggle and chance of a limb injury. Ducks should not be caught by the leg because they are prone to leg injury if handled in this way. Large, strong birds such as turkey toms can be difficult to control by grasping a limb. They can also deliver punishing blows with their wings when struggling against capture. To pick up a very large turkey such as breeder tom, grasp one wing near the base of the body and then grasp the leg on the opposite side and set the bird's breast on the floor.

Finally, proceed with restraining the bird by grasping both legs. For intermediate-sized turkeys, the base of the wing and then both legs can be grasped simultaneously while lifting the turkey off the floor. Turkeys and ducks can be driven, so catching and handling of individual birds can be minimized by judicious use of alleys, ramps, and driving techniques when flocks must be relocated. However, some birds such as older turkeys will not walk on different surfaces and therefore may have to be moved by individual handling. In many experimental and teaching situations, newly hatched birds or relatively small numbers of older birds need to be handled. In those cases, individuals can be easily caught and manipulated. Examples included wing-or leg-banding; immunization by intranasal or intra-ocular application of drops and wing-web puncture; and removing or placing birds in different groups, cages, and holding crates. Trained and experienced scientists and caretakers know that birds struggle less if they have been socialized, if the environment is relatively quiet, and if the body is fully supported in an upright position. More complex procedures; for example, obtaining blood samples, intraperitoneal and venous puncture, and artificial insemination, often require at least 2 experienced persons.

Skilled operators should adequately train personnel in such handling procedures so that stress to birds is minimal. Particular care should be exercised in handling caged layers to minimize the risk of bone fractures. When large numbers of birds housed under commercial conditions are to be moved or treated, handling methods need to be compatible with the housing systems involved. A source of major concern should be the manner in which individual birds are caught, carried, and placed in new quarters or crates. In many situations, birds are at risk of injury because they are caught and moved by grasping a single wing with subsequent exertion of excessive force in moving the bird. No types of poultry should be picked up by one wing.

Gregory and Wilkins found that when laying hens were caught by one leg and removed from cages at the end of lay, the incidence of broken bones was 12.7%; the incidence was only 4.6% when both legs were used in removing hens from the cages. On commercial broiler farms, the chickens are usually picked up by a single leg. Leg breakage can be reduced if the birds are carried a short distance to the transport cage. When research is done under commercial broiler farm conditions, it is acceptable to pickup broiler chickens in this manner.

SWINE HANDLING

Snaring by the nose is a common method for holding swine for blood testing and other procedures. Good descriptions are in Battaglia and Sheldon. Snaring is probably stressful for pigs because they will attempt to avoid the snare after they have experienced snaring. For biomedical research, small pigs can be trained to enter the Panepinto sling. The animal is fully supported in a sling and its legs protrude out through leg holes. A panel is the best device for moving pigs. Nonelectric driving aids such as cattle paddles and flags can also be used by properly trained people. Guidelines on electric prod use are in the section on driving aids. Previous experiences with handling and the amount of contact with people will affect the ease of pig movement. Pigs with previous experiences of being calmly moved may be easier to move in the future. Calm, nonthreatening movements of people will reduce stress levels in pigs and make them more willing to approach people.

VETERINARY CARE

ATTENDING VETERINARIAN

The agricultural animal health care programme is the responsibility of the attending veterinarian. The Institute for Laboratory Animal Research (ILAR), National Research Council *Guide for the Care and Use of Laboratory Animals* defines the attending veterinarian as "a veterinarian who has direct or delegated authority" and who "should give research personnel advice that ensures that humane needs are met and are compatible with scientific requirements." Animal Welfare Act regulations and the Public Health Service policy require that the attending veterinarian have the authority to oversee the adequacy of other aspects of animal care and use, including animal husbandry and nutrition, sanitation practices, zoonoses control, and hazard containment.

Research and teaching institutions must provide investigators and instructors with access to a veterinarian who has experience in the care of agricultural animals. The veterinarian can be full-time or part-time and must have authority to ensure that the provisions of the programme are met. The attending veterinarian must be provided access to all research and teaching animals and to any related documents including health care records. The attending veterinarian also must be involved in the development and oversight of the veterinary care programme, as well as in other aspects of animal care and use such as protocol review, establishment of anesthetic and analgesic guidelines, study removal criteria, training of animal users, and responsible conduct of research activities. Veterinary involvement in these activities helps to ensure animal health and well-being. The attending veterinarian is not required to be the sole provider of veterinary care and can delegate authority to another qualified veterinarian. However, the attending veterinarian must communicate with, and oversee veterinary care provided by, other veterinarians. When necessary, the attending veterinarian should utilize the expertise of other professionals when making determinations about agricultural animal care. Trained nonveterinary staff may administer treatments according to standard operating procedures approved by the attending veterinarian.

PREVENTIVE MEDICINE

Adequate agricultural animal health care in research and teaching involves a written and implemented programme for disease prevention, surveillance, diagnosis, treatment, and endpoint resolution. The objectives of such a programme are to ensure animal health and wellbeing, minimize pain and distress, maintain animal production, prevent zoonoses, provide assistance to investigators on study-related animal health issues, and avoid contaminants or residues in animal products. The programme should include training for animal users regarding animal behaviour, humane restraint, anesthesia, analgesia, surgical and postsurgical care, and euthanasia. A mechanism for direct, frequent, and regular communication must be established among personnel who are responsible for daily animal care and observation, animal users, and the attending veterinarian. This will help ensure that timely and accurate animal health information is effectively communicated.

SICK, INJURED, AND DEAD ANIMALS

Animal care personnel must be trained to recognize signs of illness and injury. In general, sick and injured animals should be segregated from the main group to protect them and the other animals, observed at least once daily, and provided with veterinary care as appropriate. When animals are separated, a mechanism should be in place to communicate to staff the status of the animals and to ensure proper daily, weekend, holiday, and emergency care.

In some circumstances, segregation is not feasible or may disrupt the social hierarchy, cause additional stress to the animal, or adversely affect research. The advantages of segregation should be weighed against its disadvantages, especially for mild illnesses or injuries that can be easily managed. Care should be taken to minimize spread of pathogens from ill animals to healthy animals by observing appropriate biocontainment measures. Incurably ill animals or ill or injured animals with unrelievable pain or distress should be humanely killed as soon as possible. Unexpected deaths should be reported to the attending veterinarian. Dead animals are potential sources of infection and should be disposed of promptly by a commercial rendering service or other appropriate means following applicable state and local ordinances and regulations. Postmortem examination of fresh or well-preserved animals may provide important animal health information and aid in preventing further losses. When warranted, waste and bedding that have been removed from a site occupied by an animal that has died should be moved to an area that is inaccessible to other animals and the site appropriately disinfected.

MEDICAL RECORDS

An important component of an agricultural animal health programme is maintaining records that can be used to monitor animal health events, both physical and behavioural health events, as well as outcomes and levels of production. Medical records should comply with the American College of Laboratory Animal Medicine (ACLAM) statement on medical records. Group health records may be appropriate for animals that are kept as cohorts, particularly when animals undergo periodic evaluation by means of examining several representative individuals of the group. The institution, under the guidance of the attending veterinarian, should determine the method(s) by which medical records are maintained. Oversight of medical records is the responsibility of the attending veterinarian and the IACUC.

When institutional representatives determine that a medical record should be created, the record typically contains the following information:

- Identification of the animal(s) or group(s);
- Clinical information, such as the animal's behaviour, results of physical examinations, and observed abnormalities, illnesses, and/or injuries;
- Immunizations and other prophylactic treatments and procedures;
- Documentation and interpretation of diagnostic tests;
- Documentation of research interventions;
- Treatments prescribed and administered;
- Clinical response and follow up information;
- Descriptions of surgical procedures, anesthesia, analgesia, and perioperative care;
- Methods used to control pain and distress;
- Documentation of resolution;
- Documentation of euthanasia or other disposition; and
- Necropsy findings if necropsy is indicated.

The record system must be structured so that information is easily collected, gathered, analysed, summarized, and available to the veterinarian, the principal scientist, and the IACUC.

The ACLAM statement on *Medical Records for Animals used in Research Teaching and Testing* suggests that:

- Notations in the medical record should be made by individuals who have administered treatments, or made direct observations or evaluations of the animal(s) or their diagnostic results, or their designee. Individuals typically responsible for making notations in the record include veterinary staff, animal husbandry staff, and research staff. All entries in the record should be dated, indicate the originator of the entry and be legible to someone other than the writer.

10

Mammals Biological in Ecological Reproduction

The biological signal field is “a total sum of mammals influence on the environment, changing its structure” (Naumov 1977: 339). The authors of the corresponding technique denote the field as “a spatial temporal continuum which determines ecosystem functioning and which is simultaneously formed by this system in its activity process” (Mozgovoy & Rosenberg 1992: 8-9). The field function is to direct animals to the condition of the environment, as well as to the state of the ecological system population. A biological signal field represents the informative-communicative process of mammals” interaction and the environment where they live, and the process is studied from the sign information recipient”s point of view. There are several signal fields: the signal field of individuals, that of populations, that of population groups (e.g. according to their age or sex), the field of co-adaptable close species complex and the bioceonosis signal field.

To develop the biological signal field theory, Mozgovoy has been, since 1961, collecting field material on the ecology and mammal behavior during the winter. The winter footprint tracking method is known in animal ecology as the “Formozov and Nasimovich technique”, it makes it possible to study the material-energetic aspects of mammal”s life activity in winter periods (Nasimovitch 1955; Formozov 1959; Oshmarin, Pikunov 1990). However, the method fails to use a very important informational aspect of the ecosystem function. This drawback may be eliminated by unifying the animals” footprints tracking method on the fixation basis applied to elementary motion acts as a response to signal field object perception and inner stimuli, determining the dominant motivation. But it”s not enough to be able “to read” animal footprints, we also need to have an articulated task and some behavior structures choice. We need to develop a conceptual basis to study animal”s behavior in the wild. The mammals biological signal field theory may be such a basis (Mozgovoy & Rosenberg 1992: 30-31). When we use such a method, the main difficulty is connected with some reinforcement of the objective approach to the investigation subject matter – mammalian activity in the environment as it is subjectively significant for them. We mustn"t allow animal outer world perception to be substituted by that of a zoologist who carries on the observation. The objective animal activity interpretation deals with two methodological problems: first, the calibration of the environment signals that cause animal reaction, i.e., with the determination of signal equivalence or non-equivalence for animals, motivated in a certain way, which could make it possible to carry out some measurements, and second, with permissible "quantum" or microscopic level reaction, taking place as a response to signal perception.

When collecting field material the researcher follows the animal footprint path and registers all the outer environment objects the animals orient themselves by and respond to by a movement. Using footprints on snow to define species, age, sex, motivation and functional state, requires, as well as the footprint path "freshness", an extensive experience of field observations. Animals possess certain species behaviour stereotypes; that is why an experienced researcher is able to define what kind of an outer environment signal and what sort of the animal"s behavior motivation guide the animal movement activity in each specific case. Wild predator mammals are very "thrifty" – they respond by a movement or by some activity to the environmental signals that are most meaningful for them. Animal ecology knowledge is a necessary condition that makes an investigation in signal field technique possible. A researcher, who has limited field observation experience, is practically unable to solve the problem.

According to the signal field theory animal behavior may be divided into discrete movement responses, determined in the following ways. On the one hand, by an individual"s species affiliation, inborn receptor delivering abilities and the animal"s genetic memory, its specific characteristics (life experience, its nervous system type, as well as its sex and age affiliation), specific motivation and in the long run, on the whole, by its behavior at a certain moment context. On the other hand, by outer environment objects, perceived by the animal, including some signals which indicate the population state. For the collection and analysis, the researcher chooses "an elementary" movement response, i.e., a complete movement fact, indivisible further without any quality loss, which may be defined by footprints. A number of examples will be given later.

The animal movement action in the wild may seem unguided by any visible landmarks. In this case its footprint path, as a rule, is twisting. Often the footprints are guided by some environment objects or events: micro relief elements, shrubs, a grass bunch, ice-covered soil patches, other animal footprint paths, a snow burrow, feeding or "comfort" animal"s behavior signs, ski-tracks, birds" "roaming" and so on. The animal makes its way directly to this object. The moving activity disposition at each object that directs the animal"s movement may differ. Let"s take, for example, four responses of fox to rodent smell or noise under snow. They are: a stoppage or pricking up of their ears, stalking, jumping and catching. Each of these elementary movement responses includes some smaller motion elements, but they have noting to do with our aim, while the elementary movement responses are stereotyped enough for the animals of the given species in similar situations. Their movements may be confidently correlated to some outer environment events.

We leave out of our account a set of things signified without any definite conformity, such as snow trace prints. It is a drawback of our method. We compare the information interaction with the environment among individuals, their age and sex groups. Therefore we believe, that we can neglect those animal perception quanta which have not made a movement print.

It"s a rather complicated task to master animal snow footprint tracking for city or town dwellers who have no experience with winter realities. Science is sometimes understood to be a prerogative of those people who live in the city and who in their majority have a rather vague idea of animal life in the wild, especially, in winter. The polluting effects of cities, including sled usage in suburban zones makes our work more complicated when we use signal field technique. All the above-enumerated facts have resulted in scarce application of this most interesting animal ecology research method — signal field technique. Besides, it"s not an easy task for an ecologist, as a rule, to further master the semiotic analytic method. Nevertheless, our experience has proved that this task may be solved.

Species, sex, age and motivation of an animal may be identified by the corresponding techniques of nature research. Such identification is based on good research observation skills. When animal motivation, sex and age characteristics cannot be determined for certain, some extra observation may be used to provide additional facts for making a choice between alternative assumptions. Formozov"s footprint tracking method has become a part of winter animal ecology study zoological practice. The method is a sensitive one, and with some due care it furnishes accurate quantitative information data.

We may easily combine all elementary movement reactions into three groups, connected with the environment objects, their meaning and value for an animal:

1) Environment events and objects orientation (code);
2) Certain events and object types search or their avoidance (meaning);
3) Movement activity connected with objects; it may be expressed by the number of elementary movement responses or by the number of drives (value).

These steady and objectively discrete elementary behavior acts are suggested as the main parameters of the mammals" biological signal field. Movement elements, behavioral reactions of similar motivation and parameters of the signal field, which represents an animal signal-information environment, may have some numerical expression and can be calculated depending on the research tasks. We should say here, that the individual itself serves as "an instrument", or a device to define the field parameters, and at the same time, it is the individual itself whose signal-information outer connections are studied. We consider that it is possible to investigate not only individual but also population-species and biocoenosis levels of sign-information organization in animals and environment interaction.

There are two methods to organize the field material collected by the animal footprint tracking method:

1) Formalization of an individual as the object of interaction with the environment, with an emphasis on the environmental objects that caused the movement reaction;
2) Formalization of elementary movement acts and the environment objects, with an emphasis on the individual behavioral type motivation affiliation.

In the first case, an individual"s behavior is reduced to some elementary movement response, and the researcher"s main attention is focused on the environmental objects as physical bearers of signals which have caused these movement reactions, as well as on the quantitative assessment of these movement responses.

The field parameters are stated, according to this approach, not in the form of physical-chemical space-time states (not in the form of reality detached from an animal perceiving outer environment objects), but in the form of typical information space and the living system time. Signal field parameters characterize its structure, i.e., the inner form of field organization as a signal-information system. This structure is revealed on the basis of interrelations between environment objects - signal bearers- and animals that perceive those signals in the process of movement activity. In the second case elementary movement responses are grouped in classes according to a form of their behavior (orienting, search-investigating, comfortable, defensive and other types). We get data, which characterize animal behavior in response to signals in the process of their movement activity (Mozgovoy and Rosenberg 1992: 27-28).

Formalization of a space-time information continuum, making up the field, presupposes a composite consideration of five parameters: the magnitude, the anisotropy, the intensity of the signal field, the equivalent distance, and the signal object value. Signal field structure, its functioning and main dynamic laws may be defined by the following characteristics:

Field magnitude is the outer environment events and objects complex, revealed through their participation in the recipient"s activity, taking into consideration the recipient"s responses in the course of perceiving the environment. The exponent of the "subjective" meaningful environment part characterizes the outer environment perception value, as well as the degree of correspondence of the outer environment to the animal"s motivated expectations;

Field anisotropy is the parameter revealed by considering repeated movement responses to similar nature events and objects. The criterion that makes it possible to define different environment events and objects as signs that possess an identical meaning for the recipient, is the same behavioral motivation. This is a selectivity index of the interaction of animals and their habitat;

Field intensity is the parameter characterized by the intensity of the movement responses in the perception of an environmental object. A certain object status index for the recipient;

Equivalent distance is measured in meters; when covering this distance the target object makes 100 elementary movement responses (100 drives). This parameter makes it possible to take into account the contribution of an individual or a group of animals to changing their habitat, it also makes possible the quantitative expression of the "information expansion" of the target object. If we reduce the field parameters and the equivalent distance, we can get comparable quantitative field parameters for animals with different body sizes and different life process tempos;

Signal object value is the quantity of elementary movement reactions in response to any signal object perception.

All studied mammals signal field parameters depend on both internal and external environment factors. But under other equal conditions, the signal field magnitude characterizes, first of all, the enrichment degree of the environment in terms of objects and events that are interesting or new for the representatives of the given species. In other words, these parameters define the form of the received information. Signal field anisotropy, first of all, characterizes animal motivation, or the information significance. Anisotropy shows the most preferable objects and events of the natural subjective sign landscape. Signal field intensity, first of all, characterizes an individual"s reactive ability to the perceived environmental objects and events. In other words, we deal with the received information value. The equivalent distance is connected with an individual or group species reference. The equivalent distance also depends on calendar time perception rate as the measure of environment changes.

Biosemiotics interprets an organism and its environmental interrelations as a meaning of the lowest sign degree (Stepanov 1971: 28). The ability to perceive environmental objects depends directly on how often and how regularly an organism and a certain object interact. Signs, which are the most regular and meaningful for the life cycle support, develop in those interrelations.

In reality both environmental objects and events differ, though in the human language, in the language of the interpreter of mammalian sign interactions, they may be called by one and the same word. How can we establish object and event equivalence when we define the signal field magnitude? When there is some difference between the objects, the problem of equivalence definition is solved through an organism and its environmental relations equivalence.

The common property we use to unite the meanings of different environment objects will be similar object and organism interaction, which may be defined by rather stereotyped behavior responses, characteristic of a certain animal species. The objects the perception of which causes the same behavior response with the similar motivation will have the equivalent significance for animals. It"s important that parameters of magnitude, intensity and anisotropy of the signal field may be calculated in two different ways: 1) the field parameters are given in accordance with the footprint path duration, expressed in meters. Studying fox behavior, for example, it is normative to carry out the field parameter calculations for a thousand meters of a footprints path; 2) the second way of calculating the signal field parameters should be used to compare different animals species behavior or to calculate signal field parameters of a group. Here we should calculate the signal field magnitude and anisotropy per the equivalent route distance. The field intensity per an equivalent route is always equal to a hundred drives, but the equivalent route length, expressed in meters, proves to be different. The most convenient technique of the statistical calculation of the information field parameters is dispersion analysis.

Figures 1 and 2 illustrate the technique of the field material collection that takes into consideration signal field parameters. The red fox *(Vulpes vulpes)* footprints are shown in Figure 1. The footprints are left during its food-search activity. The animal is moving from the left to the right. Its footprints path was oriented by the following objects: 1) a ski-track; 2) a tree; 3) again a ski-track; 4) again a tree; 5) a ski-track; 6) an elk"s footprint; 7) an elk"s footprint on the ski-track; 8) a stub; 9) a bush; 10) a stub. There are six different objects (the field magnitude): 1) a ski-track; 2) a tree; 3) an elk"s footprint; 4) an elk"s footprint on the ski-track; 5) a stub; 6) a bush. The total number of objects, actualized by the information recipient movement activity on a certain plot, i.e. field anisotropy is ten.

Elementary movement reactions number or field intensity on the certain part of the footprints path is equal to twelve: a ski-track is one response (1); plus a tree is one response (1); plus a ski-track (1); plus a tree (1); plus a ski-track (1); plus an elk"s footprint (1), plus an elk"s footprint on the ski-track (1); plus responses, connected with a stub (an approach, a territory marking, a reorientation – the beast turned round and paused) (3), plus one movement response in the directions of the bushes (1); plus a response to a stub (1); then the animal moves on. Should we consider a ski-track, an elk"s footprint and the elk"s footprint on the ski-track to be different orientation objects or maybe in the third case the object is not a new one and it is only a sum of the objects met earlier? The answer to such questions may be given only by the animals" preliminary observation practice. Our observation experience shows that an elk"s footprint on the ski-track provides quite different information from that of a ski-track and an elk"s footprint taken separately. Animals cross "dangerous" plots, connected with man"s activity, following other animals, imitating them. The figure shows that the fox follows the elk"s footprints precisely, "step by step", crosses the ski-track, but then it notices a stub and moves to the stub.

Animals often follow other animal footprints or their own which were left as an earlier footprint path.

During field material collection a researcher chooses some prearranged metric extent of a footprint path, taken as a standard meter, to get some comparable exponents of the signal field for different animals. The fox"s signal field parameters calculation was made on the animal"s 1000-meter path. This magnitude is provisional, it is defined experimentally. The thing is, that having covered about 1000 meters the fox responds practically to the whole variety of objects within its life interest sphere. If we take the footprints path longer than 1000 meters, new objects rarely appear. Besides, this distance is convenient for making the calculations, it"s comparable with the red fox"s day and night hunting plot size, and it is good for the researcher because he is able to collect some essential field material covering the distance in an hour.

Figure 2 shows the pine marten"s *(Martes martes)* track. The magnitude of the signal field is equal to four, there are four movement orienting objects: 1) a tree hash; 2) a bush; 3) a grass stem; 4) a stub. The marten field anisotropy on the footprints path plot, i. e. the total number of the objects is also equal to four, as all the objects were different. How did we define that a large forked tree in the beginning of the footprints path and a stub with a branch sticking are different objects for the marten, different "signal-words" of this creature"s thesaurus? Based on long-term field experience we conclude that there are stereotyped sets of responses to different "words" in the semiotic thesaurus of different species of animals. The marten almost always jumps on low stubs if they occur in its path as it searches for small rodents, and will as a rule, climb trees if it sees fox footprints often and for a long period of time. We may suppose that the fox footprints produce some stress influence on them. The marten signal field intensity in the situation, shown in Figure 2, is equal to ten, which is the number of "elementary movement responses", connected with the four outer environment objects, which orient its movements. As for the tree hash, there are two responses here: its approach and its gaining foothold of the tree hash (two reactions).

Then the pine marten changed its "two-set" movement for short steps without any dependence on an object (one response), one response to a bush, then grass (one response), a stub (three responses – the marten approached it, jumped on it and then jumped off the stub), pace change without an object (one response), all in all: ten elementary movement reactions. The animal crossed a hollow without any response, that"s why this micro relief element was not taken into consideration when we calculated the field magnitude, but we have marked it in our notes, since this object might be meaningful for the marten under different circumstances. Thus, this object is of different significance for the fox and for the marten, since the fox, having its short rest while hunting, sometimes lies down on a sunlit slope protected from the wind. And the fox "does it so as to be heated by direct sun rays on the one side and by the rays reflected from a snow wall or a tree stub on another side" (Formozov 1959: 22). Motivation provides the context of the message received from the environment. The motivation is based within an animal"s physiological needs such as hunger, thirst, comfort and reproductive behaviors, such as its need for a rest, its need for reproduction, etc. The animal"s emotional state adds to its motivation. The behavioral context includes an automatic stimulation effect because the behavioral action itself prolongs the duration of such activity. The environmental signals that determine another type of activity are understood as habitual, and thus, weak and average in their intensity, and therefore can"t cause any dominant behavior displacement. But such sideline signals can result in a new type of behavior, as an addition to the basic behavioral type. The new behavior represents a subdominant type. The activation of one continuous behavior type produces nervous system tension. Since the animal"s attention is very mobile, this fact reveals itself in periodic dominant and subordinate type activity alteration.

Since we register animal movement reactions, our method could seem behavioristic. This is not so. The research is focused on the signified or what is meaningful to the animal, and there is no way to access this interpretant other than through its signifier. It is the main difficulty in zoosemiotic research. Behaviorists deny the content plane. The basic problem here is the perception continuum subdivision, according to the animal"s properties, but not to those of the researcher conducting the observation. In other words, the problem remains semiotic – the problem of attributing the signifier to their hypothetical signified, proceeding from their "language" or semiotic system as well as from the peculiar features of animals treated as the objects of observation.

One of the main aims of signal field theory is to make possible the measurement and comparison of the information contribution of different species and animal life rates to their mutual habitat alteration. Field magnitude, anisotropy and intensity estimates enable us to formalize communicative processes in populations and co-adaptable close mammal species complexes in order to acquire the possibility to compare adaptive behavior responses of different individuals, populations, species and representatives of different intra–population groups of one and the same species (e.g. age and sex) (Mozgovoy 1989: 138-150).

Signal field theory substantiates the necessary set of parameters which - if taken into consideration – enable us to make a model of population dynamics of small predator mammals living near Samara (Mozgovoy 1983: 105-107). According to the population self-regulation hypothesis (Shwarts 1980: 126, 164-166; Gilyarov 1990: 105) mammalian populations are able to support their number at a level adequate to their habitat environment conditions. Apart from genetic mechanisms that ensure the dominance of more fertile genotypes depending on the number of individuals in the population, the population dynamics is based on stress mechanism or "shock disease" that changes the behavioral responses of mammals as well as the size of their ecological niche (Dajoz 1975: 245; Giller 1988: 32). The hypothesis of the behavior regulation of predator mammals number suggests that social behavior depends on the population density at a certain moment of time; endocrine predator responses to a higher density change, first of all, territory; and reproductive behavior responses through the increase of "individuals" aggression" (Rosenberg, Mozgovoy & Gelashvilly 1999: 213.)

A number of specific ecological problems had been solved with the help of signal field theory and field observation technique. For example, we compared responses of organisms and above-organism systems, living under different anthropogenic pressing factors. In Table 1 we show fox *(Vulpes vulpes)*, marten *(Martes martes)*, ermine *(Mustela erminea)* and weasel *(Mustela nivalis)* signal field parameters. The field magnitude is calculated according to these animal"s equivalent footprint distance. The field magnitude is determined by the variety of the environment objects and events to which the animal reacted. For the fox one hundred elementary movement reactions fall on about 900 meters of its path, for the marten the same number of drives occurs (in the average) on 343 meters of the footprints path, the ermine produces one hundred drives covering about 220 meters distance, and the weasel has the same if it runs 145-meter distance. The field intensity, while some equivalent distance is covered, is equal to 100 elementary movements. The field"s anisotropy is determined by the overall number of objects and events, to which the animal reacted while covering a route of some fixed length. Anisotropy may be also determined per its equivalent distance. But in the example given in Table 1, anisotropy and intensity are calculated for 1000 m of the animal"s footprints path. It was made to demonstrate different animal species tempo of their motion activity. The research was carried out in the Samara region flood-lands woods in 1978-1982.

We may see that there is a different degree of discreteness of the environment perception in different species, this fact is likely to reflect the width of their connections with the environment and the ability to adapt to the changes; it is expressed by the reflected environment objects number. The fox, possessing a larger signal field magnitude, has the maximum environment reflection abilities, assimilation and transformation, unlike other ecologically related species. We may consider it to be the dominant species of this co-adaptable complex, inhabiting the floodland woods of the Samara region. In compared species we mark different signal field intensity: the fox"s one is minimal, the weasel"s intensity is maximal, we should say, for example, that the marten"s field intensity is 2.5 - 3.0 times higher than the fox"s. One-way analysis of variance (ANOVA) has shown that individual variations of this parameter are not higher than their interspecies differences, though those of the marten are twice as large. Their interspecies variations and interspecies differences of the signal field anisotropy are similar. Let"s examine signal field parameters within the fox species, within the different variables of sex and age affiliation as well as in their behavior type. The degree of influence of those three factors on the parameters of the signal field was calculated with the help of the dispersion analysis (analysis of variance). The reliability of the influence of this factor on the sign was determined with the help of Fisher"s criterion. The data taken from J.P.Mozgovoy"s and I.V.Yudina"s work (1995) are shown in Table 2.

The accumulated material is divided into four parts characterizing the dominant motivation form. Such division is necessary, since the field parameters depend on the dominant form of behavior in the process of day and night activity. It"s easy to differentiate the dominant behavior forms, they are, as a rule, revealed in the complete investigation of an animal"s day and night activity. All parameters of the signal field increase according to the change of activity from the comfortable or "at-ease" behavior to the hunting behavior through appropriate stages.

In Table 3 we show the marten and the fox activity tempo changes with age. The same animals were observed during four winter periods in the city of Samara environs. All the animals were engaged in their food-searching activity. We may see that the individual"s activity tempo slows down with age. Scientific sources of information assume that this phenomenon is connected with the slowing down of the activity rhythms of metabolism. Research of the same character conducted during field seasons of 1993 – 2000 confirmed this regularity.

As an example of signal field technique application to animal ecology studies let"s follow some signal interrelations among the fox, the marten, the ermine and the weasel. The signal ties among the different species of this complex differ. In Table 4 you may see some signal relations hierarchy that shows in different species information dependence. The data analysis enables us to conclude that for the weasel the information value of the same species activity footprints is much higher than the information value of the signals left by the individuals of other species. Analyzing the obtained data, it is possible to make the following conclusions.

The animals belonging to close species inhabiting the same region make up one common co-adaptable complex. The species of the same co-adaptable complex have identical natural "signscapes". Their sign fields are similar in magnitude and consist of similar elements. The animals react to animal"s footprints paths more actively than to elements of a landscape. The intensity of intraspecific contacts is higher than the intensity of interspecific contacts. Males react to unusual signs of the natural environment and to anthropogenous signals more actively then females. A similar research task was set in 1993 – 2000. The conclusions drawn on the basis of the material of the previous years were once again confirmed.

The following example illustrates a comparative analysis of signal fields of the animals living in similar natural conditions, which only differ in some anthropogenic influence level. The work was carried out in the winter period in 1978-1985. These data are shown in Table 5. We examined signal fields of 12 adult pine martens *(Martes martes)* inhabiting the Volga flood-lands not far from the city of Samara, in Krasnosamarskoye forestry of the Samara region and in Bashkirsky Preserve. The anthropogenic factor influence on the animals" habitat increases from the Bashkirsky Preserve, through the Krasnosamarskoye forestry, toward the environs of the city of Samara. The field intensity calculations were carried out on 1000m animal footprint paths. The intensity gives movement activity tempo characteristics and is measured by the common number of movement responses on the distance unit.

So you can see that the pine marten"s activity is higher in the anthropogenic condition than when such influence is weaker. In anthropogenous natural signscapes parameters of the anisotropy and the intensity are higher, than in those without anthropogenous effect. The females" field intensity in the anthropogenic environment is higher than that of the males. The increase of the anisotropy and the intensity in natural signscapes testifies to the animals" stressful state.

MARINE ANIMAL ECOLOGY

Animal ecology researchers that study marine life will focus on marine plants and animals and how they interact with each other and their environment. Many marine animals and plants live in symbiotic relationships, meaning that they benefit from their relationship with each other. Marine animals and plants also have symbiotic relationships; for instance the Pompeii Worm lives within the tubes of the hydrothermal vents in the deep ocean.

The worm is able to flourish within the extreme heat of the hydrothermal vents due to the bacteria that lives on it's back. The bacteria have a symbiotic relationship with the worm which gives the worm a protective fleece-like coat. Another marine animal, the squid has a symbiotic relationship with microorganisms that produce light. The squid can scare away predators by firing off intense light from the bacteria. The bacteria are luminous and the squid can light up at will.

VAST ARRAY OF CAREER CHOICE

People that are interested in careers in animal ecology have a vast array of areas in which to work. Whether it has to do with birds, pets in the veterinary field, exotic animals in a zoo, wildlife, or marine life, there is a course of study for you. There is a career for you. As for your education, you may need to have a Bachelor of Arts or a Bachelor of Science degree. Some career choices may require degrees as high as a Master's degree or a Ph. D., depending on the field of work you have chosen. Men and women who are trained in the field of animal ecology are also trained in the fields of biology, zoology, anthropology and sociology.

TEACHING ANIMAL ECOLOGY

If you are interested in a career in animal ecology, you might want to become a teacher. Most universities require a Ph. D, but many smaller colleges require a Master's degree. If you want to teach in high school you may be able to teach animal ecology with a Bachelor's degree. Teaching is one of the most competitive jobs for animal ecology, because students training in veterinary medicine, animal science, animal conservation and other fields of study will be taught the concepts of animal ecology.

You may not want to teach; you may just want a career working with animals. You might want to work for a veterinarian as a veterinary assistant. You might want to be a care taker at a zoo. Whatever career you want to pursue in the field you may have to be certified through programs associated with animal ecology. For more information you can do a search on the Internet, or visit your local library.

DEFINITION OF ECOLOGY

Ecology is defined as 'the interdisciplinary scientific study of the distribution and profusion of organisms and their interactions with their environment.' From the German's perspective, it is defined as the 'comprehensive science of the association of the organism to the environment.' An organism's external environment includes abiotic and biotic factors such as climate and geology, and the members of the species and other species that share a territory, respectively.

The simplest definition of ecology may be given as follows. Ecology is the science of ecosystem. Ecology comes from two Greek words: oikos and logos. aikos means "house- hold" or " home" or a " place to live" or the "habitat", or the "place where one lives". Logos means a science or a study or a systematic body of knowledge. Ecology is a field study concerned with relationship between the living organisms and their environment. In other words ecology is the scientific study of animals and plants in relation to their environments. In a very broad sense ecology is the study of the Ecosystem or the Nature. The following are some of the definitions articulated by various people on ecology.

DEFINITION

Over the years many people have tried to define ecology and hence we have a number of definitions on ecology. Some of the most important ones are given here. Ernst Haeckel (1869), who coined the word ecology, defined it as the total relations of animals to both their organic and inorganic environment. Charles Elton (1927) in his book on animal ecology defined ecology as scientific natural history. According to Taylor (1936) ecology is the science of all the relations of all organisms to all their environments. Woodbury (1955) defined it as a science which investigates organisms in relation to their environment: a philosophy in which the world of life is interpreted in terms of natural processes. Odum(1963) defined ecology as study of structure and function of nature. Andrewartha (1961) defined it as the specific study of the distribution and abundance of organisms.

According to Charles J. Kreb (1972) defined ecology as the scientific study of the interactions that determine the abundance and distribution of organisms. We can see that each of these definitions is an improvement of the previous one. However the most clear and appropriate definitions of ecology seems to be the one given by Petrides (1968). He defined ecology as the study of environmental interactions which control the welfare of living things regulating their distribution, abundance and evolution.

SUH-DIVISIONS

Initially ecology was broadly divided into autecology and synecology by Kirchner and Schroter (1896,1902). Autecologyis the study of individual organisms or individual.species in relation to environment. Whereas synecology is the study of groups of organisms which are associated together as a unit in relation to environment. Ecological studies can be made with particular reference to animals or to the plants.

Hence-ecology was considered under two divisions: animal ecology and plant ecology. But again plants and animals cannot be studied alone without considering the other things in nature such as soil, water, air, light and heat which are essential for plants and animals for their survival the following are some of the most important sub-divisions of ecology. Habitat ecology: Depending upon the nature of habitat ecology is considered as (a) fresh water ecology (b) desert ecology (c) forest ecology (d) grassland ecology (e) crop ecology (1) marine ecology etc. Population ecology: The study of interrelationships of different groups of organisms comes under population ecology. The study of a number of organisms their number, distribution and the determinants also come under population ecology.

Ecosystem ecology : When the ecosystem from the point of view of the structure and function is studied it is called ecosystem ecology. Besides it also deals with the interrelationships between biotic and abiotic components. Conservation ecology: Conservation ecology deals with the conservation of the natural resources such as land, water, forests, sea, mines etc. for the benefit of human beings. Production ecology: Production ecology deals with gross and net production of different ecosystems like freshwater, agriculture etc. so that proper management is possible to get maximum yield. Radiation ecology: Radiation ecology is concerned with radioactive substances, radiation and the environment.

Ecological energetic: Energy conservation and flow in the organisms within the ecosystem is the subject matter studied under ecological energetics. Paleoecology: Paleoecology deals with the organisms of the past geo- logical environment and helps to trace the gaps in the evolutionary lines and origin of various groups of plants and animals. Gene ecology: Gene ecology is concerned with the genetic make up of species or populations in relation to environment. Space ecology: Space ecology studies the development of partially or completely regenerating ecosystems for the support of human life during prolonged space flights.

Taxonomic ecology: Taxonomic ecology deals with various taxonomic groups such as insect ecology, microbial ecology, invertebrate ecology, vertebrate ecology, etc. Ecophysiology: Ecophysiology is concerned with the functional adjustments of organism for the survival of populations. Chemical ecology: Adaptation of organisms to chemical substances is studied under the chemical ecology. Eco-geography: Eco-geography studies the role of environment in animal distribution on the land. Human ecology: Human ecology is the study of environment with man as the central theme. Resource ecology: Resource ecology is concerned with natural resources and their conservation. Community ecology: The interrelationship of environment with community of organisms is termed as community ecology. Pollution ecology: Pollution ecology studies the undesirable changes in the air, water, soil etc. affecting human beings and animals.

APPROACHES

Ecology is studied mainly under three approaches namely: (1) mathematical (2) laboratory, and (3) field. The mathematical method helps in anlysing theoretically the 'aspects of the ecology in an abstract way. Whereas through the experiments in the laboratory we can find the cause and effect of various things happening in the ecosystem. In the field level study of ecology actual things are observed or experienced and data is collected. Besides these general approaches the following are also used in the study of the ecosystem.

Botanical approach: Different concepts and laws controlling the relationships between the plants and animals are studied in the botanical approach. Zoological approach:

In the Zoological approach animals are placed in the centre of the ecosystem and rest is studied in relation to them. Ecosystem approach: Ecosystem approach is a study of the understanding of the functional aspects of the plants and the animals and the exchange of materials and energies between them. Biotic approach: Biotic approach is a very comprehensive method in which all the biological components such as plants and animals along with their interrelationships are studied.

Statistical approach: Statistical methods are applied in predicting the possible changes that can take place in the ecosystem. Besides these approaches productivity approach, population approach, habitat approach etc. also can be adopted in the study of the ecosystem. Study of the ecology also can be initiated through various ecologically oriented disciplines.

ECOLOGY ORIENTED FIELDS

The science of ecology provides sufficient guidelines regarding the conservation of the natural resources which should be the underlining principle in all the activities, technologies or applied sciences through which man intervenes and utilizes all the natural resource in the ecosystem or nature. These applied sciences are briefly explained here.

Soil and water conservation: Soil and water being the substrata as a primary requisite for all the biotic generation factors in the ecosystem or nature conservation of these natural resources is of paramount importance.

Agriculture: Besides industry and medicine, agriculture is tile field in which all the sciences are applied. Agriculture is a science of man's involvement in nature or ecosystem to produce all his ever increasing requirements for his existence and human development using his ever increasing knowledge about the various components in the ecosystem. It involves three main branches: (a) crop production, (b) animal husbandry and (c) biotechnology. Earlier agriculture included only crop production and animal husbandry. But of late due to the recent discoveries of the high potentials for generating basic human requirements such as fluid, food, fuel, fodder, fiber, fabricate, fertilizers and other processed products at the microbial and cellular level biotechnology has also come into the ambit of agricultural science. But otherwise if we look into natural system itself the order in the process of biomass generation microbial and cellular activities are prior to the production process in crop or animal production process. Hence they are explained in that order: (a) biotechnology, (b) crop production and (c) animal husbandry.

Biotechnology: Strictly speaking biotechnology means the technology which makes use of the biological organisms and their activities. But basically it refers to the activities at the microbial and molecular level. The modem technological advances in. the field of chemistry, physics and biology has made the biotechnology possible for human beings. It has opened the world of thousands and thousands of microbes and their activities in nature which can be harnessed by human beings.

Crop production: Crop production is the science of growing various crops required for human beings and animals. Excluding the flower and tree crops there are about 250 crops officially recognized and grown all over the world. The technologies applied for each crop may be similar or different depending on the agro-climatic and soil conditions.

Animal husbandry: Animal husbandry is the science of animal rearing for generating some of the basic human requirements mentioned above. There are about 25 domestic animals which are generally reared by human beings for their benefits. Forestry: The science of planning and taking care of forests is called forestry. Forests are classified into several types such as reserved, unreserved, social, farm and agroforestry. All these have their own impact on the ecosystem. Silviculture is another term used for the cultivation and caring of forest trees. Horticulture: Horticulture is the science of cultivation of fruits (pomology), vegetables (olericulture) and flowers (floriculture).

Aquaculture: Various types of cultivation practices in water are called, aquaculture. This includes fisheries, pearl cultivation, prawns, and shelled fish culture, cultivation of aquatic plants etc. Pest control: Anything that destroys crops and animals can be considered pests. The damage may be caused by disease causing organisms, insects, mammals or birds. Use of pesticides have a far reaching impact on the various components in the eco- system. Bio-geography: Biogeography is the study of the geographical distribution of the living things.

Oceanography: The branch of physical geography which deals with the ocean, currents and, marine life is called oceanography. Meteorology: It is a science dealing with the atmosphere and its phenomena including weather and climate and its effects.

Space research: Study of the outer space beyond the atmosphere of the earth is called space research. Nuclear research: Studies on nuclear power does have its impact on the environmental aspects. Public health: The health of the public depends very much on the environmental condition in which the people live. These are only few examples of the ecology oriented fields of studies. There may be other disciplines like wild life management, behavioral sciences, bio-geography, population genetics, range management, environmental physiology, lim- nology etc.

ECOSYSTEM

Most plants and animals live in areas with very specific climate conditions, such as temperature and rainfall patterns, that enable them to thrive. Any change in the climate of an area can affect the plants and animals living there, as well as the makeup of the entire ecosystem. Some species are already responding to a warmer climate by moving to cooler locations.

For example, some North American animals and plants are moving farther north or to higher elevations to find suitable places to live. Climate change also alters the life cycles of plants and animals.

For example, as temperatures get warmer, many plants are starting to grow and bloom earlier in the spring and survive longer into the fall. Some animals are waking from hibernation sooner or migrating at different times, too.

A system is a complex unit consisting of various components with various functions and roles which when performed makes the unit a whole performing a common function leading to a common good. The solar system consisting of sun and the planets and their moons, various organs in the body performing one function of other for the good of the body, a mathematical model describing the functional dynamics of the various components in any unit etc. are examples of systems. A system may be consisting of physical, chemical or biological components interrelated to each other in such a manner as to act as an entire unit. Since different components work as one unit, definite relationship exists between them which ensures the proper functioning of the system. The system may be living or non-living functioning within certain boundaries specific to their own nature. In both the living and non-living systems both energy and matter are cycled.

Eco-system etymologically means the system of houses, housing, living, living together, existing together, the system of inter-relationships etc. of various components in it, among themselves as well as to the whole as one unit. But ecosystem concretely means the nature or the cosmos consisting of major components such as soil, water, air, light, heat, microorganisms, plant kingdom, animal kingdoms and humans.

These are considered as the major components because under each of these several minor components varying horizontally and vertically. Horizontally means: there are different components at the same level equal in status. Vertically means: there are different subcomponents existing within the same major component at different levels or status. These major components can be grouped into various categories.

SIGNIFICANCE

An ecosystem is defined as a community of organisms and the environment in which they inhabit which functions as an ecological unit. Examples of ecosystems include grasslands, forests and wetlands. Plants and animals evolve and adapt to the pressures of any given ecosystem. Together, they present a picture of a problem and a solution.

IDENTIFICATION

Essential processes occur in an ecosystem to make it sustainable over time. Using non-living components of sunlight, water, and carbon dioxide, plants will use photosynthesis to produce oxygen and sugar. Nutrients are returned to the ecosystem through decomposition. To further illustrate animals' role in the ecosystem, let's look closer at the temperate forest ecosystem.

TYPES

The forest ecosystem experiences a great exchange of nutrients. Animals of the forest include microbes in the soil. Litter-feeding arthropods including insects and spiders aid decomposition. Consumers include herbivores such as rabbit and deer which feed on plant materials.

Omnivores feed on a variety of materials. They include non-predators such as raccoon and possum as well as predators such as coyotes and bear. These predators' diets will vary by season and food availability. Finally, carnivores include true meat eaters including bobcat and lynx.

CONSIDERATIONS

The relationships within an ecosystem are complex. Key to sustainability is adaptability. Animals of the ecosystem must be able to adapt to new pressures. For example, introduction of invasive species can impact food supplies. The forest ecosystem has had to adapt with such invasive plants as garlic mustard and buckthorn. Both of these plants can be extremely aggressive, crowding out native plants that form the food base for forest animals.

Animals must cope with pressures from man as well. Deer, for example, have virtually no natural predators in temperate forests. Consequently, populations have skyrocketed. While still a forest animal, deer have also adapted to suburban environments. Loss of coyote habitat has resulted in animals venturing into suburban areas too.

Categories

The major components are grouped into solid, liquid, gaseous or sub-atomic stages though they are all basically matter and energy. The same matter in the ecosystem exists in different forms of solid, liquid, gaseous and sub-atomic forms. Soil, solidified water, microorganisms, plants, animals and humans are the solid major components in the ecosystem, while water either free or bound with other solid components exists in liquid stage. Similarly air which is a mixture of various types of gases either free or trapped in the pores of the solid exists in the gaseous form. Light and heat are the subatomic stages of the matter or they can also be called the different forms of energy.

Another classification of the major components is based on whether they are living or non-living. Soil, water, air, light and heat are the major non-living components whereas the microorganisms, plants, animals and the humans are the living components in the ecosystem.

The non-living components can be divided into three parts: (a) the climatic regime and physical factors like temperature, relative humidity etc. (b) inorganic substances such as water, carbon, nitrogen, sulphur, phosphorus and so on, which are involved in the cycling of the inorganic materials (c) organic substances like proteins, carbohydrates, lipids, humic substances, etc. which are involved in the living organ- isms.

The living components are again divided into (a) producers (b) consumers and (c) decomposers. The producers are those living organisms which are capable of producing their own nourishments. They posses a substance called chlorophyll which can trap solar energy through photosynthesis in which carbon dioxide from the atmosphere and moisture from soil or air are chemically combined to produce carbohydrate. Producers are also called autotrophic. the autotrophs are again divided into photoautotrophs and chemoautotrophs. The former are the one which utilizes the solar energy and the latter are those which use the energy generated in the oxidation-reduction process. Those with chlorophyll are examples of photo- autotrophs whereas microorganisms like *Beggiatoa* and sulphur bacteria are examples of chemoautotrophs.

Consumers are those depending on the producers for their food material. They do not have chlorophyll in their body and hence they cannot trap the solar energy and use it. They may be herbivorous or carnivorous. Herbivorous live on plants whereas the carnivorous live on other animals.

Decomposers are those which depend on the dead organic matter for their food. They are chiefly microorganisms like bacteria, *actinomycetes* and fungi. These break down complex organic matter like cellulose, hemicelluloses, chitin etc. found in the plant and animal body. In the process they release simple substances used by producers. Even earth-worms, protozoa, olegochaetes which are feeding on the dead organic material also called decomposers. Some ecologists consider microorganisms as primary decomposers and the invertebrates mentioned above are secondary decomposers.

MATTER AND ENERGY

The whole ecosystem can be considered under two main concepts: (1) matter and (2).energy cycling systems. These are briefly explained here.

Matter

The whole ecosystem consists of matter which again consists of the presently known chemical elements which have different physical and chemical characters. The elements as we know can be further broken down into sub-atomic particles like electrons, protons, neutrons, X-Rays, Alpha and Beta particles etc. Ultimately somewhere down at the end of the line it is assumed that the matter is same in all the components in the ecosystem. The same matter cycles and recycles through all the components one after the other in cyclic chains. Thus the same matter comes in the nonliving and living materials, in the solid, liquid and gaseous stages.

The matter may be divided into three depending on the origin: (a) organic matter, (b) inorganic matter and (c) neutral matter. Materials that have origin from some living being is called organic matter. Whereas materials from non-living origin are called inorganic matter. Proteins, carbohydrates, enzymes, hormones, vitamins, humus are some of the important organism materials. Where all the chemical elements and their compounds are examples of inorganic materials. Water can neither be considered organic nor inorganic. It is found in the free form both in the inorganic and organic materials. Hence it is named a neutral material in the ecosystem.

The matter may be again divided into solid, liquid or gaseous states. But under normal conditions certain materials exist in solid state and water which is the combination of hydrogen and oxygen exists in liquid form and elements and compounds like nitrogen, oxygen, carbon dioxide, helium chlorine, sulphur dioxide, nitrous oxide etc. exist in gaseous stage.

Energy

Just as we can consider all the components in the ecosystem as matter so too we can consider them all packages of energy. We know any matter can be converted into energy. Burning is the simplest method of converting most of the it, materials into heat energy. Light, electricity, magnetism, chemicals, organic materials etc. are forms of energy. De- pending on whether anything is moving or not it may be possessing various degrees of kinetic energy. Similarly depending upon the position it may possessing different degrees of potential energy also. Besides all the microorganisms, plants, animals and humans are bundles of energy. In the same way all the inorganic forms of materials are packages of energy.

Recycling

In the ecosystem matter and energy are in a constant process of recycling. Based on the type of matter there are three types of recycles: (1) inorganic matter cycle (2) organic matter cycle and (3) water cycles. They are briefly explained here.

Inorganic matter cycle: All the elements in the ecosystem are in constant process of cycling and recycling. the most important inorganic cycle in the ecosystem is the carbon cycle in which the elemental carbon from atmosphere is fixed in the plants and in microorganisms. From plants and microorganisms it moves on to the animals and humans, from here it moves into soil, water and air when the living beings decompose. Again it begins the recycling process through the same major components in the nature. Another important inorganic matter cycle is nitrogen cycle in which similar to carbon, nitrogen is cycled and recycled through the various components in nature or ecosystem. Similarly there are phosphorus cycle, sulphur cycles etc. Practically speaking all the elements are cycling and recycling in the nature. Use of chemical manures in agriculture is another form of inorganic matter recycling.

Organic matter cycle: Inorganic elements form into compounds in the living beings in the ecosystem. Such compounds are called organic matter. This is cycled and recycled through the producers, consumers and decomposers. This is also called the food chain cycle in the nature. In the food chain cycle pre-forms of life becomes the food the after forms of life. For example the bacteria and other microorganisms are utilized by plants, the plants are the food for the animals and animals in turn becomes food for human beings. But when all the living beings decompose the same organic matter becomes food for the microorganisms again the food chain starts.

Water cycle: Water though a neutral substance in the sense it never undergoes any change while it is being cycled through various components in the ecosystem except during the photosynthesis. Water acts as medium for the organic matter and inorganic matter recycling in the nature. There is a constant exchange of water between soil, microbes, plants, animals, humans and atmosphere. Water has some peculiar properties which makes it a unique substance in nature. It is a universal solvent, high heat absorption capacity, high latent heat, higher freezing point, possesses surface tension and viscosity, transparency, higher density at 4°C etc. Depending on the salts dissolved in the water it may be saline, alkaline and acidic in nature.

It is fact a that without water cycle organic matter cycle does not take place. In other words both organic matter cycle and water cycle takes place simultaneously in ecosystem. In the production of natural resources this is an important factor that is to be considered.

Water cycle is also known as hydrological cycle. In the nature there are two types of hydrological cycle that is taking place: (a) rain fall or abiotic cycle and (b) biotic cycle. This is only a theoretical explanation to understand the phenomenon of water cycle. In the actual situation both abiotic and biotic cycling of water takes place simultaneously.

Rain or abiotic cycle: Hydrological cycle through the evaporation from the sea, and bigger water bodies on earth and condensation into rain, snow or dew drops is called rain or abiotic cycling of water. It is called abiotic because even before the appearance of the living beings on the earth rain was occurring on the surface of the earth. Through this process every living being on earth is provided continuously with potable water.

Evaporation from, the sea, formation of water bearing clouds moving up into atmosphere and to the land, condensation of the water vapor into tiny rain drops due to decrease in temperature and pressure, falling again on the surface of the earth are the important steps involved in the formation of rainfall. Plants on the land also contribute to the rainfall by evapo-transpiration to maintain the relative humidity sufficiently high. Through the evapo-transpiration plants on the earth give out absorbed moisture into the atmosphere. This is necessary for the plants because plants need to create a suction pressure to absorb more water into it~ body. As already mentioned nutrients are absorbed by the plants through medium of water. Therefore evapo-transpiration is a necessary evil which also contributes to the rainfall on the land.

If the relative humidity is high in an area the water vapour condensed into tiny rain droplets as they come down towards the earth's surface will gather more and more water molecules and the droplets become bigger and bigger and rainfall occurs. But if the relative humidity is low then as the droplets come down they will lose more and more water molecules from their surface until the droplets themselves will disappear into the dry and thirsty air. This is a very simplistic and common man's explanation of the complex phenomenon of rainfall occurring in the nature.

Biotic cycling: About 70-95% of the body weight of any living being is water. Thus water is an integral part of the living beings. Water is cycled through all the living beings on the earth in a continuous manner as a part of the overall hydrological cycle in the nature. Thus water is absorbed by the microorganisms and plants from the soil and atmosphere to form a substantial part of their body. When the animals and humans consume the plants water from the plants is transferred to the animal and human body. The same takes place in the case of the carnivorous animals also. Thus through the food chain cycle water is also recycled.

Just as the living beings consume the water so also they give out water in the form of waste which go back into the soil or atmosphere. Thus we see two types of hydrological cycle even in the biotic cycle: (1) hydrological cycle within each living being and (2) hydrological cycle between the living beings.

Importance of organic matter and water cycle

From the ecological point of view organic matter and water cycles are inevitable for the maintenance of the ecosystem in a congenial state for the well being of the living beings. It is through the organic matter and water cycle that the much import3nt biomass on the surface of the earth is produced. The same organic matter cycles through various living beings in the presence of the water cycle. All the requirements for human beings for their existence and development are generated through these two cycles taking together. Therefore the most important practice to preserve the ecological balance is to maintain the organic matter and water cycle in the nature.

CONCEPT OF ECOSYSTEM

The concept of ecosystem can be applied at ever so many ways and at different levels. First of all ecosystem can be applied to the whole universe consisting of galaxies and the solar system in them as sub-ecosystems. Then one can consider the solar system as an ecosystem. Thirdly one can consider the earth as an ecosystem. Further we can think of a continent as an ecosystem. Again a country can be also an ecosystem. Similarly a state, a district, a taluk, a block, a panchayat, a village, and even each house hold can also be considered a ecosystem. Strictly speaking even each plot in farm land can be treated as an ecosystem.

The most important practice to maintain the balance in the ecosystem is, ensure the maintenance of the organic matter and water cycles in all the above mentioned types of ecosystems. It all depends on how big a unit a man chooses to operate for himself. But man operates only on a small portion of the ecosystem.

CONTROLS ON ECOSYSTEM FUNCTION

Now that we have learned something about how ecosystems are put together and how materials and energy flow through ecosystems, we can better address the question of "what controls ecosystem function"? There are two dominant theories of the control of ecosystems. The first, called bottom-up control, states that it is the nutrient supply to the primary producers that ultimately controls how ecosystems function. If the nutrient supply is increased, the resulting increase in production of autotrophs is propagated through the food web and all of the other trophic levels will respond to the increased availability of food (energy and materials will cycle faster).

The second theory, called top-down control, states that predation and grazing by higher trophic levels on lower trophic levels ultimately controls ecosystem function. For example, if you have an increase in predators, that increase will result in fewer grazers, and that decrease in grazers will result in turn in more primary producers because fewer of them are being eaten by the grazers. Thus the control of population numbers and overall productivity "cascades" from the top levels of the food chain down to the bottom trophic levels.

So, which theory is correct? Well, as is often the case when there is a clear dichotomy to choose from, the answer lies somewhere in the middle. There is evidence from many ecosystem studies that BOTH controls are operating to some degree, but that NEITHER control is complete. For example, the "top-down" effect is often very strong at trophic levels near to the top predators, but the control weakens as you move further down the food chain. Similarly, the "bottom-up" effect of adding nutrients usually stimulates primary production, but the stimulation of secondary production further up the food chain is less strong or is absent.

Thus we find that both of these controls are operating in any system at any time, and we must understand the relative importance of each control in order to help us to predict how an ecosystem will behave or change under different circumstances, such as in the face of a changing climate.

MAMMALS SIGNAL FIELD ORGANISATION AS A SIGN SYSTEM

Signal field theory studies mammals living in the wild. Animals, as populations and as a close species co-adaptable complex, and using signs in their information interaction process with the environment, may be characterised by the following properties: 1) their information exchange with the environment ensures more effective adaptation of populations and of the close species co-adaptable complex; 2) individuals taking part in the sign processes possess their peculiar group and genetically fixed memory, therefore, memory of some past experience is always present in a sign, producing connotations. A sign is a reference to another significant situation in the past, therefore it becomes fixed as a part of some individual experience (either in the form of a movement response or its blocking).

Mammalian behavior in their signal field is a process during which the animals successively "read" reports without any address that deal with environmental objects and events and inform them of the environmental state. Those environmental objects that produce a result within the mammalian signal field theory are defined as signal objects or mammals sign denotations. It is not an easy task to differentiate separate signals, expressed in a movement, a pose, a sound or some other things, and, hence, it is impossible to divide "the interaction text" into its components. In an indirect interaction, by means of the environment signals in the long-term fixed text, the animal-recipient responds to every signal by its movement activity, forming the way of its behavior. This behavior may be divided into separate units – or response "words" to "the text" signal (Mozgovoy, Rosenberg, Vladimirova, 1998: 17). We should mention here that the environment objects themselves are not signs, they become such having gone through an animal-recipient perception.

One of the founders of zoosemiotics, CharlesMorris, in his work *Foundations of the Theory of Signs* noted that "not only people, but also animals respond to some things taking them as signs of something else" (Morris 1983a: 37; translation from Russian). Then he continued, "sign functioning is, in general, a way when some phenomena take into their consideration other ones by means of the third class indirect phenomena" (Morris 1983a: 43; translation from Russian). In his other work *Signification and Significance: A Study of the Relations of Signs and Values,* he introduced basic semiotic terms in the following way:

"semiosis (or a sign process) is a fine element ratio of *V, W, X, Y, Z,* where *V* arouses in *W* some predisposition to a definite response *(X)* to a definite object appearance *(Y)* (which, therefore, does not act as a stimulus) under certain conditions *(Z).* In the cases where we have this ratio, *V* is a sign, *W* is an interpreter, *X* is a thing interpreted, *Y* is a meaning (signification), and *Z* is a context where this sign exists" (Morris 1983b: 119; translation from Russian). Morris outlines his basic semiotic terms with the reservation that he is doing it "for the present work only". We support Morris" point of view completely, and we should mention the fact that he does not insist on his definitions being "objective" ones for "a sign", he "considers them to be the requirements for the recognition of signs as such" (Morris 1983b: 118-119).

It may seem that Morris" animal sign behavior notions differ from the ideas offered by the authors of mammalian biological signal field theory, but a more profound examination of the problem has shown that the differences are due to what kind of analysis - static or dynamic - is the basis of sign phenomena modelling. In the static approach, what is called a "predisposition to a definite response" (Morris 1983b: 119), is, in the dynamic approach, called "elementary movement responses to the environment objects and events" (Mozgovoy & Rosenberg 1992: 15) or "the thing interpretated" in Morris"s terms. This predisposition "may be interpreted taking into consideration the probability notion as a certain response probability under some definite conditions when a certain sign appears" (Morris 1983b: 120; translation from Russian). "Or, as we shall see further, the thing interpreted may be considered to be an intermediate variable quantity which is postulated in theoretical aims and is controlled by circumstantial empirical data" (Morris 1983b: 120; translation from Russian).

We shall now refer to the notions of "semiosis" and "sign", which, we believe, correspond to our understanding of information-sign processes in the mammalian signal field theory. Reflection over these definitions leads to a better comprehension of the peculiar approach of biological signal field theory to problems within ecology-ethology.

Zoosemiotics is a process, an energy phenomenon, and a means of adaptation, that ensures the interaction of an individual or any other bigger living system with their outer environment. The function of the notion "sign" in this approach is to denote the relative character of the signified and its environmental interrelation, and the signifier and its inner environmental relation, and, if it is possible, to bear in mind their unity in specific research. Additionally, "semiosis" is understood as some real energy phenomena, and "sign" is understood as the model of this phenomenon, oriented, first of all, to its outer environment. Von Uexküll"s "Umwelt", meaning "the semiotic world of an organism" and including "all the meaningful aspects of the world for a particular organism" (Kull 1998: 302) is used in the semoisis model, stressing the features of semiosis as a process of translation (Kull 1988: 300), as well as the "individual"s limited abilities to the outer environment perception" (Dewsbury 1981: 21), and its "dependence on its motivation and an already formed search image" (Hinde 1975: 135-136).

Sign perception as "a model, generalising the functional properties of some given object or phenomena", but not of "a real object or some reality or some reality phenomenon" (Leontjev, 1967: 37), in our opinion, does not contradict the ideas described above, since psychical mechanisms construct some adaptive - for a given function level - models including scientific ones. The division into "reality", and "reality modelling" ignores the fact that any scientific discourse implies some reality modelling. This sign interpretation is found within the works of Morris and von Uexküll, of modern biosemioticians, and aslo, of the authors of signal field theory.

"Researchers's dissension boils down to one simple technical question: what sign property should be called "meaning"? (Melnichuk 1968: 43). The field observation method based on mammalian signal field technique implies associating "meaning" first of all, with the field anisotropy. Meaning is used as "an integral sum total re-organisation operator" in Lévi-Strauss's terminology (Lévi-Strauss 1999: 127, 129), and in the signal field theory text 'integrity' is determined by the animal's biological motivation.

If in zoosemiotics we deal with such notions as "sign", "semiosis", "meaning", "sign sense", then we should describe semoisis using biological signal field parameters: an individual sign sum total (a vocabulary); we should connect with "a signal field size", we should compare text meaning for an individual with the text meaning for another individual with the help of the notion of "a signal field anisotropy", sense (value) text peculiarities for different individuals may be measured with the help of the notion of "a signal field tension". Linguistic correlation with signal field theory does not mean any contextual equivalence of these notions. Instead, it gives an opportunity to accentuate various aspects of the less differentiated sign system of animals by this analogy with human natural language. In pragmatically oriented signal field theory "field magnitude" plays the part of "a syntax information component", field intensity characterizes "pragmatic" information component, field anisotropy enables us to take into consideration the "semantic" information component (Rosenberg, Mozgovoy & Gelashvilly 1999: 115). We should again point out that these associations only emphasize some aspects within the whole mammalian semiosic process.

Wardool writes, "in the information theory any information quantity is studied irrespective of its essence. In Linguistics (wider - in Semiotics) information subjectivity is studied irrespective of its quantity" (Wardool 1967: 9). Signal field method investigations allow a researcher, we believe, to take into consideration both the quantity and essence of any sign information.

Thus, in Zoosemiotics the following definitions of the "sign" are possible:

- A sign is a thing that stands for something;
- A sign is a thing referring its user to something which differs from the sign itself;
- A sign is a thing creating a perception of something which differs from its perceived form;
- A sign is a thing causing a movement response, if the signified is correlated with the addressee"s dominating motivation;
- A sign is a movement from the perceived form (signifier) to some contents (signified) of the sign user's species or individual experience;
- A sign is a thing inspiring some activity, corresponding to the user's dominating motivation (intention) with less than 100% probability. If "a sign" simply causes an activity, we deal with a causal-consequential interaction but not with a sign one.

An elementary movement act (a drive) in the signal field theory corresponds to an animal movement division unit, which is denoted by some correlation between the signified and the signifier. A possibility of the division of expression plane and contents plane into units is preserved. The units have no correlation in their opposite planes and such division of the individual animal's movement process will be wrong. For an animal, the signified denoted objectively is their life experience element, partially corresponding to a search image.

The signal field signs equivalence problem finds its correlation in linguistics. The reduction of infinite various realisations of signs to a finite number of invariants is based on Karl Bühler's principle of "abstract relevance" (Bühler 2000: 34). "In accordance with this principle not all substantial sign characteristics are taken into consideration but only those ones, which are abstracted from the whole and carry out the semasiological function and could be defined by some system opposition since we speak of sign systems" (Buligina 1967: 8-9).

Pierce writes: "A sign or "a representamen" is something that stands for anything for somebody in certain relation and quality. It is addressed to somebody, that is, it creates an equivalent sign in this man"s mind, or maybe a more advanced sign. The sign, which he creates, is called the interpreter of the first sign. The sign substitutes something –and namely, its object. It substitutes this object not in all its manifestations but only in reference to some idea which is sometimes called "the representment ground"" (Pierce 2000: 48). This definition seems to be suitable enough for using it as the subject in mammals biological signal field research, that is in a metalanguage description of the animal sign systems peculiarities.

Since outer world objects and phenomena may or may not correspond to the expectations of motivated animals, the sign interaction of individuals with their outer environment serves as a structured system of meanings, and the scientific discourse including this interaction character description by a researcher is a social phenomenon which depends on its own structural change and reconstruction.

Let's produce some evidence in favour of an information recipient semiotics in comparison with an information sender semiotics for ecosemiotic modelling.

Sign systems study from a recipient's point of view is more adequate for ecological research aims, because in this approach a sign is always vital as something "grasped" by an individual's attention in the outer - as this individual is concerned - environment. The attention may differ only in its degree of intensity. On the one hand, the sign is required by the recipient's motivation, conditioned by its individual and species experience; on the other hand, the sign is generated by some outer - as far as the recipient is concerned - reality, if it is adequate to the recipient's intentions and its perceiving apparatus.

What will be 'marked' by an individual in its adaptive behavior as a sign? How can we define the environment or the individual functional state roles in the semiosis process? Everything may seem to become a sign in semiotics, oriented to the sign information recipient. Gestalt psychologists point to a figure and its background existence in perception: figures, in their opinion, differ from their background in their details and some definite structure. Since an actual semiosis is always less in its volume than a potential one, then in the real world that surrounds the individual, there are always objects and events not included into an individual subjective world. The outer environmental influence on an individual surpasses its abilities to perceive. Since we have no other way to penetrate into the animal inner world but our observation of them, to get some comparable objective results we should mark only such outer environmental objects that cause animal movement response.

Thus, mammalian signal field theory appeals to the recipient's semiotics much more than to the sender's semiotics. In zoosemiotics and in semiotics on the whole the opposite idea finds its supporters. Actually animals often give a signal and wait for a response. We believe that in individual ecology the opposite approach may prove to be more productive than that of the signal field theory authors, depending on the tasks set. It goes without saying that the mammalian sign field theory authors do not ignore the studies of mammalian species evolutionary experience. The other point of view must exist, it deals, first of all, with some communicative intention in animal sign activity.

Semiotics, oriented to a sign message sender makes it possible, first of all, to stress those sides of the sign function which were called "a symptom" by Karl Bühler (Bühler 2000: 34-38). In Table 7 the comparative characteristics of different sign functions is given. The mammals signal field theory concepts resemble neo-behavioral ideas, the basic difference here is that the signal field theory, created to solve some concrete ecological problems, deals with individuals and over-organism systems as its investigation objects. Besides, unlike neo-behaviorist suppositions, mammalian signal field theory treats a whole 'text' rather than a single stimulus.

The investigation of mammalian communication using mammalian signal field technique makes it possible to find particularities of basic language activities – selection and combination. Thus, surpassing the threshold level of one species sign capacity leads to individual activity to promote type changes. The two ways of mammalian signal field organization, in an analogy with textual structure – paradigmatic and syntagmatic - correlate, first of all, with a behavior self-stimulating effect, that is "behavior stimulation by means of some similar behavior that prolongs the given behavior act" and with the displacement of the dominant behavior type; we also witness "subdominant activity" appearance according to the time division principle (Mozgovoy, Rosenberg & Vladimirova 1998: 7).

The communication instrument of animals is their own behavior, perceived through immediate contacts between individuals or through the environment changed by their adapting behavior. The main problem of solitary living animal zoosemiotics is the clarification of a non-intentional, non-directed message structure "written" in the environment objects and events and organized as a "text" read in consecutive order in the course of the animals moving activity. Moving activity of animals in their own or group information sign field actualises this message. The task of a researcher is to organise the process of sign message reception in such a way as to reflect as minutely as possible the structure and organisation of the sign message received by animals.

THEORETICAL SEMIOTICS AND ECOLOGICAL SEMIOSIS

Not all theories of semiotics are able or willing to recognize semiotic aspects in organism-environment interactions. For example, F. de Saussure's

(1857-1913) anthroposemiotics is a semiotics without any ecosemiotic perspective. According to Saussure, "nothing" in the cognitive environment of humans "is distinct before the appearance of language" (1916: 111-12), and even human thought, without the shaping form of language, is an "indistinct mass", and "a vague uncharted nebula" (ibid.), in which nothing is defined by necessity. Such a linguocentric program of semiosis is bound to impede any prospectives for the study of the ecological determinants in the process of semiosis interaction of the organism and its environment (see further Nöth 1994a).

A theoretical semiotics of far-reaching ecological implications, by contrast, is the one of Charles S. Peirce (1839-1914). His interpretation of the interactions between organisms and their environment seems often to be a pansemiotic one, for example, when Peirce writes: "The entire universe is perfused with signs, if it is not composed exclusively of signs" (CP 5.448, fn.). However, Peirce distinguishes among the relations between the objects and the organisms in the environment of humans between those which are only of a dyadic and those which are of a triadic nature, specifying that only triadic relations between organisms and their environment can be of a semiotic kind. A merely dyadic and thus nonsemiotic organism-environment interaction occurs when the organism is confronted with something which presents itself as a "brute fact" or in an effect of mere chance. The environment in such a dyadic relation is experienced as "eminently hard and tangible; [...] it is forced upon us daily; it is the main lesson of life" (CP 1.358). Only when such dyadic interactions become triadic relations is the organism-environment relation transformed into a semiotic one.

In a semiotic interaction, the organism experiences its environment no longer in its immediacy as a brute fact, but interprets it with reference to a third, a "meaning", purpose, goal, or law which transcends the immediate environmental situation (see also Nöth 1994c: 3f.). Such triadic relationships of semiosis are characteristic of cognitive processes (cf. Nöth 1994b), goal-directed behavior, and more generally, any mental activity.

Semiosis in this sense is by no means restricted to processes in higher organisms, to culture and social convention. Any primitive biological organism already interacts semiotically with its environment when it selects or avoids energetic or material objects in its environment for the purpose of its own survival. Such triadic interactions of the organism with its environment constitutes a semiotic threshold from the nonsemiotic to the semiotic world. Peirce goes so far as to see the presence of mind in organismic nature when he writes: "The microscopist looks to see whether the motions of a little creature show any purpose. If so, there is mind there" (CP 1.269; see also Santaella Braga 1994).

Before such ecosemiotic guidelines began to be developed any further in the more recent history of semiotics (see below), another paradigm for the extension of semiotics to the environment of signs users was developed by

Charles Morris (1901-1979). In his behavioral semiotics, the horizon of semiotic studies is equally extended from human semiosis to processes of sign production and reception of "living organisms" in general. Morris also emphasized the necessity of going beyond the syntactic and semantic dimension of signs in order to study, in the paradigmatic dimension of semiosis, the "origin, use, and effect" of signs in the environment of the organism (cf. Morris 1971: 366 f., 302). However, pragmatics after Morris has not really fulfilled the expectations of liberating semiotic studies from their anthropo- and logocentric bias.

ANIMALS AND THEIR ENVIRONMENT

A first step to understanding individual animals, and in turn populations of animals, is to understand the relationship they have with their environment. The environment in which an animal lives is referred to as its habitat. A habitat includes both biotic (living) and abiotic (non-living) compents of the animals environment. Abiotic components of an animal's environment include a huge range of characteristics, examples of which are:

- temperature
- humidity
- oxygen
- wind
- soil composition
- day length
- elevation.

Biotic components of an animal's environment include such things as:

- plant matter
- predators
- parasites
- competitors
- individuals of the same species.

Animals require energy to support the processes of life: movement, foraging, digestion, reproduction, growth, work. Organisms can be categorized into one of the following groups:

- autotroph - an organism that obtains energy from sunlight (in the case of green plants) or inorganic compounds (in the case of sulfur bacteria)
- heterotroph - an organism that use organic materials as a source of energy.

Animals are heterotrophs, obtaining their energy from the ingestion of other organisms. When resources are scarce or environmental conditions limit the ability of animals to obtain food or go about their normal activies, animals' metabolic activity may decrease to conserve energy until better conditions prevail. The different types of metabolic dormancy or responses include:

- torpor - a time of decreased metabolism and reduced body temperature in daily activity cycles

- hibernation - a time of decreased metabolism and reduced body temperature that may last weeks or months
- winter sleep - periods of inactivity during which body temperature does not fall substantially and from which animals can be awakened and become active quickly
- aestivation - a period of inactivity in animals that must sustain extended periods of drying.

Environmental characteristics (temperature, moisture, food availability, and so on) vary over time and location and animals are adapated to certain range of values for each characteristic. The range of an environmental characteristic to which an animal is adapted is called its tolerance range for that characteristic. Within an animal's tolerance range is an optimal range of values at which the animal is most successful. Sometimes, in response to prolonged change in environmental characteristic, animals' physiology adjusts to accomodate the change in its environment, and in doing so, its tolerance range shifts. This shift in tolerance range that the animal experiences in response to an changed environment, is called acclimation.

ENVIRONMENT

The surroundings of any organism or a group of organisms may be simplest definition of the environment one can think of. Hence environmental studies are concerned with a deeper understanding of the ecosystem in relation to an organ- ism or a group of organisms. In ecology we study all the components and their interrelationships without giving any priority to anyone of the components. Whereas in the environmental studies one or some living beings are kept in the centre and all the rest are studied with reference to it.

It may be a man centered, animal, plants or microorganism centered study. Hence a humanist will look at the ecosystem as a complex reality which ultimately should lead to the direct benefit of the people living in a particular place. A zoologist may study the same for the sake of understanding the factors that contribute to the best and suitable surrounding for a specific group of animals. Whereas a botanist will approach the ecosystem from the point of view of the plants.

COMPONENTS

The environment of any organism has basically two components: abiotic and biotic. These are the same as ones explained in the ecosystem namely soil (lithosphere), water (hydrosphere), air (atmosphere), light and heat are the abiotic components. These components are characterised by physical and chemical factors such as temperature, rainfall, pressure, pH, the oxygen content, the content of various gases and so on. These factor exhibit variations during the day and night, according to seasons and year after year. The biotic components are those living organism which interact with each other and with the abiotic components. Organism interact with its own kind (intraspecific interaction) and with those of other species (interspecific interaction). Interactions may be in the form of parasitism, symbiosis, commercialism, prey-predator relationship etc. The interactions may be positive or negative depending on whether they are beneficial or harmful to an organism.

EQUILIBRIUM

Normally any organism in an environment lives in a state of dynamic equilibrium. As the environment is in constant state of flux the organism has to make internal adjustments to cope up with the changing situations. Such adjustments are needed not only for the day to day activities such as feeding, moving, resting etc. but also for the very survival of it Thus any organism adjusts itself to be in a state of equilibrium. The present state of such enormous diversity of organ- ism is the result of such evolutionary process of adjustments down the centuries. Organisms are classified according to the environment' they live, or according to the adjustments they make to achieve environmental equilibrium. The following are some of the classifications.

Homeothennic

Those organisms which maintain a steady internal situation in spite of the changes in the environment are called homeothermic organisms. This is called homeostasis. For example whatever be the fluctuation in the environmental temperature the body temperature of certain organisms(man cows, poultry etc.) remain constant.

Pikilothennic

Pikilothermic are those organisms which change the internal environment (body temperature) according to the external environment. This is also called heterostasis. For example, the body temperature of the fishes and amphibians like crocodile etc. change according to the temperature of the external environment.

Hydrophytes

Hydrophytes are plants which grow under waterlogged or submerged conditions whereas aquatic animals live in water.

Mesophytes

Mesophytes are those plants that grow where water is available abundantly.

Xerophytes

Xerophytes are plants that grow in arid and desert areas and their counter part animals are called desert animals. There are other classifications such as plants and animals in the tropical area, sub tropical area, temperate zone and arctic area. Based on the response of plants to light some are called short day, long day and day neutral plants. In the same way there are nocturnal and diurnal animals. These examples are sufficient to show how the environment affect the plants and the animals.

AGRO ECOSYSTEM

Animal agriculture can have very negative ecosystem impacts, or it can bring ecosystem benefits. In general, when animals are raised in large confinement systems and fed grain, their production uses more energy and causes more pollution than the production of field crops. When animals are raised in small groups primarily on pasture, their production uses less energy and tends to cause less pollution than field crop production. However, good management is the key in all cases. Well-managed confinement systems can minimize environmental damage, and poorly managed grazing can cause serious environmental problems. In sustainable agriculture the goal is to take advantage of ecosystem processes by designing an agricultural system that works with them.

Man is the end product of the evolutionary that has been going on for billions and billions of years in the ecosystem. Everything seems to be directed towards the benefit of the human beings. Man is the master and centre of the ecosystem the earth. He controls many functions in the ecosystem which are otherwise happening naturally.Man exercises his control over nature mainly through the agricultural operations to produce all his requirements for his existence and development. That part of the ecosystem where man engages himself in agriculture is called agro-ecosystem. In other words all the cultivated land together can be considered agro-ecosystem.

The same major components found in the ecosystem are also found in the agro-ecosystem. Man takes control of the soil, water, microorganisms, plants and animals, organises and 3franges them to produce all the things required for him.Taking control of the components in the ecosystem implies knowledge about the various components in the ecosystem as well as their interaction effect on the ecosystem itself. Knowledge is power and the more one has knowledge greater will his control over the nature and more will the production potential.

CHARACTERISTICS

Agroecosystems differ from natural ecosystems in several fundamental ways. First, the energy that drives all autotrophic ecosystems, including agroecosystems, is either directly or indirectly derived from solar energy. However, the energy input to agroecosystems includes not only natural energy (sunlight) but also processed energy (fossil fuels) as well as human and animal labor. Second, biodiversity in agroecosystems is generally reduced by human management in order to channel as much energy and nutrient flow as possible into a few domesticated species. Finally, evolution is largely, but not entirely, through artificial selection where commercially desirable phenotypic traits are increased through breeding programs and genetic engineering. Agroecosystems are usually examined from a range of perspectives including energy flux, exchange of materials, nutrient budgets, and population and community dynamics.

Solar energy influences agroecosystem productivity directly by providing the energy for photosynthesis and indirectly through heat energy that influences respiration, rates of water loss, and the heat balance of plants and animals. Nutrient uptake from soil by crop plants or weeds is primarily mediated by microbial processes. Some soil bacteria fix atmospheric nitrogen into forms that plants can assimilate. Other organisms influence soil structure and the exchange of nutrients, and still other microorganisms may excrete ammonia and other metabolic by-products that are useful plant nutrients. There are many complex ways that microorganisms influence nutrient cycling and uptake by plants. Some microorganisms are plant pathogens that reduce nutrient uptake in diseased plants. Larger organisms may influence nutrient uptake indirectly by modifying soil structure or directly by damaging plants.

Although agroecosystems may be greatly simplified compared to natural ecosystems, they can still foster a rich array of population and community processes such as herbivory, predation, parasitization, competition, and mutualism. Crop plants may compete among themselves or with weeds for sunlight, soil nutrients, or water. Cattle overstocked in a pasture may compete for forage and thereby change competitive interactions among pasture plants, resulting in selection for unpalatable or even toxic plants. Indeed, one important goal of farming is to find the optimal densities for crops and livestock. Widespread use of synthetic chemical pesticides has bolstered farm production worldwide, primarily by reducing or eliminating herbivorous insect pests. Traditional broad-spectrum pesticides such as DDT, however, can have far-ranging impacts on agroecosystems.

For instance, secondary pest outbreaks associated with the use of many traditional pesticides are not uncommon due to the elimination of natural enemies or resistance of pests to chemical control. Growers and pesticide developers in temperate regions have begun to focus on alternative means of control. Pesticide developers have begun producing selective pesticides, which are designed to target only pest species and to spare natural enemies, leaving the rest of the agroecosystem community intact. Many growers are now implementing integrated pest management programs that incorporate the new breed of biorational chemicals with cultural and other types of controls.

TYPES

Man's involvement in nature are so varying that there can as many agro-systems as there are farming families on the earth. However the broad divisions of agro-ecosystem is based on the types of crops cultivated or animals reared. The following are some of the agro-ecosystems commonly found any where in the world.

Seasonally cropped

Most of the agro-ecosystems in the world are cultivated with seasonal crops such as cereals, pulses and oil seed which fulfill the food requirements of the people. One or more crops may be sown on the same piece- of land depending on the soil moisture availability and climate.

Fibre crops takes the next place after the food crops followed by fodder and narcotic crops in the seasonally cropped area. Regular tillage is required in the seasonally cropped area and hence the chances of soil erosion and loss soil fertility are very high.

Therefore only leveled land should used for seasonally cultivated crops. If the land is not sufficiently leveled then proper soil and water conservation methods will have to be adopted before it is seasonally being cultivated.

Similarly the soil fertility of the land also will decrease quickly if a land is cultivated under the same crop for several years continuously. Hence proper soil fertility maintenance practices should be adopted along with the types of crops and the cropping pattern chosen.

Permanently cropped

Large tracts of agro-ecosystem are under the perennial crops such as, orchards, plantation crops like tea, rubber, cardamom, coffee, coconuts, areca nuts, cashew nuts, oil palms etc.

Forestry

All the man made forests are part of the agro-ecosystem. Forestry areas are least tilled compared to other forms of agro-ecosystem. Man made forest systems may be again classified into social forestry, farm and agroforestry and government forestry plantations.

Aquaculture

Man managed water bodies whether for fisheries or for i hydro-electric generation form a specific agro-ecosystem and: their management requires high expertise.

Animal farms

Animal farms such as dairy, sheep rearing, piggery, poultry, rabbitry etc. and the land on which these depend are considered as separate agro-ecosystems. These are only few examples of the major agro-ecosystems to give a fairly good idea of the type of the agro-ecosystems.

ECOLOGY AND ENVIRONMENTAL SCIENCES

Ecology and the other environmental sciences are not to be divorced from each other. In a very real sense, all the natural sciences are to some degree environmental in their application or their implications. Ecology is a legitimate contender for identification as the culmination of all the sciences. At one level, it is important to understand that physical and chemical conditions are the essence of ecology and environmental sciences. Each abiotic factor, physical or chemical, exhibits a minimum, optimum, and maximum for every biological system, from the subcellular to the ecological level. If a factor occurs below the minimum, the biological entity will be unable to function. If one occurs above the maximum, the entity will be "poisoned."

Frequently, the optimum, the quantity best serving the entity, is near the maximum tolerable. As will be discussed in greater detail in the context of transitions between the purely chemical and physical components of ecosystems and the biota, mixtures of conditions are actually affecting biological systems in rapidly altering quantitative terms, which can be difficult to follow. Thus, minima, optima, and maxima of individual components are not so readily detectable in real ecosystems as they are in isolated situations. Fortunately, the Theory of Integrative Levels serves ecology and the environmental sciences.

Within the ecosystem and its community of populations, each individual organism has the innate capacity to follow the pattern that is the life history of the species, but it will exhibit behavior patterns that, although unique, are within the constraints posed by the species and will adapt to circumstances in ways that range from momentary physiological accommodations to behavior responses. Similarly, the species itself has a life history, exhibits behavior unique to it, and can adapt to changes in the environment. So, too, do ecosystems, when studied over relatively long intervals, reveal a life history consisting more of adaptation and change than of *behavior* as that term is usually understood.

While ecosystems are structural and functional units represented by relatively stable biological communities, their boundaries are to a certain extent artificial and arbitrarily established. Aquatic ecosystems, even oceans, are inextricably linked to terrestrial systems, yet they and portions of them can legitimately be isolated for analysis without compromising the quality of the results attributed to the system as such. Similarly, although terrestrial ecosystems can be isolated and identified by several classification systems, in large part associated with a combination of latitude and altitude, there are no totally independent ecosystems.

Moreover, there are "specialists" among organisms that thrive in habitats between ecosystems. There are, in short, not just overlaps but microcosms within microcosms within (and between) ecosystems. The complex of ecosystems forms the planetary biosphere. Each can influence any or all of the others. Despite the internal reality and integrity, these systems are *inextricably* connected. The environmental professional who loses sight of that reality will almost certainly live to regret the oversight. Since everything from the physics of fundamental particles to the history of the universe is connected and is at least arguably focused in the ecosystem, it is invaluable to pause here for reflection on two extraordinarily profound aspects of the scientific endeavor: cosmology and the relationship between scientific order and the relative newcomer to science, chaos theory.

Cosmology

The whole of the natural world emerged from four basic "elements"—earth, air, fire, and water—combined with two forces-gravity and levity. This was a time when matter was deemed continuous. It could be subdivided into ever-smaller bits without limit. There would never be a point at which the material of the world was no longer divisible. Later, atoms were identified and held to be indivisible.

Centuries later, the precise relationships among atoms and molecules were detected. As recently as 1905, Einstein observed that Brownian motion—the constant joustling of protoplasm and other suspensions viewed with a light microscope—is actually the result of collisions between atoms and particles large enough to be visible. In another few years, the internal structure of atoms-the complexes of protons and neutrons surrounded by clouds of electrons-was discerned. Now we have discovered protons and neutrons to be precisely divisible into oddities known as quarks bearing features physicists whimsically refer to as "flavors" and "colors."

All of this is quite beyond ordinary powers of comprehension. Earth, air, fire, and water are far more accessible.

At the same time, gravity, if not levity, has transformed into four forces, including some associated with subnuclear particles. In addition to the familiar, but no less mysterious, gravitational force, there is the electromagnetic force as well as the weak and strong nuclear forces.

While gravity may be familiar, it is not as well understood as might be suspected. Although it is both universal and consistently a force of attraction, gravity is the weakest force and is mediated by the graviton, a virtual particle without mass.

It is this infinitesimal world of vanishingly small particles and associated forces to which cosmologists turn for explanations of the origins and destiny of the universe. In a very real sense, energy and matter are wholly interchangeable, if not actually identical. In a comparably real sense, ecological sciences are derivatives of both extremes in the scientific scale.

The biosphere is one expression of both fundamental physics and cosmological events. But this realization does nothing to advance precision in predicting events from causes, as was once a hope, if not an expectation, among scientists.

Order and Chaos

Because of the emerging simplicity and order of the natural world, a mission was advanced for at least a moment of human history. When physical phenomena were extended into the biological and then into the psychological and social realms, a kind of giddy optimism followed.

Among scientists and observers of science, there were those who sincerely believed every event explicable "in terms of antecedent events in causal chains and networks, characterizable in terms of universal laws which make no reference to the causal efficaciousness of future events or higher levels of organization.

"In the early nineteenth century, arguments were seriously advancing the concept of a complete determinism. Scientific laws would allow predictions of "everything that would happen in the universe, if only we knew the complete state of the universe at [any] one time." Since "everything" included the vagaries of human behavior, it certainly included more scientific environmental processes.

Promise or threat, such scientific predetermination has now been dismissed. Scientists and those observers of science are coming to accept that life, at the very least, is "not meant to be free from contradiction or ambiguity."

It is only in this century that determinism has lost credibility in the face of advancing science. That level of order gave way to the Heisenberg Uncertainty, which has revealed that one cannot accurately know both the position and speed of subatomic particles simultaneously. The new science of quantum mechanics arises empirically from mathematical manipulation of the components of the Heisenberg Uncertainty to predict not a single, definite result but the array of possible outcomes and the likelihood of each.

One of the resultant insights crucially important in ecology is that light, while composed of waves, behaves as if particulate. Light energy is emitted and absorbed only in the packets known as quanta. Primarily a practical branch of physics, quantum mechanics explains phenomena as wide reaching as properties of collapsed stars, conduction of electricity, structure of atoms and their nuclei, chemical bonding, and the mechanical and thermal properties of solids.

In more recent days, scientists have come to recognize that while chaos seemingly arises from the orderliness of scientific law, order is the mark of chaos. A new kind of highly mathematical science has reached the headlines and fiction, not to mention volumes intended for coffee tables. In the end, the important conclusion is that life consists of orderly and lawful behavior on the part of matter. Its tendency is not exclusively to proceed from order to disorder; living matter is based on keeping up existing order through metabolism. Not even large biological molecules like DNA escape or invalidate physics, chemistry, or the laws of probability. But none of them can adequately explain life or predict the direction of cell, species, community, or ecosystem. The reason is embedded in chaos.

THE GAIA HYPOTHESIS

Ecology could hardly remain untouched by novel scientific insights, on the one hand, and the political implications of an evolving environmental movement, on the other. There can be few in this country who do not subscribe to the concept of a healthy, diverse ecosystem in a state of dynamic balance. Within such an ecosystem, there are cycles and chains. Food chains connecting animal to plant direct energy outward, whereas death and decay restore energy to the earth. Whenever a change occurs anywhere within the circuit, the remaining parts must adjust to restore the balance of the whole.

Such a description of ecological balance might be uttered by either a practicing ecologist or an environmental professional. It could also be a political statement, for ecology has become a matter of policy and politics. This description might also be a reflection of the spiritual realm and, as such, could arise from any number of traditions, from the Judeo-Christian to the Native American to the Asian to the primal, extant as well as extinct. Ecology is no longer the sole province of the scientist working in aloof isolation.

Deep Ecology

Today, three ecologies—scientific, political, and spiritual—are merged in what is called deep ecology. Yet the proponent of deep ecology need not be a scientist or even any one of the three kinds of ecologist. *Anyone* can be a deep ecologist. In fact, scientific ecology, especially as practiced by environmental professionals, is viewed by some as the antithesis of deep ecology, which is more a discipline of philosophy expressed in poetry than any other form of science.

The mission of the deep ecologist is to cultivate individual but widespread ecological consciousness with an insight into the ubiquitous connections of the world around us. Deep ecology is holistic. Its message is one of appreciation, receptiveness, and trust. Whether one reacts to deep ecology with empathy or impatience, its tenets proffer much for contemplation by the environmental professional and the interested nonscientist:

- All life has intrinsic value.
- The richness and diversity of life have value.
- Human life is privileged only to the extent of satisfying vital needs.
- The relationship of humans to the natural world endangers life's richness and diversity.
- Maintenance of life's richness and diversity mandates a decrease in human population.
- Changes are needed to accommodate cultural diversity affecting basic economic, technological, and ideological components.
- Ecologically sensitive ("green") societies value quality of human life over quantity of human life.

How these tenets fit into the ecology of populations, especially of humans, and into the matters of the place of the biota in the strategy of ecosystems will be explored throughout this book, with special reference to the concluding chapters. Whatever the scientific realities of the ecology of the human species, deep ecologists are obligated to promote the needed sociocultural changes. Surely, even these philosopher-poets will be more effective if informed by ecological realities from the scientific realm.

Gaia Hypothesis

Ecologists, deep, scientific, or political, have come to recognize this planet's biosphere as a distinct level of organization arising from the interconnections among all the ecosystems. If an ecosystem is a biological system, logic is not strained through the perception of the biosphere as the highest of all biological systems. There are those who would take one more step, perhaps moving from science into metaphysics in doing so. Is the biosphere itself actually a biological entity—a living organism? This is the position advanced by the Gaia Hypothesis. There are valuable insights to be taken from Gaia, whether one is a believer or a skeptic content with stopping short of Gaia with the biosphere as nothing more (or less) than the highest level of organization. J. Lovelock propounds "that the entire range of living matter on Earth, from whales to viruses, and from oaks to algae, [can] be regarded as constituting a single living entity, capable of manipulating the Earth's atmosphere to suit its overall needs and endowed with faculties and powers far beyond those of its constituent parts."

An intriguing "branch" of the Gaia Hypothesis asserts bacteria to be the primary cybernetic mechanism at Gaia's command: "The environment is so interwoven with bacteria, and their influence is so pervasive, that there is no really convincing way to... say this is where life ends and this is where the inorganic realm of nonlife begins." According to the variant of evolutionary theory and of the Gaia Hypothesis, bacteria go beyond filling every known habitat on the earth's surface to maintain all life forms and to accelerate all biological cycles. In short, bacteria represent a complete planetary regulatory system. Biosphere or Gaia? Is the dominant taxon of earth the kingdom of Monera (bacteria) or *Homo sapiens sapiens* or some organism ecologists have overlooked? Are there practical differences among these distinctions? The individual reader must decide. Armed with the definition of life, the Theory of Integrative Levels, and an awareness of how science works and how the several ecologies fit into human endeavor, the reader will be provided in the chapters to follow with principles and concepts to inform a personal conclusion based in ecology.

ECOLOGY AND FUTURE

Much of the current controversy about ecology concerns the future. Will man continue to progress in knowledge, health and standards of living, or is he headed toward oblivion in the near future? Is the good life for everyone gradually spreading around the world, and is man coming into better balance with his environment, or is he already on a path of self-destruction?

It is now possible to find numerous writers and scholars expressing opposite views on these questions. Some scientists believe that man's remaining time on earth may be less than 100 years, unless major improvements occur in his basic ecologic knowledge and relationships to his environment. Many people believe that the planet earth is already dying from misuse, pollution and overpopulation—trends that must be reversed very quickly if we are to survive. They cite projections on current levels of air and water pollution which could make the earth uninhabitable within the next 50 years unless these processes are sharply controlled.

Other scientists consider these attitudes as overly emotional, fear-producing, and scientifically unjustified. They feel that ecologists cannot support many of their prophesies of doom and gloom, and that they are, in fact, raising unreasonable bogeymen. They point out the great strides in health, welfare, education and social advance which have already occurred, and they feel that there is a good deal of inaccurate sentimentalism about "the good old days." They note that the good old days had no electricity, no easy transportation, long working hours, very little educational and recreational opportunities, and plenty of diphtheria, smallpox, cholera, malaria and tuberculosis. They feel that the alarmist-type ecologists cannot recognize progress when they see it. To this the ecologist replies, "Does progress require polluted rivers and lakes, choking air, birds dying from pesticides, intolerable crowding, ulcers in children, violence on the streets, and heart attacks in young men?" Thus the controversy and arguments can continue almost indefinitely. The dichotomy of these heated arguments has been clearly pointed out by Garrett DeBell.

In general, ecologists have tended toward pessimistic views of the future for more than 30 years. The first scientific books on the ecologic imbalance of man in the world appeared in the 1930s and 1940s. Since these early warnings about the ecologic problems of man, these difficulties have generally increased. Ecologists have found ample evidence for their fears. They feel that current events show that world population growth will not be amenable to significant slowing before the world is severely overcrowded. They have found that man has not learned the lessons of history and has continued to destroy his environment. They believe that the future survival of man will be, at best, a close and hectic race between these destructive forces and an enlightened society which can find the knowledge and maturity necessary for solutions. They now see little evidence that man will really achieve these solutions before it is too late.

This ecological view leapt into world attention in 1969 and 1970 in a highly emotional fashion, further antagonizing the optimists. Ecology suddenly became the "in-thing"; the cause of students, politicians, housewives and scientists. It had many of the characteristics of a popular fashion, however, even a cult, and, as such, it clearly attracted resistance and opposition. The editor of Science, Dr. Philip Abelson, correctly pointed out that the emotional outburst of 1970 on environmental issues could not be sustained. Although it had substantial elements of fact, it also contained too many half-truths and unwarranted fears. Before 1970 was over, a definite backlash developed in the minds of many people. Speeches and articles began to appear suggesting that ecologists were much too pessimistic and the world wasn't in such bad shape after all.

In the terminology of 1970, it was obvious that the credibility of ecology was eroding fast. Much of the progress made in alerting people to environmental and population problems appeared to be fading, and a strong reaction to believe in technologic progress once again asserted itself. The optimists again pointed to the vast potential of the earth when viewed in modern terms. 'We've barely begun to capture the wealth of the ocean', they insisted, "to harness nuclear energy, to apply scientific progress to wood agriculture, to probe the wonders of the computer age, to capitalize on modern medicine, and to develop the skills and potential of human beings through better education."

Throughout it all, the future has remained fair game for everyone. The prognosticators of gloom and doom on the one hand, and of a technologic utopia for all men on the other, have continued to express their views with equal fervor.

Every conceivable arena of human activity has been considered: from the intentional genetic modeling of man to the exploration of space, from agriculture to the future of warfare, from social and educational problems to computer-driven automated industries.

Some of the difficulties in reconciling diverse points of view arise from the time and area scale of different writers. Some have concerned themselves with the next million years, considering the world as a whole, whereas others have thought only in terms of 25 to 50 years, considering just the United States. Obviously, one's opinions might differ greatly depending upon the span and extent of one's outlook.

This chapter will not deal directly in the game of forecast and prediction, but it will attempt to highlight some of the major issues and sources of controversy, and the scientific knowledge or lack thereof relating to these issues.

FUTURE ISSUES

The most difficult and essential problems for man's future lie in broad ecologic and social issues. No two questions are more fundamental or more troublesome to the future of man than the ecologists' inquiry, "What is the carrying capacity of the earth for man? In other words, what are the limits of the life support capabilities of the earth in terms of human populations?" or the behaviorists' concer, "What are the tolerance levels of man to the pressures generated by his own societies? In other words, if man is his own worst enemy, at what point, or by what stimulus, does this lead to his self-destruction?"

The carrying capacity, or life support capability, of the earth for man may be dependent upon a great variety of factors. We can readily identify oxygen, water, food, space and shelter as vital requirements for human life. There might be many others as well, such as mineral resources, energy availability, or the concentration of toxic metabolites which could reach states above human tolerance levels. Most of these, however, would operate through the media of air, water or food. Hence, it is worthwhile to examine each of these briefly.

OXYGEN

The atmosphere of the earth consists of about 78 per cent nitrogen, 21 per cent oxygen, 0.03 per cent carbon dioxide, and the remainder, other gases. This composition is remarkably stable despite the fact that oxygen is a highly reactive element which readily combines with a great many other elements in chemical processes of oxidation.

The ecologist Lamont C. Cole has pointed out that oxygen has remained stable in the earth's atmosphere because green plants recycle it in molecular form through photosynthetic processes. Approximately 70 per cent of the free oxygen produced each year is thought to come from planktonic plants in the ocean, and the remaining 30 per cent from terrestrial vegetation of forests and grasslands. Cole emphasized that if we should seriously pollute the sea, as is already happening in coastal areas, and if we should excessively denude the forests and grasslands of the earth, we shall be in danger of upsetting the oxygen balance in the atmosphere. In other words, we must look upon the oceans, forests and grasslands, as the world's oxygen tank, and we must insure their continued healthy ecologic function.

This point of view is contested by W. S. Broecker, a geochemist at Columbia University. Dr. Broecker points out that each square meter of the earth's surface is covered by 60,000 moles of oxygen gas. Plants in the, ocean and land produce only about 8 moles per square meter per year, and this is almost entirely consumed by their own respiration and that of animals and bacteria. Thus other organisms use all but 0.0004 per cent of the oxygen produced by plants. Broecker maintains, therefore, that man does not depend upon the oxygen generated by plants, and that there is no current danger at all to his oxygen supply. "In conclusion it can be stated with some confidence that the molecular oxygen supply in the atmosphere and in the broad expanse of open ocean are not threatened by man's activities in the foreseeable future. Molecular oxygen is one resource that is virtually unlimited". Broecker feels that man's existence will be threatened by other types of environmental pollution long before his oxygen supply becomes endangered, and that we need not worry about total oxygen supply.

This is typical of some of the different opinions which are unfolding between physical and biological scientists. Such differences often indicate the need for more research and better knowledge before we can fully accept one position or another.

Another atmospheric problem of long-term concern is the increase in carbon dioxide in the atmosphere. Between 1960 and 1990, the combustion of fuels increased the CO_2 content of the air by 14 per cent of its formerly stable level. Carbon dioxide tends to reflect infrared rays from the earth, and this provides a "greenhouse effect" for the whole earth; that is, it accumulates heat. This will gradually increase the temperature of the earth—an effect which may have long-term implications in climate modification. A rise of just 2 or 3 degrees in annual mean temperature would have a major melting effect on glaciers and ice caps, and this could raise the level of the seas several feet. Such a rise in sea level would inundate money of the world's major cities. Some experts predict it may require 4,000 years, and others feel it will not happen at all. The latter believe that any occurrence of the greenhouse effect due to increasing CO_2 in the atmosphere will be offset by increasing particulate pollution in the air and increasing opacity of the earth's atmosphere. Thus less light energy will enter, and we could actually have a cooling of the earth's surface. Once again, we see fundamental controversies on major issues—largely because we do not really have the complete answers.

The atmospheric problem may also become acute in terms of various toxic elements released into surface air and waters: carbon monoxide, sulfur dioxide, lead from automobile exhaust, hydrocarbons from industrial operations and numerous other products of modern technological societies. For example, 500 million pounds of lead are discharged into the atmosphere of the United States each year from automobile exhausts alone, and significant amounts of this become incorporated into living organisms. A recent study in Sweden showed concentrations of lead in mosses to be as high as 300 to 500 ppm along roadsides. Some roadside plants in the United States may have lead levels up to 3,000 ppm. This lead enters the plants via both air and water and can then enter man and animals. A hundred years ago, concentrations in roadside plants were less than 20 ppm. Lead levels over 0.5 ppm have detectable physiological effects in man and animals, and 1.0 ppm levels are often toxic.

In conclusion, there seems to be little or no immediate threat that we will run out of air for breathing, but several warnings have appeared regarding the quality of our air. We apparently have an adequate supply of total oxygen for many centuries to come, though even this is a debatable point. In some localities the situation may be critical at certain times. If stationary inversions of air trap the polluted atmosphere over some of our largest cities such as Tokyo, London, New York or Los Angeles, toxic air pollutants increase to dangerous levels.

FOOD

Nowhere is scientific controversy more evident than on the issue of world food supplies. Some scientists predict famines and mass starvation within the next 10 years. In fact, Ehrlich pointed out that we already have famine in many parts of the world, if one define famine as people dying of lack of food. Even at the height of the Green Revorution in Asia in which new strains of rice and wheat were producing phenomenally larger yields, famine conditions existed in parts of Rajasthan in India, in sections of Burma and in southern Thailand. Starvation is now a grim reality in much of the world and it may well get worse despite the Green Revolution.

Other scientists refute this pessimism and find evidence for a hopeful outlook in the world food situation. They feel that the Green Revolution which was based on new strains of rice and wheat in Asia and Africa, and which produced a doubling and tripling of yields in one or two years, shows what can be done with modern agriculture. For the first time in many decades, agricultural output increased more rapidly than population growth. India began to approach self-sufficienly in food production, and the Philippines began to export rice again for the first time since 1900. Some economists have been sufficiently impressed with agricultural potential that they feel the world can feed 45 billion people if modern technology is utilized. Boerma has pointed out that less than one-half of the world's total cultivatable land is now under agricultural production (only 512 million hectares in use in 1962 out of a total of 1.1 billion available).

Many others take a more cautious attitude and, while recognizing technologic potential, they realize the practical difficulties. These are difficulties of education, ingrained social customs, distribution and warehousing, and numerous other mundane problems which spell the difference between success and failure.

A word of caution about the Green Revolution is also necessary. If is quite true that new strains of agricultural crops can sometimes dramatically increase yeilds, but often these new strains require more careful management, more intensive care, more water, more fertilizer and more insecticides. They may be more vulnerable to plant viruses or fungi. Although the plant geneticists try to breed in every possible disease resistance these new strains do not have the centuries of natural selection and regional adaptation behind them as do the local strains which the villagers have always used. In West Bengal and Orissa, there were reports that some of the newly introduced high-yield strains of rice were succumbing to a disease that was not affecting the old traditional strains.

Another factor in the world food picture is one of pure climatic good fortune. The Green Revolution of 1968 and 1969 in India was accompanied by the best monsoon seasons in over 10 years. A long series of droughts had broken in southern Asia and adequate rains fell in the right pattern. The possibility exists, therefore, that a good part of the success of the Green Revolution was due to good weather, combined with new strains and more fertilizer. This is a question that will be more adequately answered in future years, to see if increasing agricultural production can be maintained in years of poor rainfall. In India in 1971, too much rain came and it fell too early. The wheat crops of northern India were magnificent in April and May of 1971 just before harvesting and threshing, but heavy premature rains in many areas caused the wheat to rot before it could be threshed. Bihar had serious crop losses from flooding. Once again, the was a tragic and dramatic demonstration that even the Green Revolution remains dependent on climatic factors outside the control of man.

Throughout all of these arguments on how many people the world can feed, one must ask the realistic questions: "Is it necessary that there always be a race between population and food production? Is it desirable to be teetering on the bring of starvation at all times? Is it the best representation of the human condition to be struggling in this manner to feed more and more people at a subsistence level?"

One also has the impression in reviewing the literature on world food supplies that too much emphasis is placed on future predictions, and not enough on current conditions. We already know that starvation and malnutrition exist throughout the world, even in the most advanced countries. We furthermore know that malnutrition of any kind has profound effects upon growth, development and behavior. Children growing up with malnutrition from early infancy definitely show reduced growth rates and possible retardation of physical and mental development.

They furthermore show increased susceptibility to infectious disease. Thus, we return to the issue of the quality of life, and the realization that merely preventing death by starvation does not by any means insure a quality nutritional base for adequate growth and human development.

It is apparent that the problem of world food supplies will continue for some time as a problem of both quantity and quality, and especially one of distribution. Two of the scientists who helped to achieve the Green Revolution, Dr. D. S. Athwal of the International Rice Research Institute in the Philippines, and Dr. N. E. Borlaug, of the Rockefeller heat Research Institute in Mexico, have both warned that the Green Revolution will fail to meet the world's food needs unless it is accompanied by a drastic slowing of the world's population growth.

SPACE

Paul Sears wrote an important essay entitled, "The Inexorable Problem of Space," in which he concluded that "Our future security may depend less upon priority in exploring outer space than upon our wisdom in managing the space in which we live." With a shortage of space crowding in upon us in the 1980s and 1990s, his words gain validity every year.

The earth's total surface is 196,940,400 square miles, of which about 30 per cent or 57,230,000 square miles is land surface. Of this total land surface, approximately 5,000,000 square miles are in Antarctica and are too cold to be easily inhabited except by scientists and explorers; 9,000,000 square miles are in deserts and 11,000,000 square miles are in mountainous regions. Of deserts and mountains, at least one-fourth of their land area cannot be inhabited, so this eliminates another 5,000,000 square miles of land surface for human habitation. We are left with approximately 47,000,000 square miles of land surface, at the most, for the world's population.

The world now has about 5 billion people, and will probably reach 9 billion within the next 35 years. This means we now have about 75 people for every square mile of inhabitable land surface on the face of the earth.

As with water, air and food, it is important to distinguish between the total or potential amount of any given resource on earth, and that amount which is actually utilized or practically available of man. It was pointed out in the sections on water and air that the earth's total amount is apparently adequate for many years to come, but the supply in any given city may not be of sufficient quantity or quality to support the standard of living we would like.

So it is with space. Although we theoretically have one square mile of land for every 75 people (about 9 acres per person), the human population is not evenly distributed. In the great urban concentrations of the world, densities often exceed 50,000 people per square mile. The amount of living space per person in some cities such as Calcutta is less than 20 square feet per person. Theoretically, we could redistribute these crowded people to provide more even spacing around the world. Obviously this cannot be done, and if it were attempted it might wreak havoc with agricultural production.

The economic and behavioral needs of man are such that he must cluster together, but in so doing, he creates superdensities such as Calcutta, London, New York, Paris, Tokyo, Shanghai and Buenos Aires—the slums of which are definitely deleterious to human health and welfare. Why, we might ask, does man insist on this degree of crowding and then complain about it so bitterly? Why do people continue to pour into the cities of the world when they are already known as centers of pollution, crime and illness?

Perhaps we need to know more about the real spatial and social needs of man. What are his requirements for space and privacy, and how do these interact with his needs for social stimulation and group activity? Does man become conditioned to crowding in early childhood and then seek further crowding throughout his life?

Does he require the social pressure of a crowd because he feels a compulsion to be in touch with the group, and thus be able to predict what the group is going to do next? Have we produced, in our urban centers, self-destructive systems which so modify the behavior of their inhabitants that these inhabitants exaggerate their own problems and can no longer achieve rational solutions?

These are all tough questions that cannot be answered in simple or easy terms. The answers will require the best intelligence we can muster from many disciplines. Some sorts of answers will certainly be necessary before we can even begin to solve the ecologic and behavioral problems associated with our own use of terrestrial space.

WATER

Worldwide water supplies represent a concern for the future of man in terms of both the quality and absolute quantity of fresh water. Many cities have reached or are coming close to their total available fresh water supply and are reaching further and further to obtain new supplies.

Two Russian geographers and hydrologists, Kalinin and Bykov, have pointed out that "The world's water resources form a single entity". The basic hydrologic cycle of the world (Figure 16-1) depends upon solar energy, atmospheric circulation, heat reflectivity and surface retention. The latter is strongly influenced by the biotic community. Kalinin and Bykov point out, on the assumption that the moisture content of the earth remains constant, that the total gains and losses from the land and the sea are in balance. Thus, the total precipitation equals the total evaporative loss from land and sea. However, the relative retention time and thus the total amount of water in terrestrial and fresh-water environments can change substantially in relation to the biota and terrestrial storage capacity. Table 15A shows estimates on the world's total water resources. Of 1.46×10^9 cubic kilometers of water in the world, 93 per cent is in the oceans, 4.1 per cent is in the earth's crust, 2.0 per cent is in glaciers and polar ice caps and only 0.052 per cent is in freshwater lakes, rivers and atmospheric moisture. The annual production of fresh water by evaporation and precipitation is estimated to be 37,000 cubic kilometers. At the present time, the world's total water use is less than 9,000 cubic kilometers, but this is estimated to increase to approximately 18,700 cubic kilometers by the year 2,000.

In other words, within 30 years, man will be using 50 per cent of the total annual fresh water production on the earth. This still remains a relatively small proportion of the total available fresh water in the world (less than 5 per cent) but much of this fresh water is locked into glaciers, polar ice cops and earth crust deposits where it is difficult for man to obtain. Considering the technologic potential of desalination, however, it does not seem likely that man will run short of an absolute supply of fresh water in the next few centuries.

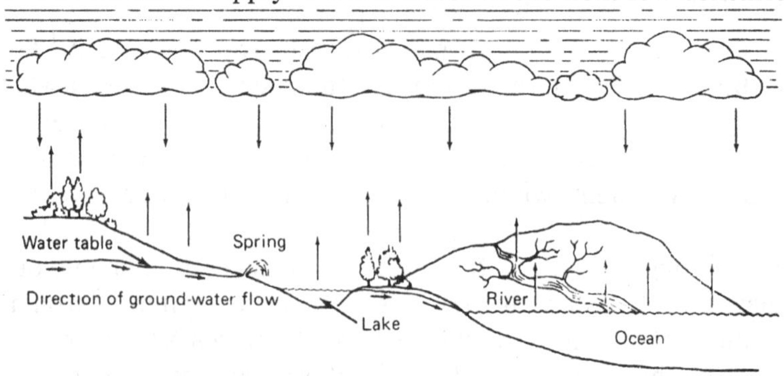

Fig. Simplified depiction of the hydrologic cycle.

This must be qualified, however, by two practical considerations, that of distribution and quality. A large proportion of the world's fresh water falls and resides in relatively unpopulated portions of the globe, particularly Siberia and northern Canada. Here, man's activities are limited by other factors, and he cannot readily obtain these vast stores of water. Secondly, the matter of water quality is of immediate concern.

The principle of water reuse is now becoming accepted, so that people recognize much of their water has been used previously by other municipal systems. Each reuse cycle, however, is increasingly costly in terms of treatment, and each reuse cycle requires disinfectants and other industrial chemicals. Combining these problems of distribution and quality, it seems that the water problem of the future is not going to be one of a global water shortage on a planetary basis, but one of local crises due to the concentrations of people, industry and water use. Certainly, the immediate concern is finding local water resources of adequate quality to meet the burgeoning needs of urban populations. To the city dweller in New York or Hong Kong whose water tap runs dry, or to the refugee in the Middle East who is dying of thirst, it will be little comfort to realize that 29,000,000 cubic kilometers of fresh water are locked in glaciers and polar ice caps.

MAMMALIAN SOCIALITY

EVOLUTION

The diverse relationships of individuals in a social network interact to create complex emergent patterns. These patterns, like the vortex that appears in an emptying sink, is not contained in the structure of a single component. Because a society represents a whole with properties different from those of its component parts, the ultimate consequences of social interactions may be remote from an observed action.

This is a fact that evolution by natural selection can take in its stride but that we, as primarily linear cause-and-effect thinkers, may find hard to accommodate. It may be clear that a lion killing a zebra is behaving adaptively, but less clear whether it is adaptive when the same lion prevents a conspecific from feeding at the kill.

The immediate effect is that the first lion may have more food to eat, but the ultimate effects reverberate through a stochastically unpredictable system of long-term consequences among the whole pride.

Denied food or coalitionary aid by an ally of the snubbed individual at a later date, the fitness consequences for the originally possessive lion may be far from advantageous.

An understanding of social dynamics offers insight into the adaptation of individual responses evolved from selection operating on them from the level of emergent systems.

CONSERVATION APPLICATIONS

Many problems in wildlife conservation and management involve humans causing changes to animal populations or their environment. In applied work, an understanding of the dynamics of a social system is a prerequisite to predicting the effect of human activities on, for example, spatial organisation, population dynamics, and dispersal. For example, attempts to control the transmission of bovine tuberculosis by killing badgers, a reservoir of the disease, clearly disrupts the society of survivors. The effects of such perturbation on social dynamics may alter the transmission of the disease, plausibly for the worse. A similar case may be argued regarding rabies control.

Translocation of elephants without regard for the social structure that provides adolescent discipline has led to problem animals in some African parks. Tuyttens and Macdonald (in press) review some consequences of behavioural disruption for wildlife management. Population control has been shown to affect the rate and pattern of dispersal, home range size, territoriality, mating system, and the nature of social interactions in a variety of species.

UNDERSTANDING OURSELVES

So much is similar in the basic biology of vertebrates, and so universal are the processes of evolution, that an understanding of non-human sociality is likely to illuminate human society. This point was hitherto neglected, but stressed by Tinbergen in the foreword to Kruuk's book, in which he concluded, "It is therefore imperative for the healthy development of human biology that studies of primates be supplemented by work on animal species that have evolved adaptations to the same way of life as ancestral man."

Following Wilson's Sociobiology, it has been widely and sometimes controversially discussed. Clearly, two routes come to mind as fruitful sources of this insight: looking at the societies of species most similar to our current condition (including some hypersocial aspects that put us in circumstances to which we have not yet had time to evolve) and focusing on those currently entering evolutionary phases through which we have already passed. The first approach has prompted (or at least its promise has funded) much primatological research. The closeness of this parallel might be diluted if, as Hinde suggested, the societies of humans differ from those of other animals in that social structure in non-humans is determined primarily by the sum of the interactions of its component individuals, whereas in human groups a structure is more often imposed from above by government or tradition in the form of Dawkins's memes.

Hinde's dichotomy may imply that the imposition of structure can cause stresses in human social systems when natural roles conflict with assigned roles. On the other hand, one could take the view that the dichotomy is not profound because the constraints of governmental ideology are loosely parallel to those imposed on all species by ecological factors such as resource dispersion. If so, a different understanding of social responses to the imposition of external constraints might be revealed by species more recently launched onto a trajectory of sociability.

Certainly, badger groups show weight reduction, higher incidences of wounding, and lower reproductive success per breeding individual as group size increases. For badgers, group living may be a social innovation facilitated by the development of agriculture; individuals may be evolving towards capitalising on this newly imposed structure (by manipulation, support, interdependence of roles, and other factors), but for the moment the stress is showing.

HOW TO DESCRIBE SOCIAL DYNAMICS

It does not detract from the excitement of behavioural, ecological, and sociobiological insights to note that recent enthusiasm for these topics has been characterised by a plethora of short, snappy papers with a clear adaptive punchline and a concomitant neglect of the empirical foundations of ethology. Historically, this arises because behavioural ecology and sociobiology were pioneered to offer ultimate functional explanations, whereas ethology embraced adaptive significance and evolution along with mechanisms and ontogeny. This vogue has led to the widespread abandonment of the ethological aspirations of the late 1970s, epitomised by Hinde's careful use of terminology and hierarchical classification to ensure compatibility between studies used for comparative work.

At its purest, this traditional ethological approach placed greater emphasis on the facility of later reinterpretation of results than on the quest for a desired result. In contrast, there is an invasive tendency to treat hard data and description as disposable assets sacrificed to analytical elegance and discussion. In a science in its infancy (such as social biology) this brings the risk that future research may be doomed to repeat previous field work solely to attempt reinterpretation of undisputed results.

ACTION, INTERACTION, AND RELATIONSHIPS

Adapting Hinde's classification, the basic units of social exchange between individual primates are action and interaction. Actions are directed towards the environment, and are often important in understanding a previous or subsequent interaction with individuals. Interactions (A attacks B) are hard to interpret without records of actions (A accidentally drops fruit, B picks up fruit). Above action and interaction in the hierarchy of social dynamics are social relationships. Relationships are quantified by the rates, frequencies, and patterning of component interactions and may be described in terms of the diversity of interactions, the degree of reciprocity or complementarity, relative frequency and pattern of interactions, synchronicity, and multidimensional qualities. In principle, relationships may be stationary or transitionary. The former do not change with prior experience (intrinsic development) or conditions (extrinsic modification) and are at most rare and perhaps non-existent in mammalian societies. Generalisations about relationships can be sought in various ways. Dyads may be assigned to predefined categories such as age, sex, kinship, or even personality. Personality, in this context, is a consistent moderator of interactions; for example, a shy animal tends to act differently from a bold animal under the same circumstances. Block model methods allow subgroupings to be isolated from sociomatrices. For example, Iacobucci compared 13 methods for recovering subgroup structure from dyadic interaction data. In general, block models are based on structural equivalence of sociomatrices.

Some individuals behave similarly in respect to their age, status, or sex. Using block models, these relationships between individuals can be extracted and further studied, for example, using tests for reciprocity and interchange of behaviours or using more detailed methods based on time structure of the processes.

In their study of capybara mating systems, for example, Herrera and Macdonald disentangled the effects of dominance on mating success. In that example, dominant males secured more matings than any other individual, but fewer matings than subordinate males as a class; this arose because while the dominant was busy driving off one subordinate, another sought quickly to mate with the female. The sum of social relationships may be compiled in a matrix of dyadic interactions to produce a social network. Analysis of sociomatrices assumes stationarity, which, as we have noted, is effectively non-existent. The solution is to divide sociomatrices into appropriately defined periods that approximate stationarity. This might involve consideration of, for example, "the first 50 interactions," "the second 50 interactions," and so forth, or "wet season interaction" versus "dry season interaction," or "simultaneous presence of dominant" versus "absence of dominant." Nested analysis is a common way to achieve this goal.

SOCIAL STURCTURE, FROM SURFACE TO DEEP

A social network provides a snapshot of one facet of society. By analogy, one analysis of a social network is akin to the view through one window into a large and labyrinthine house; the view through all windows gives the structure. It is therefore necessary to compile several networks that describe different facets of one society. This task may be made harder because different sociometric variables (*e.g.*, grooming, aggression, and play) may not follow similar patterns of stationarity; aggression may covary with age and presence of dominant, whereas grooming may not. Notwithstanding these complexities, a society's structure can be described in terms of these networks.

Indeed, there are layers of completeness to this description. The structure that prevails may vary on a circadian basis, or seasonally or annually; it may also be characteristic of a species' society in only one habitat or set of environmental conditions. At its most fundamental, elements of social structure may characterise all populations of a species. Therefore, social structure might usefully be categorised on a continuum from surface structures to deep structures. The study of social dynamics seeks to describe and explain the patterning of transitions and stability of social structures. An important goal of evolutionary biology is to identify the rules, derived from a variety of empirical and theoretical sources, that are thought to guide an individual's decisions in a social context—Axelrod's seminal question of whether to cooperate. An accurate description of structure is clearly a prerequisite to a sensible exploration of these rules.

Operationally, the point at which a thorough description of social structure is complete is probably the first point at which it is legitimate to consider exchanging data language (grooms, fights) for theory language (alliance formation, competition). These interpretative substitutions are topics for the discussion section of a paper, whereas in the results section data should be presented without such interpretation. Exploring exhaustively the layers of structure in animal societies is a major undertaking. Not least because a major objective of studying social dynamics is to contribute to the solution of practical conservation problems, it is inevitable that such studies may sometimes have to be undertaken quickly.

The obvious shortcut, within the framework of existing theory, is to use selected revealing behaviour as a guide to an overall system. As a loose analogy, this is akin to using the seating arrangement at a formal dinner as a guide to the social role of the guests in contexts beyond the dinner. Naturally, such shortcuts necessitate validation.

BEHAVIOURAL PARAMETERS

Even to a casual observer it is obvious that most behaviour patterns occur in bouts; that is, they do not occur randomly in time. Although the existence of bouts may be obvious, how best to define them is not. A review of major textbooks and many papers reveals that many prefer to avoid this issue.

The most common usages define bouts as a repetitive occurrence of the same behavioural act (states or events) or a short sequence of behavioural actions that occur in some functional pattern. States usually have durations, and states with extremely short durations are called events. The difficulties of defining the hierarchy of bouts, states, and events is illustrated by allogrooming by a mouse. This comprises a series of actions (nibbles) of short duration; an uninterrupted string of these nibbling actions might make up a bout of grooming.

However, a student of the detail of mouse grooming will see that these strings of nibbles may sometimes transfer from one body region to another (*e.g.*, from head to neck to flanks or back), and for some purposes it may be helpful to distinguish bouts at this finer scale (a bout of head grooming distinct from one of flank grooming). The problem is that the best definition of a bout depends on the purpose of the analysis in which it will be used.

Depending on the scale of resolution required, even a short sequence of nibbles at one patch on the flank might be distinguished from another bout of grooming at the next patch of fur.

Ultimately, each nibble could be defined as a state, punctuated by another state (shifting the head a fraction to grasp the next tuft of fur). At a given level of resolution it may be helpful to define states from which bouts are built up, but often, under closer scrutiny, a state will emerge to have a structure that could itself represent a bout (rather than one nibble, or one sweep of the paws, while grooming).

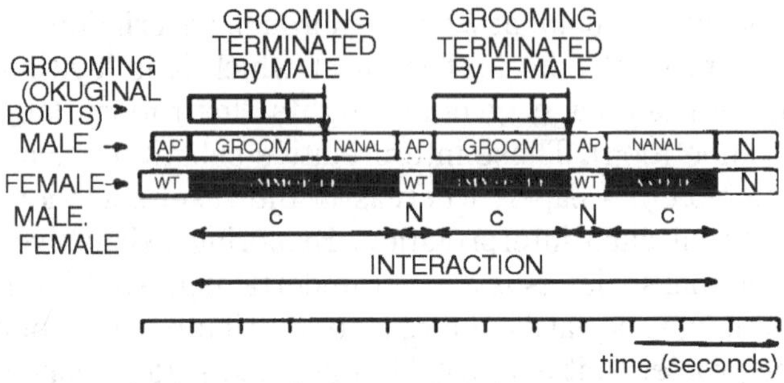

Fig. Data on the Interactions between male and Female Wood mice.

In practice, the best definition of a bout depends on the purpose of the analysis. The top row illustrates that grooming (of the female by the male) is split into a series of brief nibbles partitioned by fleeting changes of position. Each period of nibbling might be defined as an event or as a bout.

If each nibble is an event, then the sequence of them might make up a bout of grooming. Bouts might also be defined in terms of contact between the two mice, and in that case the period during which the male was first grooming and then nasoanal sniffing the females constitutes one bout of contact, during which the female was immobile.

Finally, the entire period of male—female interaction might be defined as a bout. This scheme is based on real data on the behaviour of wood mice. Depending on the model under analysis, grooming bouts could be distinguished as one continuous process or as a series of original grooming bouts in which a mouse shifts between body positions. Even an interaction can be considered a bout if several criteria are fulfilled. C = contact behaviour, N = non-contact behaviour, AP = approach, WT = wait, N-anal = nasoanal contact.

In some contexts this wracking down of the microscope to reveal more and more detail may seem merely a quest to bring into view the number of angels perched on the pinhead, but an important point nonetheless emerges: the unit of much behavioural analysis is the bout, and the usefulness of a definition of a bout is affected by the level of magnification at which the analysis is being undertaken. Bouts must be defined very carefully because their definition will have far-reaching statistical consequences for any analysis in which they are involved and because of their role as an indicator of motivation and neural processes. From the mathematical point of view, when a behaviour is modeled it is easiest to keep definitions simple, so Haccou and Meelis define a bout as a "time interval during which a certain act is performed. A bout length is the duration of such a time interval."

In the calculation of transition matrices, transitions to the same act are impossible, so diagonal elements in the matrix are treated as zero (the notion of transitions from one bout of behaviour to another of the same behaviour presupposes that the observer can distinguish a bout from an interval between two consecutive bouts).

The complexities of defining bouts seem particularly difficult to accommodate in studies of mammals, for which one action pattern often appears to slur into another. For example, although the task of defining a bout of drinking by a fox (made up of a string of lapping events) is feasible, the parallel quest of distinguishing the gulps of a rat or primate (which drink continuously) might be dubious. In comparison it would be straightforward, in a parallel study of a bird, to identify consecutive pecks and the interval between them, which can be analysed using log—survivor plots. The awkward truth is that the convenient hierarchy of bout, state, and event is often arbitrary and often concerns a continuum of lengths (clearly revealed by techniques such as the Noldus videotape analysis system, which measures even the durations of events).

To continue with the example of allogrooming wood mice and opting for Haccou and Meelis's definition of a bout as either the duration of a state or the interval between two states, it can be straightforward to recognise bouts. Wood mice, for example, often switch between two states during exploration: scanning while walking and rearing up or scanning while immobile. In this example, the behavioural elements scan, rear up, and walk each have durations and are therefore states. For example, the duration of scanning is a bout. During scanning, however, wood mice often turn their heads back for only a tenth of a second; turn-head-back is an event. In this case, one bout may include scanning interrupted by several turn-head-back events.

Sometimes, however, it is difficult to distinguish between bouts, although methods are available to do so. When behaviour is studied in sequences (*i.e.*, continuous records), the existence of bouts can be confirmed because the distribution of their lengths follows an exponential distribution as long as successive bouts comply with the assumptions of a first-order continuous-time Markov chain model. In practice, if bout durations do not follow an exponential distribution, there are two possible explanations.

First, the observer incorrectly recognised the bouts and therefore measured the wrong thing, perhaps because some bouts were only partially observed through insufficient time for observation. Second, the first-order

Markovian assumption is not upheld. In the latter case, there are again two possibilities. First, bout lengths may exhibit dependency (between successive bouts or every second or third bout). In this case it is always better to use a semi-Markovian model. Second, and more abstruse, there may be second- or third-order Markov models, which according to Haccou and Meelis are rare and intractable in ethology.

In general, bouts approximate to a first-order Markov process and therefore can be distinguished on the basis of testing their distribution or fitting a non-linear curve to the logarithm of observed frequencies of gap length. Because most behavioural studies are based on parameters such as latency, duration, and time intervals, bout length is a very important parameter to study at the outset.

STATIONARITY

Obviously, if circumstances change over a series of bouts it is confusing or misleading to lump them for analysis. Consequently, it is important to identify stationarity, during which things do not change. Plots of transition frequencies from one act to another in several consecutive periods can be used to judge whether the behavioural process is approximately stationary. Haccou and Meelis emphasise that non-stationarity can mask treatment effects and make the results of an analysis ambiguous. Quite apart from the mathematical implications of inhomogeneity in the data, the existence of the motivational change that causes non-stationarity may be the very object of study, so it is important to identify it from an ethological standpoint. The complexities of stationarity reverberate through ethological methodology. Bekoff, for example, is skeptical that the concept of stationarity can be applied in a social context and therefore concludes that Markovian analysis should be avoided.

THE ETHOGRAM

Early in any study a researcher must classify the behaviour patterns to be documented. This classification is an ethogram, and constitutes a dictionary of the researcher's language; without an ethogram, meaning is not fixed. Ethograms have become unpopular because (like dictionaries) they take up large amounts of space and are dull to read. However, they are vital reference material for those wishing to assess a study's conclusions critically. As a corollary, it is not uncommon for the brunt of reviewers' comments now to fall on statistics rather than data acquisition, reflecting the same shift in emphasis away from data, and onto interpretation, as the hard currency of behavioural science. By analogy, consider the shift from real objects to paper representations in financial systems: 50 years on, would you rather find a stash of gold or war bonds?

We propose that the Internet, with its capacity to archive and disseminate large quantities of multimedia information, will revolutionise the use and usefulness of ethograms. For example, in parallel to a written publication on badger vocalisations, we have created a multimedia vocal ethogram and another based on digital video. Ethograms are often constructed in a pretrial period during which behaviour appropriate to the study is chosen and described. However, short studies are unlikely to detect a complete catalogue of relevant behaviour and are likely to miss social behaviour characteristic of context-sensitive dyadic interactions. Fagen tentatively proposed that a sample of 50,000 acts or more might generally be necessary to estimate the repertoire of a typical carnivore or primate species.

Fagen's estimate was based on the biologically general type—token relationship. This relationship was shown by May to be a general statistical property of all catalogs in which an infinite number of objects belong to a finite number of categories. It prescribes that the logarithm of the number of types in an inventory depends approximately linearly on the logarithm of the total number of acts in the catalogue.

In practice, our badger study confirmed the point: Some antagonistic behaviours (coordinated attack on the rump of an animal after a partner has grasped its head) that we predicted might occur from their occasional appearance in ritualised play between cubs were seen for the first time in earnest between adults only after thousands of hours of direct observation. Although rare in badgers, these coordinated attacks gave an important insight into a previously undocumented realm of cooperative aggression.

What are the components of an ethogram? Ideally, each element might be purely descriptive, free of any imputed function. A heroic attempt at this purity of description was Golani's use of balletic choreographic scores to quantify the spatial and sequential organisation of body part movement, together with its qualities such as speed and force and the degrees of variation tolerated within categories.

It was intended to help solve what Golani called a blind spot in the behavioural sciences: the need for a universal language to describe animal movement.

Despite potential for universality of description, such quantitative choreography has proved impractical for most field studies. Also, focusing on the minutiae of postures may be too detailed for this purpose. A realistic option, facilitated by the Internet, is the creation of an archive of film clips and spectrographic catalogs within a taxonomic library.

However, such a "content and quality" ethogram is still denuded of context. Is a bird pecking a conspecific attempting fighting, grooming, or feeding? The answer may seem obvious from the rate of pecking, its strength, and the reaction of the other bird, but logging these contextual clues is time-consuming.

This is why many ethograms incorporate a shorthand notation that uses not only purely descriptive language but also proximate function language, derived from context and likely result. The demons of tautology and teleology lurk in such language.

BEWARE TELEOLOGY

Omnipresent dangers in the study of social behaviour are the closely allied traps of teleology and unwitting anthropomorphism. Teleology, or the doctrine of final causes, infers purpose in nature (*e.g.*, to infer the existence of a creator from the works of creation). The teleological conviction that mind and will are the cause of all things in nature is not within the scope of scientific method. In the context of animal behaviour, teleological explanation would name and account for a behaviour by its presumed ultimate effect (*e.g.*, appeasement, submission, or punishment) and not by its proximate causes or physical appearance.

It may be convenient to label as "punishment" the category of attack launched by a dominant meerkat on the only member of her group not to join in a fight with territorial trespassers. The danger lies in (inadvertently) interpreting the functional nuance of this convenient label as the proximate cause of the attacker's behaviour. We know only that one individual did not join the fight and that the dominant member of its clan then initiated an attack on it (joined by all its group-mates). It is a matter of interpretation whether this attack functioned as punishment and a matter of speculation whether the attacking meerkat had punishment (or anything else) in mind when it attacked; it is certainly unwarranted to conclude that the putatively punitive attack was launched with the ultimate purpose of increasing the fitness of the attacker (although that may well be its consequence).

Interpretation based on context again harbours the pitfalls of premature use of proximate function language. It would be folly, for example, to categorise as "supportive" an instance of a large female grooming subordinate kin but to label as "repressive" the grooming by the same female of non-kin subordinates. In such a case, proximate function language would have prematurely slipped all the way to ultimate function language. Clearly, the risk is that the very hypothesis used to make this interpretation may later be said to be supported by the observation; in this hypothetical case, the erroneously circular conclusion would be that kin selection theory is supported by the observation that females are supportive of kin and repressive to non-kin.

In fact, such theories can be tested only by following actions through to fitness consequences—a very difficult task. In the progress of a given scientific enquiry, there is no virtue in premature exchange of data language for theory language. The teleological trap arises because in humans, conscious action (and even empathy to other people's unconscious actions) often involves mental plans and objectives that stimulate or explain the performance of behaviours. But consciousness has not been proved in other species and to confuse proximate factors with ultimate factors in this way may stifle correct interpretation. As Kennedy noted, "Teleological terms such as 'searching' ... really describe the animal's presumed state of mind. ... Trying to find an objective substitute for a teleological term will always pay off in research because it forces a mental break-out and a closer look at the components of the behaviour actually observed, components which the handy teleological term leaves unnoticed or at best unformulated in the back of the mind." Kennedy concluded that scanning would be a more useful term for searching. The worst cases of teleology may use such "catchy" labels that proximate and even ultimate function are obscured in the mind of the reader (if not the writer) because of the human innuendo of the word. Rape, used as a label for resisted matings, has been widely considered a case in point.

Used correctly, "mock anthropomorphism" can be a very valuable heuristic tool to guess the function of behaviour, using our own mental processes to explain behaviour in an ultimate fitness context. Such hypotheses can be tested, but even if they are supported we must beware of unwittingly crossing the threshold of assuming that the animal has used the same mental processes when deciding on its own actions.

The temptation of teleology—to impose our mental model on others—may be greatest when dealing with other primates. Tinbergen foresaw this when he wrote, "Teleology may be a stumbling block to causal analysis in its less obvious forms. ... The more complex the behaviour systems we deal with, the more dangerous this can be." These strictures against teleology do not imply that ethologists diminish animals to the level of Descartean machina anima; rather, the objective is to be mindful of Lloyd Morgan's canon that.

In no case may we interpret an action as the outcome of the exercise of a higher psychical faculty, if it can be interpreted as the outcome of the exercise of one which stands lower in the psychological scale". This is a methodological rather than ideological stance, which may be more likely to be correct than the converse assessment. As Dawkins put it, a pragmatic aid in navigating this tricky terrain is to advance "always reassuring ourselves that we could translate our sloppy language into respectable terms if we wanted to."

CLASSIFICATIONS OF BEHAVIOURAL INTERACTIONS

How, in practice, can we impartially assign positive or negative implications to behavioural interactions such as proximity or grooming that are ambivalent, without recourse to the very theories we seek to support? One solution lies in sequence analysis, using unequivocal behaviour patterns as anchors; high-intensity attacks are certainly detrimental to the receiver's fitness, whereas allowing mating is usually beneficial to fitness.

If transition probabilities revealed grooming as a predictor of attack, then it might usefully be classed as aggressive, but if grooming often precedes acceptance of mating, it is probably amicable. Firm grounding of a behaviour in context may justify an interpretative classification. Often, however, it is impossible to establish a uniform link between ambivalent behaviours (*e.g.*, grooming) and anchors (*e.g.*, coalitionary aid or attack) until the whole social network of interactions within the group has been described. Descriptions based on ultimate function should be eschewed until such links are established. A very long list of behaviour patterns or relational types could be described and analysed at each level of the structural hierarchy of social dynamics. Here, we consider just one example at each of three levels: grooming as an interaction, dominance as a relationship, and the concept of "social group" as a structure.

- *Grooming*: Allogrooming can be abundant, observable, and clearly bidirectional or unidirectional, a combination of attributes that have made it perhaps the most frequently studied social interaction. Despite the common assumption that it is amicable or beneficent, it may also cue either dominance or submission in a ritualised context.

The style of grooming, be it simultaneous, alternating, or routinely one-sided, is often largely species typical and even a small sample may give important clues to social relations in a wider context. Grooming has been the focus of many primatological studies, among which it appears to have more to do with social bonding than with hygiene. For example, there is a significant correlation between time spent grooming and group size but not body size. The idea that primates compete for grooming access in a social setting has also been very influential.

To unravel more complex intricacies requires more probing analytical techniques, of which an especially rigourous example is Hemelrijk and Ek's study of reciprocity and interchange of grooming and agonistic "support" during conflict in captive chimpanzees. Reciprocity was defined as one act being exchanged for the same thing (grooming for grooming), whereas interchange was defined as involving two different kinds of acts being bartered (*i.e.*, grooming for support). They created an actor matrix (who initiates to whom) and a receiver matrix (who is recipient from whom) and used a correlation procedure, the K r test, to examine links between the two matrices while taking account of individual variation in tendency to direct acts.

They also attempted to retain stationarity in the data by distinguishing between periods when an alpha male was clearly established or when alpha status was in dispute. Hemelrijk had shown that grooming and support were both independently correlated with dominance rank, so whenever reciprocity or interchange was part of a triangle of significant correlations, they partialed out the third variable to see whether the remaining two retained significance. Between the females, for example, a significant interchange between grooming and support received did not depend on dominance rank. Females groomed individuals that had supported them regardless of rank, indicating a social bond.

However, the reverse was not true in that support was not given in return for grooming, so it was not possible to "buy" support with grooming. Patterns of relationships were different between the sexes. Cheney used the distribution of grooming among individuals within a group to examine whether adversity, in the form of rivalry between groups, had a uniting effect within the group; the expectation of this hypothesis was a more egalitarian spread of grooming within the group when competition with neighbours was intense.

This expectation was not upheld, perhaps because neglected individuals would suffer a greater loss of fitness by shirking in their support of their own group than by attempting to trade this support for better treatment, even assuming a lack of punishment for failure to cooperate. Even when intergroup competition was strong, marked hierarchies in grooming favouritism characterised intragroup relations. This study used the distribution of grooming to generate data with which to infer intragroup cohesion and equality. The ultimate functional explanations given depend directly on the validity of that assumption.

Our acceptance of such hypotheses may be influenced more by our intuitive anthropomorphic bias for their seeming correctness than by our purely objective assessment of the supporting evidence. This is the dilemma of being a social mammal attempting to describe the societies of other mammals. The site to which grooming is directed may have social implications. Among long-tailed macaques (Macaca fascicularis), for example, low-ranking females expose the chest, face, and belly less often to higher-ranking females than vice versa. Male—male dyads almost never groomed the face, chest, and belly. Similarly the face, chest, and belly were underrepresented in grooming between individuals that groomed each other less frequently.

One interpretation is that recipients of grooming expose less vulnerable parts of their body to, and avoid eye contact with, individuals they perceive as potentially dangerous.

Another analysis of the form, distribution, and context of social grooming was undertaken in two groups of Tonkean macaques (Macaca tonkeana) by Thierry *et al.* They found that kinship and dominance role had no effect on the form or distribution of social grooming among adult females, the most common class of individuals to be observed grooming. The caveat that no one method of disentangling social relationships is universally appropriate has been stressed by Dunbar. For example, in a study of grooming in three species of macaques, Schino *et al.* found that whereas frequency and total duration of grooming were highly correlated, there was low correlation between its total duration and mean duration, and frequency and mean duration were not correlated.

A closer inspection of the data also revealed that even this general equivalence between measures of frequency and total duration did not always hold within specific grooming relationships. In general, frequency is a measure of initiation and mean duration is a measure of continuation. In Schino *et al.*'s case, both measures were needed to interpret adequately the macaques' society. Not surprisingly, one important stimulus for grooming in rodents is soiled fur. However, because grooming can be undertaken alone or mutually, it has social implications transcending cleanliness. Stopka and Macdonald (in press) used a similar approach to Hemelrijk and Ek's analysis of grooming in captive chimpanzees to examine patterns of reciprocity in grooming among wood mice (Apodemus sylvaticus). A powerful method for investigating this involved row-wise matrix correlation and the Mantel test. Allogrooming was less common than autogrooming and was most commonly directed by male wood mice to females. Having described a social network in grooming, Markov chain analysis then revealed that the termination rate of female contact behaviour (expressed as her tendency to flee the male's attentions) depended largely on the male's tendency to terminate allogrooming. The pattern of transition rates from one behaviour to another revealed that the most common transition was from allogrooming of the female by the male to male nasoanal contact with the female. This indicates the motivation underlying the male's tendency to allogroom females: males groom a female in order to gain the opportunity to sniff her nasoanal region and, ultimately, to decrease her tendency to flee, thereby allowing them the opportunity to mate.

Females are most likely to mate with males that groom them the most. This constitutes an unusual example of the market effect in a short-lived mammal, with females essentially selling sex in exchange for grooming. Allogrooming is the clearest and most common form of cooperation among badgers. It appears to be a valuable supplement to self-grooming because it is focused on the parts of a badger (back of neck, shoulders, and upper rump) that are most difficult for an individual to reach for itself. The proportion of grooming directed to each segment of the body differs, but is complementary between self-grooming and allogrooming.

Bibliography

A. Sahoo and R.K. Singh: *Animal Health and Production*, Satish Serial Publication House, Delhi, 2013.

Adam Epstein and Andrew Jacobson: *The Familiars: Animal Wizardry*, Harper Collins Publication, Delhi, 2011.

Amarjeet Singh: *Animal Husbandry*, Rajat Publication, Delhi, 2008.

Arun Kumar Tomar, Sukhvir Singh Tomar and Rajbeer Singh: *Animal Genetics and Breeding*, Daya Publication House, Delhi, 2015.

Ashok Kumar: *Animal Husbandry,* Discovery Publication, Delhi, 2006.

Asok Mukhopadhyay: *Animal Cell Technology*, IK Publication, 2009.

B.K. Tikader: *Threatened Animals of India*, Zoological Survey of India Publication, Delhi, 2011.

Bina Mishra, B.P. Mishra, Pran P. Bhat and P.N. Bhat: *Animal Cell Culture*, Studium Press Publication, Delhi, 2011.

C.V. Singh: *Animal Breeding and Genetics*, New India Publication Agency, Delhi, 2015.

Charles Darwin: *The Expression of Emotion in Man and Animals*, Cosmo Publication, Delhi, 2004.

Gyan Deep Singh: *Animal Husbandry*, Anmol Publication, Delhi, 2008.

J.D. Murray, G.B. Anderson, A.M. Oberbauer and M.M. McGloughlin: *Transgenic Animals in Agriculture*, New India Publication, Delhi, 2005.

Jonathan P. Balcomb: e*The Exultant Ark : A Pictorial Tour of Animal Pleasure*, University Of California Press, 2011.

K.C. Agrawal: *Threatened Animals of India*, Nidhi Publication, Delhi, 2010.

M M Ranga: *Transgenic Animals*, Agrobios Publication, Delhi, 2006.

M P S Bakshi and M Wadhwa: *Animal Feeding Concepts and Practices*, Satish Serial Publication House, Delhi, 2016.

Mahendra Kumar: *Animal Byproducts Utilization Through Semi-Moist Rendering*, Daya Publication, Delhi, 2007.

Nazir Ahmad Zeerak: *The Quranic Plants and Animals*, New India Publication Agency, Delhi, 2015.

Prakash Puranik and Asha Bhate: *Animal Forms and Functions : Invertebrata*, Sarup Publication, Delhi, 2007.

R. Lydekker: *The Wild Animals of India, Burma, Malaya, and Tibet* , Natraj Publication, Delhi, 2005.

R. Spier and J. Griffiths: *Animal Cell Biotechnology*, Academic Press Publication, Delhi, 2010.

Ruskin Bond: *The Rupa Book of Great Animal Stories*, Rupa Publication, Delhi, 2005.

S. Nandi: *Animal Cell Culture and Virology*, New India Publication, Delhi, 2009.

S.H. Prater: *The Book of Indian Animals*, Oxford University, 2005.

Shivangi Mathur: *Animal Cell and Tissue Culture*, Agrobios Publication, Delhi, 2006.

Subodh K. Singh: *Animal Health*, Bio-Green Books Publication, Delhi, 2012.

T.K. Bhattacharya: *Animal Genomics for Conservation and Production: A Practical Approach*, Agrotech Publication Company, Delhi, 2013.

Varadaraju: *Threatened Animals of Sunderbans : Vertebrates*, Nature Books India Publication, Delhi, 2015.

William Arthur Hagan and Dorsey William Bruner: *The Infectious Diseases of Domestic Animal*, Agri Horti Press, 2015 .

Index